Praise for "Childhood Leukemia"

"Of all the many kinds of help we had (and we had lots) the book was the single best gift we received. It was the gift of knowledge, so we could ask intelligent questions about our daughter's care. It was the gift of security, allowing us to foresee much of what was coming, and giving us the tools we needed to cope. And it was the gift of hope, for we could see that many children do, indeed, get through this trying time, and come through the grueling treatment intact."

— Kim Warren
Mother of a leukemia survivor

· · · · ·

"Faced with a diagnosis of a life threatening disease, parents of a newly diagnosed child with leukemia often struggle to understand the facts and explanations of the disease and treatment they face, while at the same time dealing with overwhelming feelings of fear, confusion and isolation. The great value of Nancy Keene's exceptional book is that it puts the facts and explanations into understandable terms while acknowledging and dealing with the emotional aspects as only parents who have had similar experience, can. This combination of science, clinical facts and humanism is a potent weapon for both new and seasoned parents who must travel this demanding path. It is also of enormous value to those of us who try to help parents understand and cope as our professional obligation."

— Mark L. Greenberg, MD, OC, MBChB, FRCP(C)
Professor of Pediatrics, University of Toronto
Senior Staff Oncologist, Hospital for Sick Children
Medical Director, Pediatric Oncology Group of Ontario

· · · · ·

"Our 7-year-old daughter was diagnosed November, 2000, with ALL. We were immediately given a copy of your book by the hospital. Initially, we were reluctant to open it and face the information inside. However, once we decided to pull our heads from the sand, we have found Childhood Leukemia to be our absolute bible. Not only do we use it for general information, but we rely heavily on this book for reassurance in times of crisis (real or potential). I cannot imagine not having the information so close at hand and so well organized."

— Jocelyn Hillman
Mother of a leukemia patient

· · · · ·

"I am a physician in acad_____ ____ _____ _f _ _hild ___ _____ O__e of the paralyzing things about having a child wit_____ _r world is turned upside down. It is the hardest c_____ d reading the advice and wisdom of parents who h_____ trable benefit to me.

The toll that pediatric cancer takes on families is unquantified, but includes physical and psychiatric illness in the child and in family members, divorce, and tremendous financial stress. Having a resource for coping with all these hardships is the first step toward putting the world back together, and Nancy Keene's books are the best solution I have found."

— Catherine L. Woodman, MD
Departments of Psychiatry and Family Medicine
University of Iowa

. . . . .

"This book is an extraordinary resource. In its pages the reader will find clear, concise, and understandable information about childhood leukemia. And even more powerfully, the reader will "hear" the voices of parents who share their experiences in their own words: what worked, what didn't, what helped, what hurt. Families, friends, and caregivers who use this book will have information and support at their fingertips, and a powerful tool with which to help young people with leukemia get what they need to claim their lives in spite of this disease and the toll it takes."

— Kathy Ruccione, RN, MPH
Nursing Administrator
Director, LIFE Program (Long-Term Information, Follow-up and Evaluation)
Co-Director, Health Promotion and Outcomes Program
Childrens Center for Cancer and Blood Diseases
Childrens Hospital of Los Angeles

. . . . .

"I highly recommend Childhood Leukemia to all families of children with leukemia. It is an immediate help for the newly diagnosed parent and a comprehensive reference for the subsequent years of treatment. This book covers everything—and I mean everything—that a parent needs to know about the issues surrounding treatment for childhood leukemia. It amazes me that for a disease as rare as childhood leukemia, someone as talented a writer as Nancy took the time to write such a complete and useful book."

—Patty Feist
Parent a survivor of ALL
Organic chemist
Editor, Pediatric Oncology Resource Center
http://www.acor.org/ped-onc

. . . . .

"What's compelling about Childhood Leukemia: A Guide for Families, Friends, and Caregivers is the amount of useful medical information and practical advice it contains.... As the mother of a two-time survivor of ALL—yes it can recur, in my daughter's case after a 14-year remission—I

can vouch that the road to cure is bumpy, filled with life-threatening complications and requiring aggressive in-hospital care. Keene spells it all out... A valuable resource to help parents and children regain their equilibrium after diagnosis and during the two to three years of treatment."

— Patricia Dane Rogers
The Washington Post

· · · · ·

"This book is an invaluable reference for children, their family and their health care providers. It provides important information written in ways families can understands. Ms. Keene presents difficult and sometimes troubling information in a sensitive and balanced manner. I highly recommend it for patients, family members and health care providers."

— Debra L. Friedman, MD
Assistant Professor of Pediatrics
Children's Hospital Regional Medical Center
Seattle, WA

· · · · ·

"Childhood Leukemia was and is an invaluable resource for me. I discovered it a few months into my daughter's leukemia journey and have read and reread it. When Katie was first diagnosed I was told mountains of information, but was unable to absorb much of it due to the initial shock of having a child with cancer. Having all that information and much more at my fingertips has been a huge help. Sometimes it helped me just to know what questions to ask. Even now, months after treatment has ended, I continue to refer to the book for information about the different drugs that were used; I also use the book to help other parents who have questions."

— Pat Lee
Mother of a leukemia survivor

· · · · ·

"This is the most comprehensive resource available for parents and caregivers of children diagnosed with leukemia. These families must become immediate experts and Childhood Leukemia: A Guide for Families, Friends & Caregivers presents up-to-date information in understandable language. Parents find the vignettes helpful, comforting and encouraging. We believe so strongly in this book that a copy is given to each family."

— Mary McSherry, ACSW, LSW
Social Worker, Division of Oncology
The Children's Hospital of Philadelphia

· · · · ·

"Keene has written a comprehensive handbook to serve as a road map for others, from diagnosis through treatments."

— *Library Journal*, starred review
First edition was 1 of only 33 books recommended
for a core children's medical collection in 1998

· · · · ·

"Finally, a book that truly addresses what is needed, practically and emotionally, to "work" the system for the benefit of the family. No preaching! No proselytizing! No slant towards a personal experience. No nagging feeling that the book has been written by doctors. Rather, my conviction is that this book wrote itself from careful and honest listening to parents, children, siblings, doctors, and others traveling the road that is the experience of cancer in a child."

— Grace Ann Monaco, JD
A Founder of the Candlelighters Childhood Cancer Foundation

· · · · ·

"Nancy Keene, whose daughter survived childhood leukemia, offers help and support in this comprehensive guide for families, friends, and health care providers of childhood leukemia patients.

Leukemia Society staff and volunteers regularly use this guide as a valuable reference tool. 'This is an excellent guide for living and coping with childhood leukemia,' says Hildy Dillon, Director of the Information Resource Center at the Leukemia Society of America."

— *NewsLine*, Fall, 1999
Leukemia and Lymphoma Society

· · · · ·

"This is the definitive book for lay people, parents of children with cancer, and survivors of childhood cancer themselves. We routinely provide a copy to all of our patients and families who are enrolled in our long-term survivor follow-up clinic for their education. It's a treasure chest of information."

— Sharon B. Murphy, MD
Chief, Division of Hematology/Oncology
Children's Memorial Hospital
Professor of Pediatrics
Northwestern University Medical School
Chicago, IL

Childhood Leukemia

A Guide for Families, Friends & Caregivers

Fourth Edition

Nancy Keene

O'REILLY®

Beijing • Cambridge • Farnham • Köln • Paris • Sebastopol • Taipei • Tokyo

Childhood Leukemia: A Guide for Families, Friends & Caregivers, Fourth Edition
by Nancy Keene

Copyright © 2010 Childhood Cancer Guides. All rights reserved.
Printed in the United States of America.

Published by O'Reilly Media, 1005 Gravenstein Hwy N., Sebastopol, CA 95472 and Childhood Cancer Guides, P.O. Box 31937 Bellingham, WA 98228

Printing History:
　　June 1997: First Edition
　　October 1999: Second Edition
　　May 2002: Third Edition
　　February 2010: Fourth Edition

Many of the designations used by manufacturers and sellers to distinguish their products are claimed as trademarks. Where those designations appear in this book, and O'Reilly Media was aware of a trademark claim, the designations have been printed with caps or initial caps and a registration symbol.

This book is meant to educate and should not be used as an alternative for professional medical care. Although we have exerted every effort to ensure that the information presented is accurate at the time of publication, there is no guarantee that this information will remain current over time. Appropriate medical professionals should be consulted before adopting any procedures or treatments discussed in this book.

While every precaution has been taken in the preparation of this book, the publisher and authors assume no responsibility for errors or omissions, or for damages resulting from the use of the information contained herein.

This book may be purchased for educational, business, or sales promotional use. For more information, contact the O'Reilly corporate/institutional sales department: (800) 998-9938 or corporate@oreilly.com.

Library of Congress Cataloging-in-Publication Data:

Keene, Nancy.
Childhood leukemia: a guide for families, friends & caregivers / Nancy Keene. — 4th ed.
　　p. cm.
Includes index.
ISBN 978-1-4493-8043-4
1. Leukemia in children. I. Title.

RJ416.L4K44 2010
618.92'99419--dc22   2009052042

 This book uses RepKover™, a durable and flexible lay-flat binding.

To my daughters
Kathryn and Alison

Table of Contents

Foreword

EVERY YEAR IN THE UNITED STATES approximately 12,000 children and adolescents under the age of 20 years are diagnosed with cancer. Of these children, approximately 3,500 will be afflicted with acute lymphoblastic leukemia and 700 with other types of childhood leukemia. Significant progress has been made in the treatment of childhood cancer over the past half century, best illustrated by the dramatically improved cure rate for children diagnosed with acute lymphoblastic leukemia. A leading textbook on childhood cancer published in 1960[1] described leukemia in childhood as being "incurable." Today, the cure rate for children diagnosed with acute lymphoblastic leukemia is 75 percent overall, and more than 85 percent in certain groups of children with particular types of leukemia.

Not every child with leukemia, however, is guaranteed a cure; and progress in the treatment of certain types of leukemia has been definite, but slow. Long-term physical and psychological effects following childhood cancer and its treatment are now common, as more children are cured of cancer. Thus, the diagnosis of any form of cancer in a child remains devastating to a family suddenly thrust into a foreign and threatening world of new and frightening words, medical tests and treatments, uncertainty about the future and, perhaps worst of all for parents, loss of control in guiding their child's life.

The best resource to help survive this new world is knowledge. Nancy Keene has taken her experience over the past 18 years following the diagnosis of leukemia in her then 3-year-old daughter, Katy, melded this with the experiences of more than 100 other families, and produced an invaluable source of knowledge for parents of children diagnosed with cancer. Although this book focuses on leukemia, it contains information that will prove extremely helpful to parents and families coping with any type of childhood cancer. Keene writes in her introduction, "I wanted to provide the insight and experiences of veteran parents who have all felt the hope, helplessness, anger, humor, longing, panic, ignorance, warmth, and anguish of their children's treatment for cancer. I wanted parents to know how other children react to treatment, and I wanted to offer tips to make it easier." She has clearly succeeded.

This fourth edition has been updated to reflect advances in our understanding and treatment of childhood leukemia over the past decade and to ensure that this continues to

---

[1]Ariel, I.M., and A.T. Pack, eds. *Cancer and Allied Diseases of Infancy and Childhood.* Boston: Little, Brown & Company, 1960.

be the most complete parent guide available. The book describes not only detailed and precise medical information about leukemia and the various treatment options, from chemotherapy to blood stem cell transplantation, but also day-to-day practical advice including how to handle procedures, hospitalizations, family and friends, school, social and financial issues, communication, feelings and, if therapy is not successful, the difficult issues of death and bereavement. The cumulative experiences of so many families who have faced the entire spectrum of what can happen in caring for a child with leukemia, and the comprehensive bibliographies, make this such a unique and helpful resource.

This book, however, is not only for parents. It will prove equally instructive for anyone, but particularly for all healthcare professionals involved in the treatment of children with cancer. The honest and candid opinions expressed by children being treated for cancer, their siblings, and their parents serve as a reminder of the continual need for the highest standards of competence and compassion in helping families manage the difficult and sometimes overwhelming physical, emotional, social, and financial burdens they face. Chapter 6, "Forming a Partnership with the Medical Team," is an especially important chapter because it is this partnership and honest sharing of knowledge that returns as much control as possible to parents in making necessary decisions about the care of their child. Every child is different, as is every hospital; and not every physician or medical center will necessarily follow all of the guidelines described in this book. Treatments evolve and change. Nonetheless, the knowledge gained by reading this book will enable parents to ask the right questions and to become an integral part of the partnership in their child's treatment.

We still strive for the universally "truly cured child." As described by Dr. Jan van Eys, a pioneer in childhood cancer treatment: "Truly cured children are not just biologically cured, free of disease, but developmentally on a par with their peers and at ease with their experience of having had cancer."[2] Parents who read this book will have the opportunity to ensure that, as much as possible, they can give their child the very best opportunity to be "truly cured."

— F. Leonard Johnson, MD, FAAP
Emeritus Professor and Chairman, Department of Pediatrics,
Oregon Health & Science University, Portland, Oregon
Past President, American Society of Pediatric Hematology/Oncology (ASPHO)

---

[2]Van Eys, J., ed. *The Truly Cured Child: The New Challenge in Pediatric Cancer Care.* Baltimore: University Park Press, 1977.

Introduction

MY LIFE ABRUPTLY CHANGED on Valentine's Day, 1992, when my 3-year-old daughter was diagnosed with acute lymphoblastic leukemia (high-risk). At the time, I was the full-time mother of two small daughters, Katy, 3, and Alison, 18 months.

The phone call from my pediatrician informing me of Katy's probable diagnosis began my transformation into a "hospital mom." On the 2-hour trip to the nearest children's hospital, I naively thought that my background would equip me to deal with the difficulties ahead. I had a degree in biology and had worked my way through the university in a series of hospital jobs. I had experience in the blood bank, the emergency room, the coronary care unit, and the IV (intravenous) team. After college, I was a paramedic with a busy rescue squad and for several years taught emergency medical technician courses at the local community college. I understood the science and could speak the jargon; I thought I was prepared.

I was wrong. Nothing prepares a parent for the utter devastation of having a child diagnosed with cancer. My brain went on strike. I couldn't hear what was being said. I felt like I was trapped in a slow-motion horror movie.

I came home from Katy's first hospitalization with two shopping bags full of booklets, pamphlets, and single sheets containing information about a wide variety of topics. I didn't know how to prioritize what I needed to learn, so I started by researching everything that I could about leukemia. With the help of my wonderful family and hard-working friends, I began to rapidly fill several file cabinets with information about the medical aspects of the disease.

Emotionally, however, I felt lost. Because most of Katy's treatment was outpatient, I lived too far away to benefit from the hospital's support group, and I knew no local parents whose child had leukemia. I felt isolated. Then I discovered Candlelighters. (See Appendix B, "Resource Organizations.") This marked a turning point in my ability to deal effectively with my daughter's disease. I began networking with other parents of children with cancer and made marvelous friends. I soon realized that we shared many of the same concerns and were dealing with similar problems. Advice from "veteran" parents became my lifeline.

Why I wrote this book

As I approached the end of Katy's treatment, I realized that I had amassed not only a library of medical information, but scores of first-person accounts of how individual parents coped. It saddened me to think that most parents of children with leukemia would, like me, have to expend precious time and energy to collect, assess, and prioritize information vital to their child's well-being. After all, parents are busy providing much of the treatment that their child receives. They make all appointments, prepare their child for procedures, buy and dispense most medicines, deal with all of the physical and emotional side effects, cope with insurance issues, and make daily decisions about when their child needs medical attention. In a sense, this book grew out of my hope that other overwhelmed parents would not have to duplicate my efforts to gather and organize information.

What this book offers

This book is not intended to be autobiographical. Instead, I wanted to blend basic technical information in easy-to-understand language with stories and advice from many parents and children. I wanted to provide the insights and experiences of parents who have all felt the hope, helplessness, anger, humor, longing, panic, ignorance, warmth, and anguish of their children's treatment for cancer. I wanted parents to know how other children react to treatment, and I wanted to offer tips to make the experience easier.

Obtaining a basic understanding of topics such as medical terminology, common side effects of chemotherapy, and how to interpret blood cell counts can help improve quality of life for the whole family. Learning how to develop a partnership with your child's physician can vastly increase your family's peace of mind. Hearing parents describe their own emotional ups and downs, how they coped, and how they molded their family life around hospitalizations is a tremendous comfort. Just knowing that there are other kids on chemotherapy who refuse to eat anything but tacos or who have frequent rages makes one feel less alone. My hope is that parents who read this book will find simply explained medical facts, obtain advice that eases their daily life, and feel empowered to be strong advocates for their child.

The parent stories and suggestions in this book are absolutely true, although some names have been changed to protect children's privacy. Every word has been spoken by the parent of a child with cancer, a sibling of a child with cancer, or a childhood cancer survivor. There are no composites, no editorializing, and no rewrites—just the actual words of people who wanted to share what they learned with others.

How this book is organized

I have organized the book sequentially in an attempt to parallel most families' journeys through treatment. We all start with diagnosis, learn about leukemia, try to cope with procedures, adjust to medical personnel, and deal with family and friends. We all seek out various methods of support and struggle with the strong feelings of our child with cancer and our other children. We try to work with our child's school to provide the richest and most appropriate education for our ill child. And, unfortunately, we must grieve, either for our child or for the child of a close friend we have made in our new community of families dealing with cancer.

Because it is tremendously hard to focus on learning new things when you are emotionally battered and extremely tired, I have tried to keep each chapter short. The first time I introduce a medical term, I define it in the text. Because boys and girls are affected equally by leukemia, I did not adopt the common convention of using only masculine personal pronouns. Because I do not like using he/she, I have alternated personal pronouns within chapters. This may seem awkward as you read, but it prevents half of the parents from feeling that the text does not apply to their child.

All the medical information contained in this fourth edition of *Childhood Leukemia* is current as of 2009. As treatment is constantly evolving and improving, there will inevitably be changes over the next few years. However, most of the medicines now in use have been utilized for many years. Their use, in combination and with changes in dosages, have accounted for the significant increase in treatment effectiveness in the last 3 decades. Scientists are currently studying some new medications, as well as genetically-determined responses to specific drugs that may dramatically improve leukemia treatments. You will learn in this book how to discover the newest and most appropriate treatment for your child.

I have included three appendices for reference: blood counts and what they mean; resource organizations; and books, websites, and videotapes. In addition, bound in the back of the book is an indispensable health record to be filled out at the end of treatment, copied, and then given to each subsequent healthcare provider for the rest of your child's life. This personal long-term follow-up guide educates healthcare providers about the types of treatment given and the follow-up schedule necessary to maintain optimum health.

How to use this book

While conducting research for this book, I was repeatedly told by parents to "write the truth." Because the "truth" varies for each person, more than 150 parents, children with leukemia, and siblings share portions of their experiences. This book is full of these snapshots in time, some of which may be hard to read, especially by families of newly diagnosed children. Here are my suggestions for a positive way to use the information contained in this book:

- Consider reading only the sections that apply to the present or immediate future. Even if your child's prognosis indicates a high probability of cure, reading about relapse or death can be emotionally difficult.

- Realize that only a fraction of the problems that parents describe will affect your child. Every child is different; every child sails smoothly through some portions of treatment while encountering difficulties during others. The more you understand the variability of cancer experiences, the better you will be able to cope with your own situation, as well as be a good listener and helpful friend to other families you meet with differing diagnoses and circumstances.

- Take any concerns or questions that arise to your oncologist and/or pediatrician for answers (or to ask more questions). The more you learn, the better you can advocate for your family and others.

- Share the book with family and friends. Usually they desperately want to help and just don't know how. This book not only explains the disease and treatment but also offers dozens of concrete suggestions for family and friends. I have tried to keep each chapter short and the technical information easy to read.

If you want to delve into any topic in greater depth, Appendix C, "Books, Websites, and Videotapes," is a good place to start. It contains a list of reputable websites and an extensive lists of books for parents, as well as children of all ages. Reading tastes are very individual, so if something suggested in the appendix is not helpful or upsets you, put it down. You will probably find something else on the list that is more appropriate for you.

Best wishes for a smooth journey through treatment and a bright future for your entire family.

Acknowledgments

This book is truly a collaborative effort; without the help of many, it would simply not exist. My heartfelt thanks to my family and friends who supported and encouraged me while I wrote all four editions of this book. I would especially like to thank my children—Kathryn and Alison—for the joy they bring to my life each day and their patience when I work long hours in my home office. Special thanks to my first editor, Linda Lamb, whose creative instinct and gentle guidance shaped this book from its inception; to Sarah Farmer and Susan Jarmolowski for their expertise, attention to detail, and unfailing good cheer; and to Tim O'Reilly for his belief and support of Childhood Cancer Guides. Alison Leake proofread every word and updated the index.

The book wouldn't be done if not for you! Huge thanks to Cathy Nell who provided the information on Australian resource organizations, which are included for the first time in this book. Thank you all for helping to make this a comprehensive, up-to-date resource for people affected by childhood leukemia.

Many well-known and respected members of the pediatric oncology community, and professionals in related fields, graciously carved time out of busy schedules to make invaluable suggestions and help ensure that the information contained in this book is factually correct. I am deeply grateful to Dr. Len Johnson for updating the foreword he wrote many years ago and for reviewing and improving several chapters of this fourth edition. I also appreciate the patient and thoughtful answers to my many phone calls and e-mails over the years to the following knowledgeable professionals. Thank you: Peter C. Adamson, MD; Nancy Bunin, MD; Bruce Camitta, MD; William Carroll, MD; Barbara Clark, MD; Lynne Conlon, PhD; Max Coppes, MD, PhD; Connie DiDomenico, CRNP; Debra Ethier, RTT; Patty Feist; Debra Friedman, MD; Daniel Fiduccia, BA; Mark Greenberg, MD; Wendy Hobbie, RN, MSN, PNT; Ruth Hoffman, MPH; JoAnne Holt, MA; F. Leonard Johnson, MD; Anne Kazak, PhD; Susan J. Leclair, MS, CLS (NCA); Grace Ann Monaco, JD; Mark Newman, MD; Ann Newman, RN; Mary Relling, PharmD; Mary Riecke, pharmacist; Susan Shurin, MD; Sheryl Lozowski Sullivan, MPH; Heidi Suni, MSW; and David Unger, MD.

The text of various editions of *Childhood Leukemia: A Guide for Families, Friends & Caregivers* was read by many people from disparate backgrounds, whose comments proved extremely helpful. Thank you, Belinda Buescher, Wendy Corder Dowhower, Mary Ellen Keene, Patricia Keene, Cynthia Krumme, Alison Leake, Christina O'Reilly, Hazel Reed, Donna Santora Vovcsko, Ralene Walls, and the many parents of children with cancer who graciously took time from their families to review and improve this book. The fourth edition especially benefited from the many talents of Karen McClure—who rewrote some sections and shared inspired ideas for reorganizing the chapters and their content—and Patty Feist, who read, researched, and offered excellent suggestions about many chapters of the book, as well as updated all of the appendices. In addition, my family of cyber-friends on PED-ONC, ALL-KIDS, and PED-ONC SURVIVORS (*www. acor.org*) supplied innumerable suggestions, great stories, and years of both support and fun. Thank you all.

To all of the parents, children with cancer, and their siblings, whose words form the heart and soul of this book, thank you: Brenda Andrews; Robin B.; Jan Barber; Naomi Bartley; Barbara Bradley; Jocelyne Brent; Betty Bright; Sue Brooks; Ann Olson Brown; Nancy and Ernie Bullard; Michelle Caldwell; Edie Cardwell; Paulette Carles; Ricky Carroll; Alicia Cauley; Naomi Chesler; Priscilla Cooperman; Cheryl Coutts; Jennifer Crouse; Carol Dean; Beth Devery, mother of Allison Devery (cancer survivor); Allison E. Ellis; Lisa N. Ellis; E. B. Engelmann; Dana Erickson; Mel Erickson;

Patty Feist; Tamra Lynn Sparling Fountaine; Faith Franzen; Alana Freedman; Jenny Gardner; Shirley Enebrad Geller; Denise M. Glassmeyer; Roxie Glaze; Melanie Goldish; Susan Goldhaber; Elizabeth Guanch; Kris H.; Alicia Hall; Lisa Hall; Erin Hall; Daphne Hardcastle; Denise Glassmeyer Hendler; Kathryn G. Havemann; Connie Herron; Douglas L. Herstrom; Connie Higbee-Jones; Honna Janes-Hodder; Ruth Hoffman; Margaret Huhner; Chris Hurley; Cheryl Putnam Jagannathan; Kelly Janzen; Theresa T. Jeniene; Karen and Brian Jordan; Fr. Joseph; Susan Kalika; Winnie Kittiko; C. J. Korenek; Cynthia Krumme; Madeline LaBonte; Marie Lappin; Joel Layfield; Missy Layfield; Bob Ledner; Pat Lee; Suzanne Lee; Kathryn C. Lim; Julie Macedo; Wies and Julie Matejko; Caitlin McCarthy-King; Deirdre McCarthy-King; Karen McClure; Sara McDonnall; Maria McNaught, mom to Trevor (leukemia survivor); Kimberly Mehalick; Wendy Mitchell; Amanda Moodie; Jean Morris; Leslee Morris; Laura Myer; Cathy Nell; Berendina Norton; M. Clare Paris; Jeff Pasowicz; Donna Phelps; Bev Phipps; Mary Riecke; Jennifer M. Rohloff; Joy Rollefson (mom to Patrik); Maria and William Sansalone; Steve and Shirlene S.; Carole Schuette; Donna Schumacher; Judith Mravetz Schumann; Mark W. Schumann; Sharon A. Schuster; Susan Sennett; Lori Shipman; Mark A. Simmons, DDS; Lorrie Simonetti; Cathi Smith; Carl and Diane Snedeker; Marlene Sorota; Anne Spurgeon; Anabel Stehli; Becky Stephan; Kim Stimson; Dawni Summitt; Megan Thomas; Gigi N. Thorsen; Robyn Thurber; Lisa Tignor; Laura Todd-Pierce; Kathleen Tucker; Brigit Tuxen; Mike and Stacey Vasquez (parents) and Darla Cain (proud Grandma); Annie Walls; Ralene Walls; Tami Watchurst; Sheri White; Helen Wilder; Jean Wilkerson; Jan Williamson; Catherine Woodman; Amy Wright; Erika Zignego; Ellen Zimmerman; Ann; K.F.; and those who wish to remain anonymous.

Also, thank you to Mitzi Waltz. Some of the material in Chapter 15, "School," was adapted from her book, *Pervasive Developmental Disorders: Finding a Diagnosis and Getting Help* (O'Reilly & Associates, Inc., 1999).

Despite the inspiration and contributions of so many, any errors, omissions, misstatements, or flaws in the book are entirely my own.

Chapter 1

Diagnosis

A journey of a thousand leagues begins with a single step.
— Lao-tzu

"WE HAVE THE RESULTS of the blood work back. I'm afraid it's bad news. Your child has leukemia." For every parent who has heard those words, it is a moment frozen in time. In one shattering instant, life forever changes. Many parents equate cancer with death and are staggered by the thought of possibly losing their beloved child. Strong emotions will batter every member of the family. However, with time and the knowledge that most children survive childhood leukemia, hope will grow.

Signs and symptoms

Leukemia is cancer of the blood-forming tissues that make up the bone marrow inside large bones. The diseased bone marrow floods the body with abnormal white cells. These cells do not perform the infection-fighting functions of healthy, mature white cells. The diseased cells also crowd out the other blood cells that are needed to nourish the body's organs and control bleeding if a person is injured. Chapter 2, "Leukemia," provides an in-depth explanation of the various leukemias, their causes, and their treatments.

Parents are usually the first to notice that something is wrong with their child. Occasionally, a pediatrician sees a problem during a well-baby visit, or the disease is discovered by chance on a routine blood test. Unfortunately, because some of the signs and symptoms of leukemia mimic other conditions, diagnosis can be difficult.

The onset of the disease can be slow and insidious or very rapid. Initially, children begin to tire easily and rest often. Frequently, they have a fever that comes and goes. Interest in eating gradually diminishes, but only some children lose weight. Parents usually notice pale skin and bruising. Some children develop back, leg, and joint pain, which makes it difficult for them to walk. Often lymph nodes in the neck or groin become enlarged, and the upper abdomen may protrude due to enlargement of the spleen and liver. Children become irritable, and may have nosebleeds.

Usually parents have an uneasy feeling that something is wrong, but they cannot pinpoint the cause for their concern.

> Preston (10 years old) had an incredible diagnosis. We were very lucky. We were at our beach cabin for Thanksgiving. Preston was tired and listless and had a low-grade fever (99–100°) that had persisted for several days. We were bringing his younger sister into town to attend a birthday party, so we decided to bring Preston in to have him checked by the pediatrician on call. The doctor asked Preston what was wrong, and he said, "I don't know, I just feel awful." The doctor ordered blood work and a chest x-ray, and within 30 minutes I was told that he had a "blood cancer." I wanted to take Preston back to the cabin, but was told we needed to go immediately to the hospital, where Preston was admitted, and treatment began.

Most parents react to their concerns by taking their child to a doctor, as Preston's parents did. Usually, the doctor performs a physical exam and frequently orders blood work, including a complete blood count (CBC). Sometimes the diagnosis is not so easy or fast as Preston's.

> I had been worried about Christine (3 years old) for 2 weeks. She was pale and tired. She ate nothing but toast, and had developed bruises on her shins. At preschool, she was unusually irritable, and would utter a high-pitched scream whenever upset. She told me that she didn't want to go to preschool anymore, and when I asked why, she said, "It's just too much for me, Mommy."
>
> When I took her to the doctor, he measured Christine's weight and height, pronounced them normal, and described her lack of appetite as "nothing to worry about." I told him that all she was doing was lying on the couch and asked why she would have bruises on her legs. He said bruises on shins always take a long time to heal. When I pointed out how pale she was, he stated that all children are pale in the winter.
>
> I grew more and more concerned and took her back the next week. The doctor discovered an ear infection and prescribed antibiotics. I asked why her eyelids were puffy and he thought it was from sinuses. When I told him of Christine's withdrawal from preschool, he suggested that I read a book entitled "The Difficult Child."
>
> Things continued to deteriorate, and I called 3 days later to say that she seemed to be sicker. Her prescription for antibiotics was changed without the doctor seeing her. I was starting to feel frantic, and went to talk to my neighbor who had recently retired after 40 years of nursing. I told her I was afraid Christine had leukemia, and I cried. She said I should take her back to the doctor and insist on blood work. When I took her in that afternoon, her white count was over 240,000 (normal is 10,000, the rest were cancer cells) and her hematocrit (percentage of oxygen-carrying red cells) was 12, far lower than the normal 36.

Where should your child receive treatment?

After a tentative diagnosis of leukemia, most physicians refer the family for further tests and treatment to the closest major medical center with expertise in treating children with cancer. It is very important that the child with leukemia be treated at a facility that has a full complement of specialists who are experienced in treating children with cancer, who know the latest treatment and research advances, and who work together as a team on behalf of the child. An effective treatment team will include pediatric oncologists, oncology nurses, surgeons, pathologists, pediatric nurse practitioners, pediatric nurses, child life specialists, radiologists, rehabilitation specialists, education specialists, and social workers. State-of-the-art treatment is provided at these institutions, offering your child the best chance for remission (disappearance of the disease in response to treatment) and ultimately, cure.

> When we were told that Katy had leukemia, for some reason I was worried that she would miss supper during the long road trip to Children's Hospital. Why I was worried about this when she wasn't eating anyway is a mystery. The doctor told us not to stop, just to go to a drive-through restaurant. I was so upset that I only packed Katy's clothes; my husband, baby, and I had only the clothes on our backs for that first horrible week.

Usually the child is admitted through the emergency room or the oncology clinic, where a physical exam is performed. An intravenous line (IV) is started, more blood is drawn, and a chest x-ray is obtained. Early in your child's hospitalization, the oncologist will perform a spinal tap to determine if any leukemia cells are present in the cerebrospinal fluid and a bone marrow aspiration to identify the type of leukemia. Details of these procedures are described in Chapter 5, "Coping with Procedures."

Physical responses

Many parents become physically ill in the weeks following their child's diagnosis. This is not surprising, given that most parents stop eating or grab only fast food, normal sleep patterns are a thing of the past, and staying in the hospital may expose them to illnesses. Every waking moment is filled with excruciating emotional stress, which makes the physical stress so much more potent.

> The second week in the hospital, I developed a ferocious sore throat, runny nose, and bad cough. Her counts were on the way down, and they ordered me out of the hospital until I was well. It was agony.

That first week, every time my son threw up, so did I. I also had almost uncontrollable diarrhea. Every new stressful event in the hospital just dissolved my gut; I could feel it happening. Thank God this faded away after a few weeks.

Parental illness is a very common event. To prevent this, it is helpful to try to eat nutritious meals, get a break from your child's bedside to take a walk outdoors, and find time to sleep. Take care not to overuse drugs, tobacco, or alcohol in an attempt to control anxiety or cope with grief. Whereas physical illnesses usually end or improve after a period of adjustment, emotional effects continue throughout treatment.

Emotional responses

The shock of diagnosis results in an overwhelming number of intense emotions. Cultural background, individual coping styles, basic temperament, and family dynamics all affect an individual's emotional response to stress. There are no set "stages" of response and parents frequently find themselves vacillating from one extreme of emotion to another. Many of these emotions reappear at different times during the child's treatment. All of the emotions described below are normal responses to a diagnosis of cancer in a child.

Confusion and numbness

In their anguish, many parents remember only bits and pieces from the doctor's early explanations about their child's disease. This dreamlike state is an almost universal response to shock. The brain provides protective layers of numbness and confusion to prevent emotional overload and to allow people to examine information in smaller, less threatening pieces. Pediatric oncologists understand this phenomenon and are usually quite willing to repeat information as often as necessary. Most children's hospitals have nurse practitioners and nurses who can translate medical information into understandable language and answer questions. Do not be embarrassed to say you do not understand something or that you forgot what you were told.

It is sometimes helpful to write down instructions, record them on a small tape recorder, or ask a friend to help keep track of all the new and complex information.

The doctor ordered a CBC from the lab. All the while I'm still convinced my son's bleeding gums were caused by his 6-year molars. The rest happened so fast it's hard to recount. We ended up at the hospital getting a bone marrow test. My husband and I tried to tell the doctor that we would go home and let Stephen rest and that when we came back in the morning they could do another CBC. We were positive that his cell counts would go up in the morning. He said that we didn't have until morning. He said Stephen was very, very sick. After the bone marrow test, the doctor called us in a room and said that Stephen had leukemia. After that word I couldn't hear a thing. My ears were ringing, and my body was numb. There were tears in my eyes. It was actually a physical reaction. I asked him to stop explaining because I couldn't hear him. I asked for a book and went back to the hospital room to read and to cry.

• • • • •

For the longest time (in fact still, 3 years later) I can hear the doctor's voice on the phone telling me that Brent had leukemia. I remember every tiny detail of that whole day, until we got to the hospital, and then the days blur.

• • • • •

I felt like I was standing on a rug that was suddenly yanked out from under me. I found myself sitting there on the floor, and I just didn't know how to get up.

Denial

Denial is one way human beings shield themselves from terrifying situations. Parents simply cannot believe that their child has a life-threatening illness. Denial helps parents survive the first few days after diagnosis, but a gradual acceptance must occur so the family can begin to make the necessary adjustments to cancer treatment. Life has dramatically changed. When parents accept what has happened, understand their fears, and begin to hope, they will be better able to advocate for their child and family.

After our daughter's diagnosis, we had to drive 2 hours to the hospital. My husband and I talked about leukemia the entire trip and, I felt, started to come to grips with the illness. However, after the IV, the x-rays, and the blood transfusions, he became extremely upset that they were going to admit her. He thought that we could just go home and it would be finished. I had to say, "This will be our life for years."

• • • • •

My husband and I sat and waited in silence until the doctor came back with the test results. The next thing I knew we were in his office with a primary nurse, a social worker, and a resident listening to the sickening news that our son had leukemia. I couldn't stop crying, and just wanted to grab my 2-year-old son and run far, far away.

Guilt

Guilt is a common and normal reaction to childhood leukemia. Parents often feel that they have failed to protect their child, and they may blame themselves for their child having the disease. It is especially difficult because the cause of their child's cancer cannot be explained. There are questions: How could we have prevented this? What did we do wrong? How did we miss the signs? Why didn't we bring her to the doctor sooner? Why didn't we insist that the doctor do blood work? Did he inherit this from me? Why didn't we live in a safer place? Why? Why? Why? Nancy Roach describes some of these feelings in her booklet *The Last Day of April*:

> Almost as soon as Erin's illness was diagnosed, our self-recrimination began. What had we done to cause this illness? Was I careful enough during pregnancy? We knew radiation was a possible contributor; where had we taken Erin that she might have been exposed? I wondered about the toxic glue used in my advertising work or the silk screen ink used in my artwork. Bob questioned the fumes from some wood preservatives used in a project. We analyzed everything—food, fumes, and TV. Fortunately, most of the guilt feelings were relieved by knowledge and by meeting other parents whose leukemic children had been exposed to an entirely different environment.

It may be difficult to accept, but parents need to understand that they did nothing to cause their child's illness. Years of research have so far revealed little about what causes childhood leukemia or how to prevent it (see Chapter 2, "Leukemia").

Fear and helplessness

Fear and helplessness are two faces of the same coin. Nearly everything about this new situation is unknown, and the only thing the parents really do know—that their child has a life-threatening illness—is too terrifying to contemplate. Each new revelation about the situation raises new questions and fears: Can I really flush a catheter or administer all these drugs? What if I mess something up? Will my boss fire me if I miss too much work? Who will take care of my other children? How do I tell my child not to be afraid when he can see I am scared to death? How will we pay for this? The demands on parents' time, talents, energy, courage, and strength are daunting.

> Sometimes I would feel incredible waves of absolute terror wash over me. The kind of fear that causes your breathing to become difficult and your heart to beat faster. While I would be consciously aware of what was happening, there was nothing I could do to stop it. It's happened sometimes very late at night, when I'm lying in bed, staring off into the darkness. It's so intense that for a brief moment, I try to comfort myself by thinking that it can't be real, because it's just too horrible. During those moments, these thoughts only offer a second or two of comfort. Then I become aware of just how wide my eyes are opened in the darkness.

A child's leukemia diagnosis instantaneously strips parents of control over many aspects of their lives and can change their entire world view. All the predictable and comforting routines are gone, and the family is thrust into a new world that is populated by an ever-changing cast of characters (interns, residents, fellows, pediatric oncologists, IV teams, nurses, and social workers), a new language (medical terminology), and seemingly endless hospitalizations, procedures, and drugs. This transition is especially hard on parents who are used to a measure of power and authority in their home or workplace.

> *My husband had a difficult time after our son was diagnosed. We have a traditional marriage, and he was used to his role as provider and protector for the family. It was hard for him to deal with the fact that he couldn't fix everything.*

Until adjustment begins, parents sometimes feel utterly helpless. Physicians they have never met are presenting treatment options for their child. Even if parents are comfortable in a hospital environment, feelings of helplessness may develop because there is simply not enough time in the day to care for a very sick child, deal with their own changing emotions, begin to educate themselves about the disease, notify friends and family, make job decisions, and restructure the family schedule to deal with the crisis. The sense of helplessness often diminishes as parents gain a better understanding of the new environment and accept it as their new reality.

Many parents explain that helplessness begins to disappear when a sense of reality returns. They begin to make decisions, study their options, learn about the disease, and grow comfortable with the hospital and staff. As their knowledge grows, so does their ability to participate constructively as members of the treatment team. For further information, see Chapter 6, "Forming a Partnership with the Healthcare Team."

However, do not be surprised if feelings of fear, panic, and anxiety erupt at varying times throughout your child's treatment.

> *A friend who had lost her husband to cancer called soon after my daughter's diagnosis with acute lymphoblastic leukemia (ALL). I told her that I felt helpless, confused, overwhelmed, and teary. I cried, "When will I be my usual competent self again?" She assured me that the beginning was the worst, but to expect to be on an emotional roller coaster for the entire 2 years of treatment. She was right.*

Anger

Anger is a common response to the diagnosis of a life-threatening illness. It is nobody's fault that children are stricken with cancer. Because parents cannot direct their anger at the cancer, they may target doctors, nurses, spouses, siblings, or even their ill child. Because anger directed at other people can be very destructive, it is necessary to devise ways to express and manage the anger.

> *We were sent to the emergency room after my son's diagnosis with leukemia. After the inevitable delays, an IV was started and chest x-rays taken. I struggled to remain calm to help my son, but inside I was screaming NO NO NO. A resident patted me on the shoulder and said, "We'll check him out to make sure that everything is okay." I started to sob. She looked surprised and asked what was the matter. I said, "He's*

not okay, and he won't be okay for a long time. He has cancer." I realized later that she was trying to comfort me, but I was very angry. Surprisingly, by the end of my son's hospitalization, we trusted and felt very close to that resident.

Expressing anger is normal and can be cathartic. Attempting to suppress this powerful emotion is usually not helpful. Some suggestions from parents for managing anger follow.

Anger at healthcare team:

• Try to improve communication with doctors.

• Discuss your feelings with one of the nurses or nurse practitioners.

• Discuss your feelings with social workers.

• Talk with parents of other ill children, either locally or by joining an online support group.

Anger at family:

• Hold family meetings.

• Exercise a little every day.

• Do yoga or relaxation exercises.

• Keep a journal or tape-record your feelings.

• Cry in the shower or pound a pillow.

• Talk with friends.

• Talk with parents of other ill children.

• Join or start a support group.

• Try individual or family counseling.

• Live one moment at a time.

Anger at God:

• Share your feelings with your spouse or close friends.

• Discuss your feelings with clergy or church members.

• Talk to a hospital chaplain.

• Re-examine your faith.

• Know that anger at God is normal.

• Pray.

• Give yourself time to heal.

It is important to remember that angry feelings are normal and expected. Discovering healthy ways to cope with anger is a vital tool for all parents.

Sadness and grief

No one is prepared to cope with the news that their child might die. Intense feelings of sorrow, loss, and grief are common, even when the prognosis is good. Parents describe feeling engulfed by sadness. They fear that they may simply not be able to deal with the enormity of the problems facing their family. Parents grieve the loss of normalcy, the realization that life will never be the same. They grieve the loss of their dreams and aspirations for their child. They may feel sorry for themselves and may feel ashamed and embarrassed by these feelings.

> *Even though my daughter's prognosis was good, I would find myself daydreaming about her funeral. Certain songs especially triggered this feeling. I invariably burst into tears because I was ashamed to be thinking/planning a funeral when I just could not imagine my life without her. When these feelings washed over me, I could actually feel a physical sensation of my heart ripping.*

Cynthia Krumme's book *Having Leukemia Isn't So Bad. Of Course It Wouldn't Be My First Choice* describes a message tacked on the Massachusetts General Clinic's bulletin board:

> *How do I feel? Don't ask!…aside from nervousness, irritability, exhaustion, faintness, dizziness, tremors, cold sweats, depression, insomnia, muscle pains, mental confusion, internal trembling, numbness, indecisiveness, crying spells, unsocial, asocial, and anti-social behavior…I feel fine…Thank you.*

Parents travel a tumultuous emotional path where overwhelming emotions subside only to resurface later. All of these are normal, common responses to a catastrophic event. For many parents, these strong emotions begin to become more manageable as hope grows.

Hope

After being buffeted by illness, fear, sadness, grief, guilt, and anger, most parents welcome the growth of hope. Hope is the belief in a better tomorrow. Hope sustains the will to live and gives one the strength to endure each trial. Hope is not a way around, it is a way through. The majority of children conquer childhood leukemia and live long and happy lives. There is reason for hope.

Many families discover a renewed sense of both the fragility and beauty of life after the diagnosis. Outpourings of love and support from family and friends provide comfort and sustenance. Many parents speak of a renewed appreciation for life and consider each day with their child as a precious gift.

A Japanese proverb says: "Daylight will peep through a very small hole."

> *Some people don't get it when I say that there were many good things about our journey through leukemia. I wouldn't wish it on anyone, but my daughter and I both learned that we have strengths we did not suspect; we found love and support and compassion in places we never expected it; we were honored to know people who dedicate their lives to helping children survive this disease; I found joy in the tiniest of pleasures; and I discovered that the world is unbelievably beautiful when we look at it through grateful eyes.*

The immediate future

You are not alone. Many have traveled this path before you and they will share their wisdom and support with you. The next several chapters will help you understand your new reality and make the decisions you will face at each stage of your journey. In their own words, parents will explain the choices they made and how they adjusted, learned, and became active participants in their children's treatment. Sharing experiences with parents and survivors of childhood leukemia may help your family develop its own unique strategy for coping with the challenges ahead.

A Mother's View

Memory is a funny thing. I'd be hard pressed to remember what I had for dinner last night, but like many people, the day of the Challenger explosion and, even further back, the day of John Kennedy's death, are etched in my mind to the smallest detail.

And like a smaller group of people, the day of my child's cancer diagnosis is a strong and vivid memory, even 7 years later. Most of the time, I don't dwell on that series of images. It was, after all, a chapter in our lives, and one that is now blessedly behind us. But early each autumn, when I get a whiff of the crisp smell of leaves in the air, it brings back that dark day when our lives changed forever.

Many of the memories are painful and, like my daughter's scars, they fade a little more each year but will never completely disappear. While dealing with the medical and physical aspects of the disease, my husband and I also made many emotional discoveries. We sometimes encountered ignorance and narrow-mindedness, which made me more sad than angry. Mistakes were made, tempers were short, and family relations were strained. But we saw the other side, too. Somehow, our sense of humor held on throughout the ordeal, and when that kicked in, we had some of the best laughs of our lives. There was compassion and understanding when we needed it most. And people were there for us like never before.

I remember two young fathers on our street, torn by the news, who wanted to help but felt helpless. My husband came home from the hospital late one night to find that our lawn had been mowed and our leaves had been raked by them. They had found a way to make a small difference that day.

Another time, a neighbor came to our house bearing a bakery box full of pastries and the message that his family was praying for our daughter nightly around their supper table. The image of this man, his wife, and his eight children joining in prayer for us will never leave me.

A close friend entered the hospital during that first terrible week we were there to give birth to her son. I held her baby, she held me, and we laughed and cried together.

Sometimes, when I look back at that time, I feel as though everything that is wrong with the world and everything that is right is somehow distilled in one small child's battle to live. We learned so very much about people and about life.

Surely people who haven't experienced a crisis of this magnitude would believe that we would want to put that time behind us and forget as much of it as possible. But the fact is, we grew a little through our pain, like it or not. We see through new eyes. Not all of it is good or happy, but it is profound.

I treasure good friends like never before. I view life as much more fragile and precious than I used to. I think of myself as a tougher person than I was, but I cry more easily now. And sure, I still yell at my kids and eagerly await each September when they will be out of my hair for a few hours each day. But I hold them with more tenderness when they hop off the school bus into my arms. And I like to think that some of the people around us, who saw how suddenly and drastically a family's life can change, hold their children a little dearer as well.

Do I want to forget those terrible days and nights 7 years ago? Not on your life. And I hope the smell of autumn leaves will still bring the memories back when I'm a grandmother, even if I can't remember what I had for dinner last night.

— Kathy Tucker
CURE Childhood Cancer Newsletter
Rochester, NY

Chapter 2

Leukemia

*The world breaks everyone and afterward
many are strong at the broken places.*

— Ernest Hemingway
A Farewell to Arms

THE WORD LEUKEMIA literally means *white blood*. Leukemia is the term used to describe cancer of the blood-forming tissues known as bone marrow. This spongy material fills the bones in the body and produces blood cells. With leukemia, the bone marrow creates an overabundance of abnormal white cells. As the bone marrow becomes packed with these abnormal cells, they crowd out all the healthy cells that are needed for blood to do its work, and symptoms of the disease begin to develop.

This chapter first looks at the function and composition of blood. Then it describes risk factors for leukemia, signs and symptoms, and features of the main types of leukemia. Detailed information about the treatment for each type of leukemia is provided in Chapter 4, "Choosing a Treatment."

Leukemia is a blood disease

Blood is a vital liquid that carries oxygen, food, hormones, and other necessary chemicals to the body's cells. It also removes toxins and other waste products from the cells. Blood helps the lymph system fight infections and carries the cells needed to repair injuries.

Whole blood is made up of plasma—a clear fluid—and many other components, each with a specific task. Blood also contains three types of blood cells (red blood cells, platelets, and white blood cells), all of which are affected by leukemia.

Red blood cells (erythrocytes or RBCs) contain hemoglobin, a protein that picks up oxygen in the lungs and transports it throughout the body. RBCs that contain oxygen give blood its red color. When leukemia cells in the bone marrow slow down the production of RBCs, anemia develops. Anemia can cause tiredness, weakness, irritability, pale skin, and headaches—all due to decreased oxygen being carried to the body tissues.

Platelets (thrombocytes) are tiny, disc-shaped cells that help form clots to stop bleeding. Leukemia can dramatically slow down the production of platelets, causing children with the disease to bleed excessively from cuts or from the nose or gums. Children with leukemia can develop large bruises (ecchymoses) or small red dots (petechiae) on their skin.

Healthy white blood cells (leukocytes or WBCs) destroy foreign substances in the body, such as viruses, bacteria, and fungi. WBCs are produced and stored in the bone marrow and lymph nodes. They are released when needed by the body. If an infection is present, the body produces extra WBCs. There are three main types of WBCs:

- **Lymphocytes.** The two types of lymphocytes are T cells and B cells.
- **Granulocytes.** The three types of granulocytes are neutrophils, eosinophils, and basophils.
- **Monocytes.**

The different types of leukemia are cancers of a specific WBC type. For instance, acute lymphoblastic leukemia affects only lymphocytes. The most common types of childhood leukemia are explained later in this chapter.

Definition of a blast

Blast is a short name for an immature WBC, such as lymphoblast or monoblast. Normally, less than 5 percent of the cells in healthy bone marrow at any one time are blasts. While in the bone marrow, normal blasts develop into mature, functioning WBCs and are then released into the bloodstream. Therefore, in healthy people, blasts are not usually found in the bloodstream. Leukemic blasts remain immature, multiply continuously, provide no defense against infection, and may be present in large numbers in the bloodstream and bone marrow.

When leukemia begins

When abnormal blasts appear in the bone marrow, they multiply rapidly and lose their ability to develop into normal WBCs. They begin to crowd out the normal cells that grow from healthy blasts into mature WBCs. After accumulating in the bone marrow, leukemic blasts spill over into the blood and, if left unchecked, may invade the central nervous system (CNS), which includes the brain, spinal cord, and other organs.

When leukemic blasts begin to fill the marrow, production of healthy RBCs, platelets, and WBCs cannot be maintained. As the number of normal blood cells decreases, symptoms appear. Low RBC counts cause fatigue and pale skin. Low platelet counts may result in bruising and bleeding problems. And if mature neutrophils and lymphocytes are crowded out by blasts, the child will have little or no defense against infections.

Leukemia is described as either acute (progressing quickly) or chronic (progressing slowly and usually involving more mature cells). The acute leukemias, which comprise about 95 percent of all childhood leukemias, are further divided into acute lymphoblastic leukemia (ALL), in which the cancerous cells are lymphocytes, and acute myeloid leukemia (AML), in which the granulocytes or monocytes malfunction.

> *Our 3-year-old daughter Charlotte changed from a quiet but friendly preschooler to a fearful, withdrawn one in just a few months. She didn't want to go to preschool, see her friends, or play outside. She would lie on the couch a lot. She had bruises, and we didn't know why because she hadn't been playing. She didn't look well but the doctor couldn't find anything wrong. She became pale and didn't sleep well. Finally, the doctor took a blood sample, and when he called me on the phone to tell me she had leukemia, I dropped to my knees and couldn't get up.*

Who gets leukemia

Leukemia is the most common childhood cancer. Often thought of as strictly a childhood disease, leukemia actually afflicts many more adults than children. Each year in the United States, approximately 4,200 children are diagnosed with leukemia.

Childhood leukemia is most commonly diagnosed in children ages 2 to 5. In the United States, leukemia is more common in Caucasians than African Americans, boys have a slightly higher incidence than girls, and the incidence is highest in Hispanic children. Children with certain genetic diseases also have a higher risk of developing leukemia than children in the general population.

Leukemia is not contagious; it cannot be passed from one person to another.

Although the exact cause of childhood leukemia is a mystery, certain factors may increase a child's risk of developing the disease.

Genetic factors

Children with extra chromosomes (genetic material contained in cells) or certain chromosomal abnormalities have a greater chance of developing leukemia. See the section in this chapter called "Genetics." Children with Down syndrome, Klinefelter's syndrome, germline BRCA2 mutations, Beckwith-Wiedemann syndrome, neurofibromatosis, Shwachman-Diamond syndrome, Bloom syndrome, Fanconi syndrome, and ataxia telangiectasia have a higher risk of leukemia than children without these genetic disorders. However, most children with these syndromes do not develop leukemia.

Two-year-old Levi has Down syndrome. He started being a little fussy and wasn't sleeping well. We thought that maybe he was getting an ear infection or something because he would act that way sometimes with an ear infection. But within a few days, his eye was swollen; he looked like "Rocky." Thankfully, Levi has the best pediatrician ever! He could not really figure out why Levi's eye would be swollen but since Levi has Down syndrome, he wanted to do a blood test just to see if everything looked okay. Levi's counts were low so they re-checked his counts in less than a week. When those counts were still low, his pediatrician immediately referred us to the hematology clinic at our local Children's Hospital where they did a bone marrow test because unfortunately, as you know, with Down syndrome, leukemia was suspected. Levi's counts at diagnosis were ANC 594, WBC 3.3, hemoglobin 9.7, and platelets 116,000. Once ALL was confirmed, they immediately admitted Levi to the cancer floor and started his chemo that same night. He is low risk because his MRD (minimum residual disease) was good within the first 15 days.

If one identical twin is diagnosed with ALL before the age of 6, the other twin has about a 25-percent chance of developing the disease. This risk is highest if the first twin develops leukemia in infancy; however, the risk for the other twin diminishes with age. After age 7, the risk for the other twin is the same as for any child in the general population (very, very low risk). In fraternal (non-identical) twins, there is minimal, if any, increased risk of ALL developing in both twins.

If one identical twin develops AML, the risk of the other twin also developing it is extremely high. However, the risk decreases with age and is the same as the general population after the age of 6 (very, very low risk).

Environmental factors

Exposure to ionizing radiation and certain toxic chemicals may predispose individuals to leukemia and other problems involving the bone marrow. Many Japanese citizens who were exposed to atomic bomb fallout during World War II, and some of the people living near the Chernobyl nuclear reactor accident in 1986 in the Ukraine, have developed leukemia. However, children who were born and raised in the United States have rarely been exposed to these levels of ionizing radiation.

Also, prenatal exposure to x-rays, or radiation given to children for conditions such as ringworm of the scalp or thymus enlargement, can increase a child's risk of developing leukemia. Chronic exposure to benzene (an industrial chemical) has been associated with leukemia in adults. Most children, however, are not exposed to radiation before birth or to high levels of industrial chemicals.

Certain types of chemotherapy (e.g., etoposide, cyclophosphamide, and ifosfamide) or radiation treatments for prior cancers can significantly increase a child's risk of developing AML.

Evidence is mixed about whether any of the following exposures increase a child's risk of developing leukemia: electromagnetic fields, emissions from nuclear power plants, exposure to herbicides and pesticides, household radon, chemical contamination of groundwater, exposure of fathers to Agent Orange or other chemicals during military service, or mothers' use of alcohol when pregnant. However, the evidence is stronger for increased risk of developing AML from exposure during childhood to organophosphate pesticides, which is more likely in children of migrant workers or children who live on farms. For more information about possible environmental causes of childhood leukemia, visit *www.acor.org/ped-onc/diseases/leukcauses.html#nrpb*.

Summary

Researchers currently suspect that a complex interaction among genetic, environmental, and immunologic factors predisposes certain individuals to leukemia. The most important point for parents to remember is that at present there is no way to predict or prevent leukemia in children.

Genetics

Treatment for childhood leukemia is increasingly based on genetic changes that can be identified in cancer cells. Thus, having a basic knowledge of genetics will help you understand some of the terms healthcare providers will use when discussing your child's type of leukemia and proposed treatment.

Cells, DNA, genes, and chromosomes. Our bodies are composed of cells, trillions of them. Each of these cells carries all the biochemical information the cells need to reproduce and keep our bodies functioning. Within the nucleus of every cell are the genes, the basic physical and functional units of heredity, which provide all the instructions the body needs to live and to pass certain traits from a parent to a child. Genes are composed of DNA (deoxyribonucleic acid) which comes in strands of various lengths that resemble a twisted ladder. The genes (and the DNA in them) are located in X-shaped structures called chromosomes. Chromosomes come in pairs, and a normal human cell contains 46 chromosomes. For more information on this topic, visit *www.ghr.nlm.nih.gov/handbook/basics/gene* and *www.chromodisorder.org/CDO/General/IntroToChromosomes.aspx*.

A mutation is a permanent change in the DNA of a gene. Genetic changes happen all the time within our cells, but the body possesses sophisticated tools for detecting and repairing the changes. A change only becomes a mutation when a repair cannot be made or is made incorrectly.

Hereditary mutations. These are mutations that are passed from parent to child. In most cases, these mutations are present in every cell in the child's body. Children with certain chromosomal abnormalities have an increased chance of developing leukemia. The hereditary syndromes linked to childhood leukemia were mentioned earlier in this chapter. However, most children with these syndromes do not develop leukemia, and inherited genetic disease accounts for only a very small percentage of childhood leukemias.

Somatic mutations. Mutations that occur after conception are called somatic or acquired mutations and may or may not be passed on to children. For more information on the difference between hereditary and acquired mutations, visit *www.ghr.nlm.nih. gov/handbook/mutationsanddisorders/genemutation.*

Chromosomal mutations. These mutations come in four main varieties:

- Duplications, in which some genes are repeated on the chromosome.

- Deletions, in which part of a chromosome is lost.

- Translocations, in which there is a break in the DNA and some genes from one chromosome attach to a different chromosome.

- Inversions, in which a break occurs and the sequence of genes is reversed.

Scientists have identified many genetic markers (DNA sequences associated with a certain trait or gene) of childhood leukemia. Some of these markers are associated with development of the disease. Others predict which therapies will be most effective for a particular child or relate to metabolic conditions that may cause a child to react atypically to certain drugs. For these reasons, when a child is diagnosed with leukemia, doctors immediately perform numerous genetic tests to gather as much information as they can about how the child should be treated and how he or she is likely to respond to treatment. This genetic knowledge has greatly improved doctors' ability to identify the best treatment for each child diagnosed with leukemia. As more information is gathered and understood, therapies in the future will be tailored or customized for each child with leukemia. For more information about this topic, visit *www.acor.org/ped-onc/ diseases/ALLmolchar.html.*

Diagnosing leukemia

A tentative diagnosis of leukemia is made after a physical examination of the child and microscopic analysis of a blood sample. Physical findings may include pale skin; bruising or unusual bleeding; enlarged liver, spleen, or lymph nodes; weakness; and fever. The child may also be experiencing irritability, night sweats, fatigue, bone pain, and loss of appetite. Blood tests may show too few RBCs, too few platelets, and either abnormally low or high WBC counts.

Our first trip to the oncologist occurred only about 5 weeks into the quest for answers, after our pediatrician grew weary of our frequent visits. Although Nikki had symptoms of leukemia, her white count was nearly normal and other blood values suggested an inflammatory process, so the oncologist referred us to an immunologist. The immunologist tested her for everything, including AIDS, then referred us to a pediatric rheumatologist. By then, Nikki could not walk. She had lost nearly 15 pounds and was fragile, pale, and weak.

The rheumatologist told us on the first day he saw us that Nikki didn't have arthritis, but said he wanted to repeat the CBCs (complete blood counts) weekly for a while to see if anything developed. I thought it was weird, but I was grateful that he was taking it seriously. He also referred her for a bone scan that showed increased activity in the growth plates, but the radiologist said he could not interpret the results.

Early one morning, 6 weeks later, the rheumatologist called me and said, "I wish things were different, but I just got the latest blood work and it confirms what I have been suspecting. I am quite sure Nikki has leukemia. They are waiting for you at the oncology clinic. I'm so sorry."

With the T-cell type of ALL, which is described later in the chapter, the thymus gland in the neck may be affected. Enlargement of the thymus can cause pressure on the nearby trachea (windpipe), causing coughing or shortness of breath. The superior vena cava (SVC), a large vein that carries blood from the head and arms back to the heart, passes next to the thymus. In some children with leukemia, an enlarged thymus gland compresses the SVC and causes swelling of the head and arms.

Some children with leukemia have the disease in their CNS at diagnosis; but less than 10 percent of children with leukemia have symptoms of CNS disease, such as headaches, poor school performance, weakness, seizures, vomiting, blurred vision, or difficulty maintaining balance.

Children with AML are sometimes diagnosed after developing a chloroma—a tumor arising from myeloid tissue and containing myeloperoxidase (a pale green pigment). These tumors are most often found under the skin near the eyes but may occur at any site in the body.

To confirm a diagnosis of leukemia, bone marrow is sampled and tested (see Chapter 5, "Coping with Procedures"). The bone marrow is examined under a microscope by a pathologist (a physician who specializes in body tissue analysis). The diagnosis of leukemia is confirmed if more than 25 percent of the blood cells in the marrow are blasts. A portion of the bone marrow (and the chloroma biopsy, if done) is sent to a specialized laboratory that analyzes many other features of the leukemic cells (e.g., chromosomes, proteins on the cell surface).

Types of leukemia

The two broad classifications of leukemia are acute (rapid progression) and chronic (slow progression). The acute leukemias are characterized by abnormal numbers of immature WBCs, or blasts. In chronic leukemia, mature WBCs are more prevalent.

Acute leukemia is the most common type of cancer found in children. The two most common forms of acute leukemia are acute lymphoblastic leukemia (ALL) and acute myeloid leukemia (AML). More than 95 percent of all childhood cancers are acute, with the majority being ALL.

The two types of chronic leukemia are chronic myeloid leukemia (CML) and juvenile myelomonocytic leukemia (JMML), and they account for less than 5 percent of all childhood leukemia. The following table shows the types of childhood leukemia and the percentages of each type.

Table 2.1: Types and Percentages of Childhood Leukemia

Acute		Chronic	
ALL (75%)	AML (20%)	CML (3.5%)	JMML (1.5%)

Acute lymphoblastic leukemia (ALL)

Seventy-five percent of all children with leukemia have ALL. It is caused by a rapid increase of immature lymphocytes (lymphoblasts), which would normally have developed into mature WBCs. There are several subgroups of ALL, which are based on whether the cancer cells developed from cells that would have become B cells or T cells.

The first sample of bone marrow taken is analyzed to identify characteristics of the leukemia cells in order to help plan the best therapy and predict how the child will respond to treatment. Different subtypes of leukemia require different types of treatment; some can be cured with less chemotherapy, while others require aggressive treatment.

> *I was walking around the hospital looking shell shocked the day after my daughter was admitted to Children's Hospital with leukemia. One of the other mothers came up, introduced herself, and asked what we were in for. I told her leukemia. She told me that her son had just relapsed again from a brain tumor. She looked wistful and said how much she wished that her son had ALL. She said, "You might think that's strange, but I see those kids come, get better, and go home. We are still here."*

Prognosis for children with ALL

Treatment of childhood ALL is one of the major medical success stories of modern medicine. As recently as the early 1960s, children with ALL usually lived only for a few months. Currently, 95 percent of children receiving optimal treatment attain remission, and 75 to 85 percent of children who receive optimal treatment are cured (defined as remaining in remission for at least 5 years after diagnosis). The appropriate treatment for each child with ALL is determined by analyzing several features related to the child and to the leukemia cells. Children who have high-risk disease need more aggressive treatments than children with average-risk disease. Below are some of the factors doctors consider when determining treatment. For more detailed information about prognostic factors, visit the National Cancer Institute (NCI) website at *www.cancer.gov/cancertopics/pdq/treatment/childALL/HealthProfessional*.

Age. Children ages 1 to 9 typically do better than infants, older children, or teens. As a result, more aggressive treatments are usually needed for infants and children older than age 9. Approximately 80 percent of infants with leukemia have cancer cells with parts of the *MLL* gene (at chromosome segment 11q23) rearranged. These infants have a higher risk of relapse than other infants with the disease.

WBC count at diagnosis. Children with a WBC count lower than 50,000 per cubic milliliter have a better prognosis than those with a higher WBC count. Most institutions place children with high WBC counts on more intensive treatment plans (also known as protocols).

Central nervous system (CNS) status at diagnosis. If leukemia is suspected, a sample of the cerebrospinal fluid (CSF) is obtained during a lumbar puncture (also called spinal tap). Children who do not have leukemia blasts in the cerebrospinal fluid at diagnosis have a better prognosis than those who do. The results of the first lumbar puncture (described in Chapter 5, "Coping with Procedures") at diagnosis will be described as:

- CNS1: No leukemia blasts found.
- CNS2: Fewer than five leukemia blasts (per microliter) found.
- CNS3: Five or more blasts (per microliter) found.

Around 19 percent of children diagnosed with leukemia fall into the CNS2 category. It is not yet known whether this number of blasts in the CNS affects prognosis. Approximately 5 percent of children are classified as CNS3, which means their leukemia has spread to the CNS and requires more aggressive treatment.

Chromosome translocations. Sometimes genetic material is exchanged (translocated) between chromosomes in leukemia cells. Translocations are extremely common in childhood ALL, and some of these are known to affect prognosis. Examples are:

• Movement of the *TEL* gene on chromosome 12 to the *AML-1* gene on chromosome 21. Commonly called *TEL-AML-1* or t(12;21), this translocation is found most often in children between the ages of 2 and 9. Hispanic children have a lower incidence of this translocation than Caucasian children. Children with this translocation usually have very good outcomes.

> *When Liza was diagnosed in July 2007, our oncologist told us that at the initial bone marrow aspiration he would be able to determine if she had leukemia or not, and then the other sample would go for cytogenetic testing. It took about 15 days to get the results back and Liza had hyperdiploidy, with triple trisomies 4, 10, 17. She was MRD (minimal residual disease) negative and an early responder (day 7–8). So she followed the standard-low risk arm without additional PEG-asparaginase.*

• The Philadelphia chromosome, called t(9;22), is found in approximately 3 percent of children with ALL. It is associated with a poor prognosis, especially in older children with high WBC counts who have a slow response to treatment.

• Translocations involving the *MLL* gene are found in 8 percent of children with ALL. The most common *MLL* translocation is t(4;11), which occurs most often in infants with leukemia cells in the CNS and high WBC counts at diagnosis. Another *MLL* translocation is t(11;19), which is associated with a poor outcome in infants but a favorable outcome in older children with T-cell leukemia.

• The t(1;19) translocation occurs in 5 to 6 percent of childhood ALL and is more likely to occur in African American children than Caucasian children. Children with this translocation usually require more intensive treatment.

Leukemia cell characteristics. There are two types of leukemia cells in ALL: B cells and T cells. B-lineage ALL has four subgroups, and at diagnosis the cells are tested to help determine the best treatment.

• **Pro B ALL.** Approximately 5 percent of children with ALL are in this group. It is most commonly seen in infants and is often associated with a t(4;11) chromosome translocation.

• **Common precursor B cell.** The majority of children with B-lineage ALL have this type, which carries the best prognosis of all types of ALL.

• **Pre-B cell.** About 25 percent of children with pre-B ALL have the t(1;19) translocation. Although pre-B ALL used to signal a poor prognosis, with more aggressive modern treatments children with this subgroup appear to fare as well as those with common precursor B leukemia.

- **Mature B cell.** Approximately 2 percent of children with B-lineage ALL have this subgroup. It is the leukemic stage of Burkitt's lymphoma and requires a completely different treatment than other types of ALL.

Around 15 percent of children with ALL are in the T-cell group. Many chromosomal translocations have been identified in this type of ALL, some of which are used to determine the best treatment. Often, children with T-cell ALL are male, have high WBC counts at diagnosis, have masses in their chests, and are older than 10. T-cell ALL requires more intensive therapy than B-cell, but outcomes after intensive therapy are similar to those for B-lineage ALL.

> We were told the exact cytogenetics at the end of induction. At the time (October 2004), based on the fact that my son was T-cell with a high white cell count at diagnosis, he was stratified as high risk. The cytogenetics results were neither a good nor bad prognostic factor, so they continued to treat him as high risk. We were told that the only change they would have made was if he had cytogenetics that put him into a very high-risk category. For T-cell kids that typically means straight to transplant.

Chromosome number. Normal cells have 46 chromosomes (22 pairs and the sex chromosomes—XX for females or XY for males). There are two ways to evaluate the number of chromosomes: counting them (karyotyping) or measuring the DNA content of cells (DNA index). Some leukemia cells contain extra copies of entire chromosomes and thus can contain more than 46 chromosomes; this is called hyperdiploidy, and it is found in approximately 20 to 25 percent of children with ALL. Children with 53 or more chromosomes per cell or a DNA index greater than 1.16 have a very good prognosis.

Extra copies of particular chromosomes also seem to have an extremely favorable prognosis. Children with extra copies of chromosome 4, 10, and 17 (called trisomies) have an especially favorable prognosis.

> Our daughter, Isabel, was placed in the low-risk category within protocol AALL0331 because she had triple trisomies and the tail end of TEL-AML-1 translocation. The cytogenetics results were given to us in the hospital clinic by our main oncologist at the end of induction.

Around 6 percent of children with ALL have fewer than 45 chromosomes in the leukemia cells. This condition is called hypodiploidy and carries a poor prognosis.

Response to treatment. One factor in a child's prognosis is how quickly the leukemia cells disappear after starting treatment. Some institutions test the bone marrow on the 7th and 14th days of treatment. If a rapid reduction of blasts in the marrow has occurred within the first 2 weeks of treatment, the child is considered an "early rapid responder" and may be given a less intensive treatment plan.

Scientists are now using special biochemical techniques to measure the amount of leukemia remaining in the bone marrow after 4 weeks of chemotherapy. This measure of residual leukemia (called minimal residual disease, or MRD) is 1,000 times more sensitive than looking at the bone marrow with a microscope. The measurement of MRD after the early phase of treatment is being evaluated in clinical trials to determine how it can be used to help choose the intensity of the remaining treatment.

> *The reports we received were: molecular diagnostics, cytogenetics, and surface markers. The molecular diagnostics report provided information on translocations, the cytogenetics report on karyotype (hyper/hypodiploidy), and the surface markers report gave results on B-lineage markers, T-lineage markers, myeloid lineage markers, stem cell markers, and other markers. We received the surface marker report very quickly, the cytogenetics report about 1 week after diagnosis, and the molecular diagnostics about 3 weeks after diagnosis. The reports showed that Tom had pre-B ALL with high hyperdiploidy and the presence of the triple trisomy 4, 10, 17, but without any translocations. The fact that he had the triple trisomy was supposed to carry a good prognosis. However, he was still MRD+ at the end of induction and consolidation and relapsed in the bone marrow 2 months after his treatment ended.*

Summary. All of the above information is used to determine what treatment is most appropriate for your child. Children at low or average risk of relapse need fewer and less toxic drugs than those at high risk. However, most children with high-risk ALL do very well when given more intensive treatment.

Acute myeloid leukemia (AML)

AML (also called acute myelogenous leukemia or acute nonlymphocytic leukemia) is cancer of the blood cells that would otherwise develop into granulocytes and monocytes. Because treatments for AML and ALL are very different, it is crucial that sophisticated laboratory studies are performed on the bone marrow samples to determine whether your child has AML or ALL. In addition, chromosomal abnormalities, present in the blasts of approximately 75 percent of children with AML, should be identified for all children with AML to determine the best treatment.

Approximately 1,000 children are diagnosed with AML in the United States each year, with almost equal numbers of boys and girls being affected. AML accounts for 15 to 20 percent of all cases of childhood leukemia. African American children have a higher incidence of AML than Caucasian children, and Hispanic children have the highest incidence.

The World Health Organization devised a new classification system for types of childhood AML, and it was updated in 2008 to include specific gene mutations. The seven basic categories are:

- AML with recurrent genetic abnormalities
- AML with myelodysplasia-related features
- Therapy-related myeloid neoplasms
- AML, not otherwise specified
- Myeloid sarcoma
- Myeloid proliferations related to Down syndrome
- Blastic plasmacytoid dendritic cell neoplasm.

> *My 6-year-old daughter had been getting bad headaches. The school would call me to pick her up, and she would throw up all the way home. She had an appointment with the optometrist, who noticed an odd-looking vein in her eye and that she looked pale and had some bruising. He recommended taking her in for blood work. We did, and she was diagnosed with AML.*

A subtype of AML that is treated quite differently is acute promyelocytic leukemia (APL). The chromosomal abnormality associated with APL is t(15;17). Excessive bleeding is usually present at diagnosis and can complicate treatment. This type of leukemia has an extremely low incidence of spread to the CNS.

Prognosis for the child with AML

Treatment for AML has improved in the last decade. Today, 75 to 85 percent of children who receive optimal treatment at a major pediatric medical center achieve a complete remission. Of the children who achieve remission, 40 to 50 percent remain in remission for 5 years and are considered cured.

The WBC count at diagnosis is the most important predictor of response to treatment. Children with WBC counts higher than 100,000 per cubic milliliter at diagnosis do not do as well as children with lower WBC counts. Other factors that might predict more difficulty reaching remission are:

- Secondary AML (develops after treatment for another cancer)
- Monosomy 7 chromosome abnormality
- Children with CNS disease at diagnosis.

Factors that predict a high likelihood of achieving remission are:

- Rapid response to treatment

- Leukemia cell chromosomal abnormalities t(8;21) and inv(16)
- Down syndrome.

For more information about AML prognostic factors, visit the NCI website at *www. cancer.gov/cancertopics/pdq/treatment/childAML/HealthProfessional.*

Chronic myelogenous leukemia (CML)

CML is rare in children, accounting for less than 3.5 percent of all childhood leukemias. It is characterized by a very large spleen, a high WBC count of mostly neutrophils and other types of granulocytes, and a high platelet count. Other symptoms of CML are fatigue, weakness, headaches, irritability, fevers, night sweats, and bone pain. Some children have no symptoms and the cancer is only diagnosed after a routine blood test is done for other reasons.

In more than 90 percent of children with CML, analysis of bone marrow cells shows a genetic abnormality called the Philadelphia chromosome. This chromosome contains a translocation or swap of genetic material involving chromosomes 9 and 22, t(9;22).

Phases of CML

Despite its name, CML can progress rapidly, but it generally has three phases:

- Chronic (less than 5 percent blasts in the peripheral blood or bone marrow), which generally lasts 3 to 5 years.
- Accelerated (greater than 5 percent but less than 30 percent blasts in the peripheral blood or bone marrow). This phase can begin gradually or abruptly. Symptoms include fever, night sweats, weight loss, and an increase in WBC counts.
- Blastic (greater than 30 percent blasts in the peripheral blood or bone marrow). Symptoms of blastic phase (also called blast crisis) include fever, fatigue, and an enlarged spleen.

> *Leah, 11 years old, enjoyed participating in basketball, soccer, and gymnastics. She developed severe hip joint pain, and we brought her back to the doctor three times in an unsuccessful attempt to find out what was wrong. The last time, my husband had to carry her in because she couldn't walk. They did blood work, and her white count was 176,000 and her platelets were 1 million. A bone marrow test confirmed that she had CML.*

For information about CML prognostic factors, visit the NCI website at *www.cancer.gov/ cancertopics/pdq/treatment/childAML/HealthProfessional* and click on "Chronic Myelogenous Leukemia" on the left navigation bar.

Juvenile myelomonocytic leukemia (JMML)

JMML accounts for less than 1.5 percent of childhood leukemias. It is usually diagnosed in children younger than 2 and is more common in boys than girls. Hispanic children are at increased risk of developing this form of leukemia.

JMML affects monocytes, and although it is classed as a chronic leukemia, the symptoms are similar to those of acute leukemias: pale skin, fever, headaches, sweating, and recurrent infections. Also usually present are enlarged lymph nodes, enlarged spleen and liver, skin rash, and an elevated WBC count. The course of JMML is unpredictable; but once diagnosed, progressive deterioration usually occurs. Infants with JMML can survive for several years, but children older than 1 usually have rapidly progressive disease.

> *My daughter was diagnosed with JMML in 1993 at the age of 27 months. Although it is a chronic leukemia, it is particularly fast moving. It is also vastly different from the adult CML. My daughter had a mismatched (5/6) related (my husband's sister as donor) BMT (bone marrow transplant) 4 months after she was diagnosed. Today, she is 8 years post-transplant, is in the fourth grade, and is the absolute joy of my life.*

A strong link exists between certain genetic mutations and JMML. About 80 percent of children with JMML have an identified mutation at diagnosis. Twenty-five percent of these children have a mutation in the RAS gene family and another 35 percent have a *PTPN11* mutation. Another 15 to 20 percent of children with JMML have an inherited genetic disease called neurofibromatosis 1 (NF1).

Best treatments for leukemia

At diagnosis, many parents do not know how to find the best doctors and treatments for their child. Excellent care is available from physicians who participate in the Children's Oncology Group (COG). This group, comprising pediatric surgeons and oncologists, neurologists, radiation oncologists, researchers, and nurses from approximately 230 hospitals that treat children with cancer, provide state-of-the-art treatments for leukemia and conduct studies to discover better therapies and supportive care for children with all types of cancer. In addition, several individual centers of excellence (e.g., St. Jude Children's Research Hospital) provide excellent care and design their own clinical trials. Chapter 4, "Choosing a Treatment," provides detailed descriptions of the current treatments for the leukemias described in this chapter.

> *I am at work, an ordinary day. The phone rings, "Hello?" "Can I speak to Patty?" "Speaking." "This is Anne at the University Medical Group Practice. I hate to tell you over the phone, but we think your son has leukemia."*

I need to back up just a bit, to the day before. I had taken my son, James, to a nurse practitioner, Anne. James had been a little tired for several weeks, and he also spoke of muscle pains in varying places, such as his shoulders, back, and legs. This in itself was not unusual for him because he was in weight training. But he just didn't have his usual energy: he could not do a 25-mile bike ride anymore without getting tired. It bothered us; he was kind of acting like an old man, too tired to run up the stairs two at a time.

Anne checked him and said he looked just fine; his oxygen levels were great and his lung capacity was great. But she drew some blood for analysis—just in case— thinking mono. Thank you, Anne!

James was a junior in high school and we were turning our thoughts to colleges and dealing with him leaving home to go to college. I only took him to see Anne to set my mind at ease. After we left, I completely forgot about the visit.

The blood samples were sent off to the University Health Sciences Center and the diagnosis came back: leukemia. As Anne told me over the phone, she was in tears herself, apologizing for not telling me in person. She wanted James at the hospital ASAP. She had already booked a room for him.

Shock set in and survival instincts took over. I knew I couldn't drive safely, so a wonderful friend at work drove me the 23 miles home. There, luckily, were my son and husband, by chance home from school and work early. Back into the car for the 55-mile drive to Children's Hospital, not knowing even exactly where it was.

We were checked into Children's Hospital in Denver within 27 hours of visiting the nurse practitioner. I had an awful time opening the door that said "Oncology" and escorting my son through it. The oncology docs re-ran the tests, and 2 hours later, we know, yes, it is leukemia. Shock. What can you do? You deal with it, somehow. You grieve. You find out what you have to know and have to do to help him.

Your life stops and starts again.

Chapter 3

Telling Your Child and Others

To name things is to tame them.
— Tim O'Brien
Tomcat in Love

YOU HAVE JUST LEARNED how gravely ill your child is. There is so much to take in, so much to do, and all you really want to do is wake up and end this nightmare; but you are the only one who knows this news. You must think of what to tell your sick child. And what can you say to her siblings? Or her grandparents? Should you tell your friends and neighbors? What can you possibly say?

Telling your child

It is important now to defy any urge you have to shield your child from the truth, because honesty is one of the most important gifts you can give him now. Your child needs to know what is happening to him. You must prepare him for what is to come. Because you are coping with a bewildering array of emotions yourself, sharing information and providing reassurance and hope may be difficult. In the past, shielding children from the painful reality of the disease was the norm. Most experts now agree that children feel less anxiety and cope with treatments better if they have a clear understanding of leukemia. It is important to provide age-appropriate information soon after diagnosis and to create a supportive climate so children feel comfortable asking questions of both parents and the medical team. Sharing strengthens the family, allowing all members to face the crisis together.

When to tell your child

You should tell your child as soon as possible after diagnosis. Sick children know they are sick, and all children know when their parents are upset, frightened, and withholding information. In the absence of the truth, children imagine—and believe—scenarios far more frightening than the reality. With no warning, they have found themselves in strange surroundings; all of their normal patterns have been abandoned; total strangers are performing scary and painful procedures on them; their parents are upset; and everywhere they look, they see sick or disabled children. They may not be talking about their fears, often in an effort to protect their parents, but they know something is very wrong. The most loving thing a parent can do is to tell the truth before the child is overwhelmed by the fear of what he has imagined. Staying silent also has another side effect: it undermines the credibility of the parent with the child. This will be a very long and frightening journey, and your child must believe you are in this together and that he can always count on you to support him and tell him the truth.

> We feel that you have to be very honest or the child will not be able to trust you. Meagan (5 years old) has always known that she has cancer and thinks of her treatments and medications as the warriors to help the good cells fight the bad cells.

Who should tell your child

This is purely a personal decision, influenced by ease of communication within the family, age and temperament of the child, religious beliefs, and sometimes physician recommendation. Children ages 1 to 3 primarily fear separation from parents, so the presence of strangers in an already unfamiliar situation may increase their anxiety. Many parents tell their small child in private, while others prefer to have a family physician, oncologist, social worker, clergy, or other family members present.

Children from 4 to 12 sometimes benefit from having the treatment team (oncologist, nurse, social worker, or psychologist) present. It provides an opportunity for the staff to strengthen their bond with the child and to promote the sense that everyone is united in their efforts to help the child get well. Staff members can answer the child's questions and provide comfort for the entire family. Children in this age group frequently feel guilty and responsible for their illness. They may harbor fears that the cancer is a punishment for something they did wrong. Social workers and nurses can help explore unspoken questions, provide reassurance, and identify the needs of parents, the sick child, and siblings.

> My 6-year-old son Brent was sitting next to me when the doctor called to tell me that he had leukemia. I whispered into the phone, "What should I tell him?" The doctor said to tell him that he had a disease in his blood and needed to go to a special children's hospital for help. As we were getting ready to go to the hospital, Brent asked if he had AIDS (it was right after Magic Johnson's announcement), if he was going to die, and what were they going to do to him. We didn't know how to answer all the questions, but told him that we would find out at the hospital. My husband told him that he was a strong boy and we would all fight this thing together. I was at a loss for words.
>
> At the hospital, they were wonderful. What impressed me the most was that they always talked to Brent first, and answered all his questions before talking to us.

When Zac (Brent's 8-year-old brother) came to the hospital 2 days later, the doctors took him in the hall and talked to him for a long time, explaining and answering his questions.

I was glad that we were all so honest, because Brent later confided to me that he had first thought he got leukemia because he hadn't been drinking enough milk.

Adolescents have a powerful need for control and autonomy that should be respected. At a time when teens' developmental tasks include becoming independent from their families, they are suddenly totally dependent on medical personnel to save their lives and on parents to provide emotional support. Teenagers sometimes feel more comfortable discussing the diagnosis with their physician in private. In some families, a diagnosis of cancer can create an unwelcome dependence on parents and can add new stress to the already turbulent teen years. Other families report that leukemia helped forge closer bonds between teenagers and their parents.

When my daughter went into the hospital to get the mediastinal mass diagnosis done, I told her doctor if she got a bad report that I wanted him to tell her father and me and not give her any such news. Her doctor, who I really didn't know before this encounter, informed me that she was 15 years old and would be the one dealing with cancer and it was very necessary that she be told everything and that nothing be kept from her. I thought that was so mean of him, but I liked him and had never shown any disrespect for a doctor before, so I decided since he had dealt with kids with cancer before and I hadn't that he must know something I didn't know. He did! There have been so many times I have been so thankful that he had the wisdom to tell me that right off the bat.

Children and teens react to the diagnosis of cancer with a wide range of emotions, as do their parents. They may lapse into denial, feel tremendous anger or rage, or be extremely optimistic. As treatment progresses, both children and parents will experience a variety of unexpected emotions.

We've really marveled as we watched Joseph go through the stages of coping with all of this just as an adult might. First of all, when he was diagnosed in April and May, he was terrified. Then in May and June he was alternately angry and depressed. When we talked to him seriously during that time about the need to work with the doctors and nurses against the cancer no matter how scary the things were that they asked him to do, he looked us right in the eye and screamed, "I'm on the cancer's side!" Then over the course of a few weeks he seemed to calm down and made the decision to fight it, to cooperate with all the caregivers as well as he possibly could and to live as normal a life as he could. It's hard to believe that someone could do that at 4 years old, but he did it. By his 5th birthday on July 26th, he'd made the transition to where he is now: hopeful and committed to "killing the cancer."

What to tell your child

Children need to be told that they have leukemia and what that means, using words and concepts appropriate to their age and level of emotional development. The sooner they are comfortable with the word leukemia, the less mysterious it will seem and the more powerful they will feel in dealing with the disease. Very young children might be satisfied to hear, "Leukemia is a disease that makes part of your blood sick and we need to go to the hospital for medicine to make it better." Older children may benefit from reading books, alone or together with a parent, surfing reliable Internet sites, or asking the hospital staff many questions to gain the information that matters most to them.

Key concepts to convey include:

- The disease is called leukemia and this is what it means (supply age-appropriate description).

- No one knows what causes leukemia, and it is not the child's fault she got sick.

- Most children are cured, but treatment takes a long time and can sometimes be scary or painful.

- It may be necessary to spend a lot of time in the hospital.

- There will be some unpleasant side effects, such as hair loss and weight gain or loss, but these are temporary.

- Leukemia is not contagious; friends and family cannot catch it.

- The parents, the child, and the healthcare team all have jobs to do to help the child get well and everyone will work together to make that happen.

- Some things about leukemia are scary—for the child and the parents—and it is okay to feel afraid, confused, angry, or sad.

- Questions or worries are normal, and the child should feel free to ask a parent or someone on the healthcare team any questions she wants to ask.

- There are many things the parents cannot control, but the parents will never lie to their child and will always try to make sure there are no surprises.

- School-age children should be told they may not be able to go to school for a few months, but that there are ways they can still keep in touch with their classmates while they are out of school.

> My daughter Kathleen Rea knew she had cancer when she was three. She knew that her motor oil wasn't running her engine right—but she called it cancer. Young children need to be reassured that they did nothing to cause the disease. It is important that they understand the disease is not contagious and they cannot give it to their siblings or friends. They need to have procedures described realistically, so that they can trust their parents and medical team.

My 4-year-old daughter told me very sadly one day, "I wish that I hadn't fallen down and broken inside. That's how the leukemia started." We had explained many times that nothing she did, or we did, caused the leukemia, but she persisted in thinking that falling down did it. She also worried that if she went to her friend Krista's house to play that Krista would catch leukemia.

Children will have many questions throughout their treatment. Parents must assure the child that this is normal and that they will always answer the child's questions honestly. Gentle and honest communication is essential for the child to feel loved, supported, and encouraged.

When I told Christine (3 years old) that she had a disease in her blood, her first concern was that I might leave. Over the years, I have repeated many times that I would always be with her, and that I would make sure that there were never any surprises. (This is difficult sometimes in the hospital setting, but it can be done.) She is very artistic and wanted me to draw a picture of the cells that were a problem. We drew lots of pictures of white cells being carried off by chemo drugs to be "fixed." Although many of the other parents successfully used images of good cells killing off bad cells, I thought that would upset my extremely gentle daughter. So we imagined, drew pictures, and talked about chemo turning problem cells into helpful cells.

When your child asks a question, take a moment to be sure you heard and understood it correctly and to formulate a thoughtful answer that your child will understand. Parents are under tremendous stress at this time and have many things on their own minds. In this distracted state, it is easy to toss off an easy answer or answer a question the child did not ask; but doing this can increase the child's confusion and undermine their trust in the parent as a source of information. Barbara Sourkes, PhD, explains the importance of understanding the child's question before responding:

Coping with the trauma of illness can be facilitated by a cognitive understanding of the disease and its treatment. For this reason, the presentation of accurate information in developmentally meaningful terms is crucial. A general guideline is to follow the child's lead: he or she questions facts or implications only when ready, and that readiness must be respected. It is the adult's responsibility to clarify the precise intent of any question and then to proceed with a step-by-step response, thereby granting the child options at each juncture. He or she may choose to continue listening, to ask for clarification, or to terminate the discussion. Offering less information with the explicit invitation to ask for more affords a safety gauge of control for the child. When these guidelines are not followed, serious miscommunications may ensue. For example, an adult who hears "What is going to happen to me?" and does not clarify the intent of the query may launch into a long statement of plans or elaborate reassurances. The child may respond with irritation, "I only wanted to know what tests I am going to have tomorrow."

Telling the siblings

The diagnosis of cancer is traumatic for siblings. Family life is disrupted, time with parents decreases, and a large amount of attention is paid to the ill child. Brothers and sisters need as much knowledge as their sick sibling. Information provided should be age appropriate, and all questions should be answered honestly. Healthcare providers (physicians, nurse practitioners, child life specialists, and social workers) can help parents educate the well siblings. Siblings can be extremely cooperative if they understand the changes that occur in the family and their role in helping the family to cope. Maintaining open communication and respecting their feelings helps siblings feel loved and secure.

> We always, always explained everything that was happening to Brent's older brother Zac (8 years old). He never asked questions, but always listened intently. He would say, "Okay. I understand. Everything's all right." We tried to get him to talk about it, but through all these years, he just never has. So we just kept explaining things at a level that he could understand, and he has done very well through the whole ordeal. The times that he seemed sad, we would take him out of school and let him stay at the Ronald McDonald House for a few days, and that seemed to help him.

· · · · ·

> We have tried to spend one-on-one time with each of the other kids. These are some other things that have been good for us:
>
> - The kids have been going to the hospital with Ethan one at a time, and getting a sense that this is no picnic, what he is going through.
>
> - If one of us is out of town and Ethan is in the hospital, I have hired a babysitter to be with him in the evening and have done something special with the other kids for one of the nights. This works great if you live close enough to the hospital where your child is being treated.
>
> - My husband and I have each taken the older kids on the traditional summer trips. This has been hard on Ethan, but none of this is perfect.
>
> - My husband and I have each taken one school subject for the kids and have really spent time with them on it. I did reading with Tucker (I read everything he does and we talk about it), French with Abe, and Spanish with Jake. My husband has different topics, and we do something every day. We were too dysfunctional to be able to do more than one subject, so we decided to focus, and it has been a lot of fun for us.
>
> We talk about lots of things as a family and help the kids where needed, but these are "special" things. This has been a long year for us, but I think these things helped.

Even with optimum communication and support, parents may see siblings experiencing difficult emotions, such as anger, guilt, jealousy, and sadness, and changes in behavior, such as regression, school problems, and symptoms of illness to gain attention. These result from the stress of living with a brother or sister diagnosed with cancer. Chapter 14, "Siblings," explores sibling issues in detail and contains many suggestions from both parents and siblings who have gone through this experience.

Notifying the family

Notifying relatives is one of the first painful jobs for the parent of a child newly diagnosed with cancer. Depending on the family dynamic, the family may be a refuge or a source of additional stress.

> *I called my mom and told her to make all the phone calls to family and friends. I couldn't choke out the word leukemia yet. Then I called our pastor.*

> • • • • •

> *I called my sister and asked her to take care of telling everyone. She called my other sister, and together they told my frail mother.*

> • • • • •

> *I waited 3 days after the diagnosis to call anyone. The doctors had trouble determining whether it was ALL or AML, and I wanted to be able to give the prognosis on the first call. I called my mom and asked her to notify everyone else but to request that they not call me for a week. I felt too fragile, and didn't want to continually cry in front of my daughter.*

Family members will often react in surprising ways, with unexpected help coming from some people and a disappointing lack of support from others. Parents must be prepared for these unexpected results and try not to take them personally. Usually, the other person is struggling to process this difficult news in his or her own way and may be trying to spare the parent from more stress by not asking too many questions.

Notifying friends and neighbors

The easiest way to notify friends and neighbors is to delegate one person to do the job. Calling only one neighbor or close friend prevents you from having numerous tearful conversations. Most parents are at their child's bedside and want to avoid more emotional upheaval, especially in front of their child. Parents need to recognize that friends' emotions will mirror their own: shock, fear, worry, helplessness. Because most friends want to help but don't know what to do or say, they will welcome any clues you can give about what might be helpful.

Tell the trusted friend exactly what information you want him or her to pass on and, most importantly, whether you would welcome visits, phone calls, or cards. The more clarity you can provide, the less stress you will experience and the better your friends can support you. If you want visitors, for example, let people know when visiting hours are and whether there are any restrictions set by the hospital (or by you or your child) about who can come and for how long.

Not everyone you know will want or need the same level of detailed information. You may wish to encourage visits from close acquaintances but ask others to wait for phone or e-mail updates. However, think twice before leaving anyone off the notification list. Many parents report that individuals they barely knew ended up being some of their most helpful and supportive resources.

Many families set up phone trees to provide ongoing updates—the parent calls one person, who calls a designated group of people, who then call others. More information about this topic is available in Chapter 12, "Family and Friends."

Notifying your child's school

You should notify the principal as soon as possible about your child's diagnosis. It is a good idea to do this in writing, in part because it is a less emotional way to convey the news, but also because it enables you to be certain you pass along all the relevant information. In this first contact, it is helpful to include the following information:

- The diagnosis and a brief description in layman's terms of what it means.

- A very brief outline of what is expected to happen next and how that will impact your child's ability to attend school.

- The address, e-mail address, and phone number where you can be reached.

- A brief description of the educational resources available at the hospital or any other educational information you have been given by the hospital social worker or child life specialist and their contact information if they wish to be contacted.

- How your child's teacher or classmates can reach your child, especially while she is in the hospital.

You can also express your hope that you, the school, and the hospital will work together to ensure that your child's education sustains as few interruptions as possible. You may wish to ask the principal to share your letter with the teacher or teachers or you can send them a separate note. If you want to ask the teachers and students to stay in touch with your child, inform them that she may sometimes feel too tired to answer right away. Personal visits may not be feasible or welcome, at least at first, but cards, letters, pictures, classroom videos, or other updates will make your child feel less isolated and will remind her that there are people who care for her outside of her immediate family and the hospital staff. The wishes of teens about notification of school and friends should be respected. (More information is available in Chapter 15, "School.")

> *Ashlee was in kindergarten when she was diagnosed. As soon as they heard the news, the class sent her a huge card. She loved studying that card and talking about how much she looked forward to her return to school. She also sent a handmade thank you card back to them. The kindergarten class made a very big deal of everyone's birthday, but when Ashlee's birthday came, her class did nothing. Several days later, I stopped at the school to tell the teacher how sad Ashlee was (and how angry I was) that no one from her class recognized her birthday. The teacher said the students had asked to do something for Ashlee, but the teacher had ruled it out, saying that Ashlee probably would not want to be reminded of all the fun everyone else was having. I was flabbergasted by how badly this otherwise kind and thoughtful woman got it wrong.*

Using technology to communicate

After the initial contacts have been made, the people in your life will be eager for updates. During those first few weeks of treatment, parents have very little time to chat and often lack the energy to carry on lengthy or meaningful conversations. The nights can be long, however, and nighttime provides an excellent opportunity to use modern technology to keep people informed about what is happening and to express your own feelings in a way that might not be comfortable in person.

Many metropolitan hospitals now have free wireless Internet access (Wi-Fi) in the room, in the parents' lounge, or in a communal room. Some Internet service providers, such as Verizon, offer their own Wi-Fi adapters that can be plugged into a laptop to provide access anywhere there is cell phone service. Blackberries®, iPhones®, and other personal data devices also all have Internet access.

Once connected to the Internet, many options exist for keeping in touch, including blog sites, MySpace, Twitter, and Facebook. Others establish an e-mail group and send regular updates to the list. One of the easiest and safest ways to communicate with your friends and family is to use CaringBridge (*www.caringbridge.org*). CaringBridge offers free websites to families and friends of critically ill individuals. Its templates make it easy to set up an attractive site and the software allows you to add text and photos. Parents, siblings, or the sick child can create journal entries that track the progress of treatment, and discuss fears, inspirations, hopes, or needs. There is a guest book where well-wishers can post words of love and encouragement. Finally, you can make the site as public or private as you wish and link your site to other places, such as a blog or Facebook page. The CaringBridge websites do not have annoying pop-ups or advertisements of any kind.

The following passage was written by Jenny Gardner and is reprinted with permission from *Candlelighters Youth Newsletter*, Spring 1995, Vol. XVII No. 2. Jenny was diagnosed with ALL in 1984. A resident of New Jersey, she is an accomplished horsewoman and also enjoys singing and acting.

When I was diagnosed with leukemia, I felt like I was trapped in a room with no windows or doors, and the walls were closing in on me. I thought that I would never be able to smell my grandmother's hand cream, or feel the way my dad's face felt in the morning before he shaves, or the way my mom's silk blouse feels when I hug her. I thought that I would never have the sensation of turning one year older again. I thought that I would never again be able to feel how I feel after it rains, when it smells so fresh and clean like the whole world just took a bath. I thought that I would never be able to taste my first glass of champagne on New Year's and feel all bubbly and warm like I was flying in a hot-air balloon. And all of a sudden my dream popped, and I realized that this wasn't a dream, it was reality.

Right now there are thousands of kids like me across the country who are feeling the same way I felt 8 years ago, and I would just like to wish them good luck. Because it's a long, hard journey full of needles, blood tests, and chemotherapy, but when you finally get to the end, you feel like you've been freed after years and years of darkness, and I'll tell you one thing—that is the greatest feeling you could have!

Chapter 4

Choosing a Treatment

*The challenge in pediatric oncology remains clear: to strive for the cure
and health of all children through the development of more effective yet
less damaging treatment for our young patients.*

— Daniel M. Green, MD and
Giulio J. D'Angio, MD
*Late Effects of Treatment for
Childhood Cancer*

THE FIRST FEW weeks after diagnosis are overwhelming. In the midst of confusion, fear, and fatigue, you must make an important and sometimes difficult decision: whether to choose the best known treatment (standard treatment) or enroll your child in an experimental treatment (clinical trial).

This chapter explains helpful things to know before deciding on a treatment course for your child, including the difference between standard treatment and clinical trials. The standard treatments (at the time this book was updated in 2009) for the most common types of leukemia are described. Also included are a description of clinical trials, discussion about the importance of informed consent, the pros and cons of selecting a clinical trial, and stories from parents about the decisions they made.

Treatment basics

To receive the best available treatment, it is essential that the child with leukemia be treated at a pediatric medical center by board-certified pediatric oncologists with extensive experience treating the disease. For most leukemias, intense treatment begins within days of diagnosis and requires aggressive supportive care. The goal of treatment is to achieve complete remission by obliterating all leukemia cells as quickly as possible. Complete remission occurs when all signs and symptoms of leukemia disappear and abnormal cells are no longer found in the blood, bone marrow, or cerebrospinal fluid (CSF).

Treatment of childhood leukemia always includes one or more of the following:

- Chemotherapy (drug treatment)
- Stem cell transplant (SCT)
- Radiation therapy.

Nearly every treatment for leukemia begins with a course of chemotherapy, usually involving several different drugs in carefully controlled combinations. For most children, the only treatment will be chemotherapy, although the treatment can be complicated and may last for many months or years. For certain leukemias, such as juvenile myelomonocytic leukemia (JMML), an SCT is usually done after one or more courses of chemotherapy. Doctors try to avoid radiation therapy unless it is necessary, because of the potential for permanent damage. Radiation is normally used only when leukemia cells are found in the CSF or testes at diagnosis, if the child is at very high risk of central nervous system (CNS) relapse, or prior to an SCT.

Standard treatments

The standard treatment (or standard of care) for each type of leukemia is the treatment that has worked best in the most patients up to that point in time. The current standards of care are the result of decades of clinical research studies. As researchers analyze the results from ongoing or completed clinical trials, they accumulate knowledge and make changes in standard treatments. In the 1980s, for example, most children with acute lymphoblastic leukemia (ALL) received cranial radiation as standard care. Carefully controlled clinical trials later demonstrated that the majority of children with ALL do not require cranial radiation, and even those who do can be given a lower dose than was used in the 1980s. Thus, the standard of care was changed.

Following are brief, general descriptions of the standards of care for the four most common types of childhood leukemia. In some cases, standards of care vary by institution. To learn more about current treatments, contact the National Cancer Institute's (NCI) Physician's Data Query (PDQ) by calling (800) 422-6237 (800-4-CANCER) or by going to the pediatric section of its website at *www.cancer.gov/cancertopics/pdq/pediatrictreatment*. PDQ provides free fact sheets that explain the disease, state-of-the-art treatments, and ongoing clinical trials. Two versions are available: one for patients that uses simple language and contains no statistics, and one for professionals that is technical, thorough, and includes citations to the scientific literature.

Standard treatment for ALL

ALL is one of the most curable forms of childhood cancer. Over the years, it has become possible to determine risk categories for newly diagnosed children, based on several criteria, such as age at diagnosis, white blood cell (WBC) count at diagnosis, location and type of leukemia cells, and certain genetic and molecular characteristics of the cancer cells. Most children in the low- or average-risk categories are cured using the standard treatment. The primary treatment for ALL is chemotherapy.

Some very high-risk patients may require radiation to the brain or spinal cord. Children with an extremely high risk of relapse or those who have relapsed are often given an SCT from cord blood or bone marrow from an HLA-matched sibling. (For more information, see Chapter 21, "Stem Cell Transplantation.")

Treatment for ALL is usually divided into phases: induction, consolidation, and maintenance (sometimes called continuation). Throughout treatment, children are given treatment in the CNS to prevent the disease from spreading. Some protocols include a reinduction, reconsolidation, or delayed intensification phase of treatment. Children with extremely high WBC counts at diagnosis may require leukapheresis (removal of the WBCs) before starting chemotherapy.

Induction. Induction is the initial phase of treatment and usually lasts 4 weeks. Its purpose is to induce a complete remission (absence of any sign of disease) in the shortest amount of time possible. Most induction protocols allow the treatments to be administered in an outpatient setting, although children often need to be readmitted to the hospital on more than one occasion due to fever or infection. Some higher-risk induction protocols require children to be hospitalized for portions of the treatment for monitoring and transfusions.

Chemotherapy is most effective if three or four drugs are used simultaneously. In 2009, the majority of standard-risk ALL induction programs included vincristine, prednisone or dexamethasone, and asparaginase. An anthracycline (usually daunorubicin, but sometimes idarubicin or epirubicin) is often added to high-risk protocols. In 2005, a new pro-drug (a substance that metabolizes in the body into a drug) called nelarabine was approved for use in children with T-cell ALL who have relapsed or who are slow to enter remission.

Chemotherapy drugs are given in five ways:

- Intravenously (IV)—through a needle or tube in the vein
- Intramuscularly (IM)—by injection in muscle
- Subcutaneously (SQ)—by injection under the skin
- Orally (PO)—by mouth in liquid or pill form
- Intrathecally (IT)—through injection into the CSF.

Chemotherapy drugs can cause numerous side effects. (See Chapter 9, "Chemotherapy," for an in-depth discussion of each drug, its side effects, and parent suggestions.)

Complete remission—the absence of any signs of disease—is determined by analyzing bone marrow samples for leukemia cells. In the 1990s, technicians could only measure the number of leukemia cells to an accuracy of 1 cell in 100 cells, and at that time, complete remission was defined as less than 5 percent leukemia cells. By 2009, tests at the molecular level for minimum residual disease (MRD) could detect the number of leukemia cells to an accuracy of 1 cell in 10,000, or 0.01 percent. Increasingly, researchers are incorporating the concept of MRD into their definition of remission for several types of leukemia in the hope that earlier identification of children at high risk of relapse will result in treatment modifications that have better outcomes.

Current treatment plans for ALL incorporate both a "traditional" definition for remission of less than 5 percent leukemia cells and a definition of remission using MRD values. In 2009, the Children's Oncology Group (COG), Dana Farber Cancer Institute, and St. Jude Children's Research Hospital were evaluating new ways that incorporate MRD-defined remission values to classify response to induction and direct the intensity of each child's treatment after induction.

Children who achieve remission in the first 7 to 14 days have an extremely good chance of long-term survival. Those who are slow to respond to treatment or who do not achieve remission within 30 days have a poorer prognosis and their treatment is modified, usually to include more drugs at higher doses. For these children, doctors are increasingly recommending an allogeneic SCT (stem cells received from a matched donor) as soon as they attain remission. See Chapter 21, "Stem Cell Transplantation," for more information.)

Central nervous system (CNS) prophylaxis. The CNS is composed of the brain and spinal cord, which are bathed in a fluid called cerebrospinal fluid (CSF). When leukemia invades the brain, leukemia blasts are found in the CSF. Less than 5 percent of children have leukemia cells in the CSF at diagnosis. However, before it became standard practice to use CNS prophylaxis (prevention), 60 to 70 percent of children with ALL eventually developed leukemia in the CNS. This statistic suggests that at the time of diagnosis, microscopic amounts of leukemia are already present in the CNS. Therefore, CNS prophylaxis is now an essential part of ALL treatment.

Because a blood–brain barrier exists that prevents most chemotherapy drugs from crossing into the CNS to destroy leukemic cells, chemotherapy drugs are injected directly into the CSF (called intrathecal medication) during spinal taps. Intrathecal medication is given periodically throughout treatment.

Interim maintenance (IM) occurs between consolidation and delayed intensification, and long-term maintenance (LTM) follows the delayed intensification phase in current standard risk protocols. Unfortunately, the treatments can sometimes cause long-term disabilities such as decreased attention span, short-term memory problems, and lowered abilities in spatial and mathematical skills, particularly when radiation is used (see Chapter 15, "School," for information about managing learning disabilities caused by treatment). Researchers continue to search for CNS treatments with fewer risks for long-term side effects.

Standard-risk patients receive intrathecal methotrexate, intrathecal cytarabine, or triple intrathecal therapy—methotrexate, hydrocortisone, and cytarabine—for CNS prophylaxis. Some children with a high risk of CNS relapse (e.g., children with T-cell ALL and a high WBC count or children who are slow to enter remission) are given cranial radiation, either in place of intrathecal drugs or in addition to them. However, this practice is controversial because cranial radiation significantly increases the chance of lasting neurological damage and may not confer any greater protection than drugs alone.

Consolidation. Even though more than 95 percent of children with ALL achieve remission during induction, without further therapy most of them would quickly relapse. The goal of consolidation therapy is to continue killing the remaining leukemic cells and stop new diseased cells from forming. This process is trickier than it sounds because cancer cells, which by definition are very unstable, tend to mutate frequently and can become resistant to the drugs that initially kill them. As a result, consolidation therapy consists of new combinations of drugs designed to destroy the cancer cells that survived induction and to stop the development of new cancer cells.

In 2009, the most common drugs used in consolidation were methotrexate, cyclophosphamide (Cytoxan®), cytarabine (ARA-C), mercaptopurine (6-MP), dexamethasone (Decadron®), asparaginase, and thioguanine (6-TG). (See Chapter 9, "Chemotherapy," for detailed descriptions of these drugs.)

Reinduction and reconsolidation. A second induction (commonly called delayed intensification or reinduction) and a second consolidation may be administered prior to maintenance in some protocols. Children who were slow to respond to induction treatment may benefit from these additional treatment phases.

Maintenance. Maintenance (also called continuation therapy) can occur between induction and reinduction (and is, in that case, called interim maintenance); or in cases when children do not require more intensive treatment, it follows induction and is the final phase of treatment for ALL. This phase is sometimes called long-term maintenance or LTM, and it consists of lower-dose chemotherapy given for 2 years (for girls) or 3 years (for boys) to kill any remaining leukemia cells. This portion of treatment is less toxic and sometimes easier to tolerate than induction and consolidation.

Most children will receive oral doses of mercaptopurine (6-MP) every evening and weekly methotrexate. In addition, other drugs such as vincristine, prednisone, or dexamethasone are given periodically given. Most protocols also give intrathecal methotrexate during maintenance therapy. During maintenance, children are monitored for effects on blood counts and drug-related toxicities.

Some children have an inherited trait (deficiency of an enzyme called thiopurine methyltransferase, or TPMT) that makes it difficult for them to break down two chemotherapy drugs—6-MP and 6-TG. These children can only tolerate small doses of these medications; at conventional doses, the children may have profound and life-threatening drops in their blood counts. (See Chapter 9, "Chemotherapy," for more information about TPMT.)

> It's a dance...keep the chemo high enough to do its job without causing system failure, so to speak. We had a really rough first few months on maintenance. Marielle was tested for TPMT but it came back normal. She also had liver problems (more than 20 times higher than the numbers should have been) and we had to hold chemo for that. I felt like we'd get her on chemo, push it up a bit, she'd crash, and it would take forever for her to come back up (we had holds of 21 days and 28 days). It was a matter of finding the right mix.

> After a few months, we found the right amount that kept her ANC (absolute neutrophil count) right around 1,000 and didn't make her crash. Remember, the numbers are for "the average child," yet every child is unique. For many, it may work fine to get the "average" amount of chemo; for some, it won't. It will get better; just give it more time as they adjust the chemo dosage. I know, everyone thinks that LTM is a walk in the park...it's not; it's just not nearly as difficult as the earlier phases of the protocol. That said, once they got the chemo mix right, we went 10 months without an ER visit or inpatient stay. Life really was much more normal.

More intensive regimens. Protocols for high-risk ALL usually contain more drugs at higher doses and sometimes involve cranial radiation. These treatments have increased toxicity, but they are more effective for the small percentage of children with very high-risk features.

Stem cell transplantation (SCT). SCT may be recommended after first remission in some children at extremely high risk of relapse, such as infants younger than 1 year who have MLL gene rearrangements, children with the Philadelphia chromosome, or children who are slow to achieve remission. (See Chapter 21, "Stem Cell Transplantation," for more information.)

Newest treatment options. Researchers are attempting to maintain cure rates using less-toxic therapies, and the following two strategies are particularly promising. Targeted therapy, in which doctors use drugs to target specific reproductive processes in the cancerous cells, may make it possible to minimize the toxicity of treatments. Risk-adapted therapies, in which doctors tailor the treatment to fit an individual's risk profile, could significantly reduce the length or severity of treatment for patients who are at low risk of relapse.

To learn about the most current standard treatments for each risk category of ALL, visit the NCI website at *www.cancer.gov/cancertopics/pdq/treatment/childALL/HealthProfessional/ page4* and *www.cancer.gov/cancertopics/pdq/treatment/childALL/HealthProfessional/page5*.

Standard treatment for acute myeloid leukemia (AML)

Children with AML have a high risk of relapse, so their treatment is very intense. However, treatment usually does not last longer than 1 year. To receive the best chance of complete remission and minimize risks from treatment side effects and complications, children with AML should be treated at a major pediatric hospital with expertise in treating acute leukemias. The goal of treatment is to achieve a complete remission by obliterating all cancer cells as quickly as possible and to prevent the disease from returning. The information in the ALL section about MRD also applies to AML treatment.

Combination chemotherapy is the primary treatment to induce remission in children with AML. For most children, treatment usually consists of two or three phases: induction (to achieve remission), postremission consolidation, and/or postremission intensification.

Radiation of the brain and sometimes the spinal cord is used infrequently. Increasingly, children with AML receive SCTs, either from matched unrelated donors (allogeneic transplants) or by harvesting cells from the child, freezing them, then reinjecting them (autologous transplant) after the child has received chemotherapy or after a relapse. (See Chapter 21, "Stem Cell Transplantation," for more information about transplants.)

Certain groups of children with AML—those with Down syndrome and those with the translocation t(15;17)—are treated on different protocols.

Before induction. Children with AML are often extremely sick when they arrive at the hospital and may require immediate treatment for complications of their disease before induction can begin. Many children have a disturbance in the blood-clotting system and may need transfusions of platelets or other blood factors to improve blood clotting. Some AML patients are very anemic and require blood transfusions before therapy can begin. At least one-third of newly diagnosed AML patients are admitted with extremely low levels of neutrophils (an infection fighting WBC) and a fever. These children may need to be treated for infection before beginning chemotherapy. Some children with low neutrophil counts are given cytokines, proteins that stimulate the body to fight infection.

The huge number of cancer cells growing and dying can sometimes overwhelm the kidneys, causing tumor lysis syndrome; this rare but serious complication can occur during treatment or may be found at AML diagnosis. Children with this syndrome are given intravenous fluids and other substances to restore proper kidney function and output. Extremely high WBC counts (greater than 200,000 cells per milliliter of blood) may cause other rare but serious side effects, such as respiratory problems, confusion, severe headaches, hemorrhage, or coma. Children with extremely high WBC counts at diagnosis may require leukapheresis (removal of the WBCs) before treatment with chemotherapy begins.

Induction. Induction is the most intense part of treatment; its purpose is to kill as many cancer cells as quickly as possible. As with ALL, chemotherapy drugs for AML are more successful if two or three are used simultaneously. Most treatment regimens combine cytarabine (ARA-C) with daunomycin and either etoposide or thioguanine (6-TG) or both. Sometimes, idarubicin, gemtuzumab, and/or dexamethasone are also used. Children with acute promyelocytic leukemia (APL) receive tretinoin (also called all-trans-retinoic-acid or ATRA) in addition to chemotherapy. A form of arsenic, called arsenic trioxide, has been used successfully outside of the United States, alone and in combination with other drugs, to treat AML in children. Clinical trials are underway in the United States to evaluate its effectiveness as a standard therapy.

Chemotherapy drugs are given in five ways:

- Intravenously (IV)—through a needle or tube in the vein
- Intramuscularly (IM)—by injection in muscle
- Subcutaneously (SQ)—by injection under the skin
- Orally (PO)—by mouth in liquid or pill form
- Intrathecally (IT)—through injection into the CSF.

Most AML chemotherapy is given intravenously. (See Chapter 9, "Chemotherapy," for an in-depth discussion of each drug, possible side effects, and parent suggestions.)

Therapy for AML is most successful if the second phase of treatment is given without waiting for full recovery from the first portion of treatment (called timed treatment). Because this approach is so intensive, the child normally must spend several weeks in the hospital and receive supportive care. The chemotherapy drugs damage both normal cells and leukemic cells, leaving the child susceptible to infections and excessive bleeding. Bone marrow growth factors such as granulocyte-macrophage colony-stimulating factor (GM-CSF) or granulocyte colony-stimulating factor (G-CSF) are sometimes used to shorten the duration of neutropenia (low WBC counts). It is often necessary for the child to have blood or platelet transfusions or intravenous feeding (hyperalimentation). Anti-fungal drugs are sometimes given to reduce the risk of certain virulent infections.

With current timed treatments, 85 to 90 percent of children with AML achieve remission during induction, although the long-term cure rate depends upon the particular biological subtype of AML.

Central nervous system (CNS) prophylaxis. The CNS is composed of the brain and spinal cord, which are bathed in a fluid called cerebrospinal fluid (CSF). When cancer invades the CNS, cancer cells are found in the CSF. CNS prophylaxis (prevention) is a component of standard treatment for AML.

Because a blood–brain barrier exists that prevents many chemotherapy drugs from crossing into the CNS to destroy leukemia cells, chemotherapy drugs are injected directly into the CSF (called intrathecal medication) during spinal taps. Intrathecal medication is given periodically throughout treatment.

CNS prophylaxis has decreased the risk of developing leukemia in the nervous system. Unfortunately, the treatments sometimes cause long-term disabilities such as decreased attention span, short-term memory problems, and lowered abilities in spatial and mathematical skills, particularly when radiation is used (see Chapter 15, "School," for information about managing learning disabilities caused by treatment). The role of CNS prophylaxis in AML is less clear than in ALL. Current clinical trials are intended to determine how much and what type of treatment is necessary to prevent CNS relapse while minimizing the risk of long-term side effects.

Postremission therapy. Even when a child is in complete remission, residual cancer cells may multiply rapidly without additional treatment. Consequently, after a short period of recuperation from induction, children with AML usually receive further intensive treatment, with an allogeneic SCT (if a matched family donor is available) or more chemotherapy, called postremission therapy. However, children in first remission with favorable prognostic factors are currently not given an SCT unless they relapse.

Therefore, postremission therapy may consist of an SCT or chemotherapy, which includes the drugs cytarabine (in high or standard doses), etoposide, an anthracycline (doxorubicin, daunorubicin, or idarubicin), thioguanine, amsacrine, azacytidine, and cyclophosphamide. Children with APL also are given a medication called tretinoin (also called all-trans-retinoic-acid or ATRA), and in some cases, mercaptopurine and methotrexate, during postremission therapy.

In the past, another phase of treatment, called maintenance, was used. This phase consisted of low-dose chemotherapy given for a number of years. Studies have shown that additional therapy after intensive induction and consolidation does not lengthen remission for children with AML; so only children with APL receive maintenance therapy at this time.

Stem cell transplantation. Stem cells are immature cells that can grow into blood cells. In the past, the only way doctors could harvest stem cells was by removing marrow from a person's bones and extracting the stem cells through an arduous process. It is now possible to harvest stem cells from circulating blood or from the placenta or cord blood after the birth of a baby. Depending on the source of the cells, the transplant may be called a bone marrow transplant, a cord blood transplant, or a peripheral blood SCT.

Increasingly, research suggests that SCTs from closely matched donors, such as siblings, may provide the best postremission protection for children with AML. However, it is not always possible to find a suitable donor quickly, so doctors may employ chemotherapy in postremission to reduce the chance of relapse before a suitable donor can be found. (See Chapter 21, "Stem Cell Transplantation," for types of transplants, procedures, side effects, and coping suggestions from parents and SCT survivors.)

Treatment for chloromas (also called granulocytic sarcoma). Chloromas are tumors made up of large clusters of leukemia cells. Chloromas usually disappear with standard AML treatment. However, if the location of a chloroma may cause a serious problem, such as vision loss or spinal cord damage, radiation therapy may be given.

Newest treatment options. To learn more about the newest treatment options for AML, visit the NCI's website at *www.cancer.gov/cancertopics/pdq/treatment/childAML/ HealthProfessional/page5.*

Standard treatment for chronic myelogenous leukemia (CML)

CML occurs in three phases: chronic, accelerated, and blast (or blast crisis). Treatment is generally much more successful if it begins in the early chronic stage. The only treatment that can cure CML with certainty is a stem cell transplant (SCT) from a matched related donor or a matched unrelated donor. Very long remissions (more than 5 years) are now being observed with a new treatment, Gleevec® (see below), but further follow-up of patients is necessary to know for certain if this treatment is curative.

While awaiting transplant, there are three treatment goals for children with CML: lower the WBC count, reduce the size of the spleen and liver, and prolong the chronic phase of the disease. The three drugs routinely used to accomplish these goals are hydroxyurea, interferon-alpha, and more frequently imatinib mesylate (STI-571 or Gleevec®).

Hydroxyurea is given by mouth daily to keep the WBC count in check. Interferon-alpha lowers the white count and helps reduce inflammation in the spleen. It can also extend the duration of the chronic phase when paired with hydroxyurea or with low-dose cytarabine (ARA-C), especially in the early stages of the disease. Some children on this regimen have survived long enough to be considered cured. However, interferon-alpha is expensive and has many side effects, some of which, such as systemic lupus erythmatosus or hemolytic anemia, can be deadly.

By far the most promising drug is Gleevec®—a molecule that is engineered specifically to block the activity of a protein (bcr/abl) that causes a chromosome abnormality called the Philadelphia chromosome. This chromosome is commonly associated with CML. By interfering with the activity of the bcr/abl protein, Gleevec® significantly reduces the number of cancer cells. Gleevec® was first used in adults and had remarkably successful results when administered before the disease progressed to the accelerated or blast phase. Gleevec® induces remission in more than 90 percent of patients, but the length of remission varies, causing uncertainty about the best time to transplant. Dasatinib or nilotinib may be given to children who relapse while on Gleevac®.

Currently, the best hope for cure remains allogeneic transplant from a matched donor or a syngeneic transplant (from a twin). The highest cure rates (60 to 80 percent) occur when the child is transplanted with marrow or blood stem cells from a closely matched family member less than 1 year from initial diagnosis and during the chronic phase. Use of a well-matched unrelated donor gives similar results. (See Chapter 21, "Stem Cell Transplantation," for detailed information.)

The accelerated phase of CML is usually brief. The number of both immature WBCs and blast cells in the bloodstream increases, and the number of red blood cells drops, and platelets may increase or decrease. The treatment options remain largely the same as during the chronic phase but have a lower success rate. Between 20 and 40 percent of children who have an SCT at this stage achieve complete remission.

During the blast phase, WBCs fail to mature and immature cells flood the bloodstream. Children in this phase respond poorly to standard chemotherapy. SCT in blast crisis has a low cure rate (10 to 20 percent). Gleevec® has shown some promise for inducing remission in children with blast crisis and is now commonly used for this purpose; but few children in blast crisis achieve remission and those who do usually relapse. Other drugs that have shown some modest success are troxacitabine and decitabine, both of which have been able to return small percentages of patients to the chronic phase. Once there, these children are usually considered for an SCT using the best available donor.

Newest treatment options. To learn more about the newest treatment options for CML visit the NCI's website at *www.cancer.gov/cancertopics/pdq/treatment/childAML/ healthprofessional* and click on "Chronic Myelogenous Leukemia" on the left bar.

Standard treatment for juvenile myelomonocytic leukemia (JMML)

The course of JMML is unpredictable. Infants can survive for several years, but older children usually have rapidly progressing disease. The prognosis for JMML has traditionally been grim, with less than 10 percent of children surviving. With the advent of stem cell transplantation (SCTs), the survival rate has jumped to approximately 50 percent for children who can be treated by allogeneic SCT.

There is no standard treatment for JMML, but most children in the United States are treated with chemotherapy—etoposide, cytarabine, thioguanine (6-TG), mercaptopurine (6-MP), tretinoin (also called all-trans-retinoic-acid or ATRA), and isotretinoin—followed, when possible, by an SCT. The success rate is highest if the donor is a matched related marrow donor or a matched unrelated umbilical cord donor.

> *My daughter was diagnosed with JMML in 1993 at the age of 27 months. Although it is a chronic leukemia, it is particularly fast moving, and there is no treatment besides transplant. It is also vastly different from the adult CML. My daughter had a mismatched (5/6) related (my husband's sister as donor) BMT (bone marrow transplant) 4 months after she was diagnosed. Today, she is 8 years post-transplant, is in the fourth grade, and is the absolute joy of my life.*

Newest treatment options. To learn more about the newest treatment options for JMML visit the NCI's website at *www.cancer.gov/cancertopics/pdq/treatment/childAML/ healthprofessional* and click on "Juvenile Myelomonocytic Leukemia" on the left bar. The JMML Foundation also keeps up with advances in JMML research and treatments; information is available on its website at *www.jmmlfoundation.org*.

The protocol

If your child is receiving standard treatment, you will receive a written copy of the treatment plan, called a protocol. Just like a recipe for baking a cake, a protocol has a list of ingredients, the amounts to use, and the order to use them in so the protocol has the best chance for success. The protocol lists the drugs, dosages, and tests for each segment of treatment and follow-up. If your child is enrolled in a clinical trial, you will receive a copy of the short protocol but can obtain the entire protocol document by asking for it (see later section called "The entire clinical trial document").

> *The clinical trial that my child was enrolled in had three arms—A, B, and C. He was in the A portion, so we only referred to the A section of the protocol, which clearly outlined each procedure and drug to be given for the duration of the trial. It also listed the follow-up care required by that particular clinical trial.*

The portion of the protocol devoted to the schedule may be longer than 20 pages. The family may also be given an abbreviated version (one to two pages) for quick and easy reference on a daily basis. This abbreviated part of the protocol is frequently called the "roadmap." Parents and teenage patients should review these documents carefully with the oncologist to be certain they understand them. It is the parents' responsibility to make the appropriate appointments and give oral medications at the correct times.

Clinical trials

Parents are often asked to enroll their child in a clinical trial within days or weeks of arriving at a major pediatric medical center with a child newly diagnosed with leukemia. These trials are carefully controlled research experiments that use human volunteers to develop better ways to prevent or cure diseases. Pediatric clinical trials attempt to improve upon existing treatments. In fact, the enormous advances in treating childhood leukemia are the direct result of clinical trials.

A clinical trial can involve a totally new approach that is thought to be promising, or it may entail fine-tuning existing treatments, improving the results or reducing the toxicity of known treatments, or developing new ways to assess responses to treatments. Many patients are needed in each clinical trial for the results to be statistically meaningful.

In some cases, such as with low- or average-risk ALL, the standard treatment has a very high likelihood of success and most children on the standard treatment achieve complete and lasting remission. In other cases, such as with high-risk AML or infant ALL, the prognosis is poor on the standard treatment, and parents may be more motivated to choose a clinical trial. Occasionally, parents choose to enroll their child in a clinical trial because they want to contribute to better treatments in the future. Other parents may be wary of participating in an experimental program and may opt for standard treatment. There is no "right" choice. Obtain all the information you can, weigh the pros and cons, and make a decision based on your values and comfort with the choice.

You may also be invited to participate in other studies that are sponsored by pharmaceutical companies, especially those designed to support patients through the effects of treatment. Such supportive care trials evaluate antibiotics, anti-nausea drugs, and new agents to raise blood counts, minimize pain, or control other symptoms. The oversight and control of these trials involves an entirely different mechanism than the oncology treatment studies discussed in this chapter. Ask your doctor or nurse to discuss these studies with you if your child is invited to participate in one.

Types of clinical trials

There are three main types of clinical trials offered to children with leukemia.

Phase I. Drug studies begin in laboratories, where the drugs are evaluated using chemical or biological models, tissue samples, and other methods to see if there is a chance the drug might be effective at treating disease. If laboratory evidence suggests a drug may work in humans, it is first tested in a Phase I study. These studies examine how the body processes (metabolizes) the drug, establishes the highest dose that can safely be given to a patient (the maximum tolerated dose, or MTD), and evaluates the side effects.

In pediatric Phase I trials, the dose of a new drug is gradually increased in small groups of children until it becomes too toxic; essentially, one small group of children gets a low dose, the next small group gets a slightly higher dose, and so on, until an unacceptable number of children experience unacceptable toxicities. Phase I studies are true experiments and their purpose is not to cure the participants. The true beneficiaries of Phase I studies are future patients. In most cases, parents are not asked to enroll their child in a Phase I study unless all other treatment options have failed. Parents often enroll their children in these trials in the hope that a new and untried drug will be effective against their child's disease, but they need to recognize that the chances of achieving remission are low.

Phase II. Phase II trials refine the safety parameters and evaluate new drugs' effects on specific tumors. This is the stage at which many drugs fail, meaning they are not as effective as originally predicted or they have unexpected or serious side effects in many patients. Sometimes patients are enrolled when they have relapsed after other therapies. Occasionally, Phase II trials are designed to test an exceptionally promising agent against a cancer for which other effective therapies exist.

Phase III trials. These clinical trials determine if a new treatment is better than the usual or standard therapy. Some Phase III trials are designed solely to improve survival; others try to maintain survival rates while lowering toxicity of treatment. In pediatric Phase III studies, some children will receive the standard therapy, while others receive some modification, such as higher or lower doses, different combinations of drugs, or shorter or longer treatments. Some children will derive direct benefit if a new modification proves superior to standard therapy. Others will receive the same therapy they would have received if not enrolled on the study (the standard arm). To ensure the results are accurate, Phase III studies require thousands of participants and several years to complete.

The NCI offers parents several resources to help them understand the clinical trial process. You can call the NCI at (800) 422-6237 or visit its clinical trials website at *www. cancer.gov/clinical_trials*.

The information below pertains to Phase III trials that are reviewed and funded by the NCI. Issues for enrolling in Phase I and Phase II trials are very different, as are concerns when enrolling in trials sponsored by private companies.

Design of clinical trials

In 2000, four pediatric cancer research groups merged to form a single pediatric cancer research organization called the Children's Oncology Group (COG), which is supported by the NCI.

Children's Oncology Group
440 East Huntington Drive, #300
Arcadia, CA 91006
(800) 458-6223 (United States and Canada)
www.childrensoncologygroup.org

Approximately 230 institutions that treat children with cancer are members of COG. Researchers from each institution contribute to the design of COG clinical trials for children with cancer. The NCI and some individual institutions (e.g., St. Jude Children's Research Hospital, Dana-Farber Cancer Institute, and Memorial Sloan-Kettering Cancer Center) also design their own trials for children treated at those institutions. COG has also partnered with the National Children's Cancer Foundation to form CureSearch (*www.curesearch.org*), an online resource for parents.

Study arms

Phase III studies have multiple arms, which means participants are sorted into different arms (groups) that receive different treatments. Every Phase III trial has one arm that is the current standard of care. Each of the other arms contains one or more experimental components, such as:

• New drugs

• Old drugs used in a new way (e.g., different dose or new combinations of old drugs)

• Duration of treatment that is shorter or longer than standard care

• The addition or deletion of certain treatments (such as radiation therapy)

• The use of new supportive care interventions, such as preventative antibiotics or new drugs to control nausea.

When the trial is completed and all the data is analyzed, the effectiveness of each experimental arm is compared to the "standard of care" arm. When designing pediatric clinical trials, the first priority is to protect the children from harm. Researchers are ethically bound to offer treatments they think will be at least as safe and effective as the standard of care.

> *In the early 1990s, my daughter's clinical trial for high-risk ALL had three arms. One arm was the standard treatment of four drug rotations of chemotherapy with a delayed intensification and consolidation, and 1,800 cGy of cranial radiation. The second arm was identical, except radiation was replaced with more frequent doses of intrathecal methotrexate. The third arm was for children who had CNS disease at diagnosis or who were slow responders to initial therapy. They received a very aggressive chemotherapy regimen plus cranial radiation.*

Randomization

Phase III trials for childhood leukemia require a process called randomization, meaning that after parents agree to enroll their child in a clinical trial, a computer randomly assigns the child to one arm of the study. The parents will not know which treatment their child will receive until the computer assigns one. The purpose of computer assignment is to ensure patients are evenly assigned to each treatment plan without bias from physicians or families. One group of children (the control group) always receives the standard treatment to provide a basis for comparison to the experimental arms. At the time the clinical trial is designed, there is no conclusive evidence to indicate which arm is superior. Thus, it is impossible to predict if your child will benefit from participating in the study.

> We decided not to participate in a study for several reasons. One arm would require extra spinal taps, and our son was just so little that we couldn't bear the thought of any more treatments than were required in the standard arm. Another arm contained a second induction, and since we were on Medicaid, we just didn't feel it was right for the taxpayers to pay for anything extra. We felt we were only entitled to basic healthcare.

· · · · ·

> We had a hard time deciding whether to go with the standard treatment or to participate in the study. The "B" arm of the study seemed, on intuition, to be too harsh for her because she was so weak at the time. We finally did opt for the study, hoping we wouldn't be randomized to "B." We chose the study basically so that the computer could choose and we wouldn't ever have to think "we should have gone with the study." As it turned out, we were randomized to the standard arm, so we got what we wanted while still participating in the study.

Researchers closely monitor ongoing studies and modify the study if one arm is clearly identified as superior during the course of the trial or if an arm has unacceptable side effects.

Supervision of clinical trials

The ethical and legal codes ruling medical practice also apply to clinical trials. In addition, most research is federally funded or regulated (all COG trials are), with rules that protect patients. COG also has review boards that meet at prearranged dates for the duration of a clinical trial to ensure the risks of all parts of the trial are acceptable relative to the benefits.

The treating institution is required to report all adverse side effects to COG, which reports them to the U.S. Food and Drug Administration. If concerns are raised, the study may be temporarily halted while an independent Data Safety and Monitoring

Board (DSMB) and the study committee review the situation. If one arm of the trial is causing unexpected or unacceptable side effects, that portion is stopped, and the children enrolled are given the better treatment.

> When Brian first entered the CCG-1922 protocol, there were four arms. One was to see which had the best response in treatments between prednisone versus Decadron® and 6MP versus 6TG. After Brian completed this protocol, in December 1996, we were told that the patients who were on 6MP and prednisone were to be switched to 6MP and Decadron®. There seemed to be a better outcome. We were told in the beginning of the protocol that if one arm was doing better than the other arm, the patients would be switched to the better arm.

All institutions that conduct clinical trials also have an Institutional Review Board (IRB) or an ethics committee that reviews and approves all research taking place there. The purpose of such boards and committees—made up of scientists, doctors, nurses, and citizens from the community—is to protect patients. Before a child is enrolled in a COG trial, the trial must be reviewed and approved by the NCI and COG. In addition, the IRB at the hospital where the child is being treated must also approve the trial.

Questions to ask about clinical trials

To fully understand the clinical trial that has been proposed, here are some important questions to ask the oncologist:

- What is the purpose of the study?

- Who is sponsoring the study? Who reviews it? How often is it reviewed? Who monitors patient safety?

- What tests and treatments will be done during the study? How do these differ from standard treatment?

- Why is it thought that the treatment being studied may be better than standard treatment?

- What are the possible benefits?

- What are all possible disadvantages?

- What are the possible side effects or risks of the study? What are the side effects of the study compared to those of standard treatment?

- How will the study affect my child's daily life?

- What are the possible long-term impacts of the study compared to the standard treatment?

- How long will the study last? Is this shorter or longer than standard treatment?

- Will the study require more hospitalization than standard treatment?

- Does the study include long-term follow-up care?

- What happens if my child is harmed as a result of the research?

- Compare the study to standard treatment in terms of possible outcomes, side effects, time involved, costs, and quality of life.

- Have insurers been reimbursing for care on this protocol?

After discussing the clinical trial with the oncologist, you will need a copy of the information to review later. Many parents bring a tape recorder or a friend to take notes; others write down all the doctor's answers for later reference.

Pros and cons of clinical trials

Making the decision whether to have your child participate in a clinical trial is sometimes difficult. The following list of reasons why some families chose whether or not to enroll may help clarify your feelings about this important decision.

Why some families choose to enroll:

- Children receive either state-of-the-art investigational therapy or the best standard therapy available.

- Clinical trials can provide an opportunity to benefit from a new therapy before it is generally available.

- Children enrolled in clinical trials may be monitored more frequently throughout treatment.

- The IRB has reviewed the protocol for protection of patients' rights, as well as for scientific soundness.

- Review boards of scientists oversee the operation of clinical trials.

- Participating in a clinical trial often makes parents feel they did everything medically possible for their child.

- Information gained from clinical trials will benefit children with cancer in the future.

Reasons why families choose not to enroll:

- The experimental arm may not provide treatment as effective as the standard, or it may generate additional side effects or risks.

- Some families do not like the feeling of not having control over choosing the child's treatment.

- Some clinical trials require more hospitalizations, treatments, clinic visits, or tests that may be more painful than the standard treatment.

- Some families feel additional stress about which arm is the best treatment for their individual child.

- Insurance may not cover investigational studies. Parents need to carefully explore this issue prior to signing the consent form.

> When we were struggling with the decision of whether to join the study, I asked the oncologist how would we ever know if we made the right decision. He said something very wise: "You will never know and you should never second-guess yourself, no matter how the study turns out. Statistics are about large groups of kids, not your child. Your child might relapse no matter which arm she is on, and she might be cured on an arm where most of the other kids relapse. Statistics for you will be either 100 percent or zero because your child will either live or die. I can't tell you which will be the better treatment; that is why we are conducting the study. But no matter what, we will be doing absolutely the best we can."

Informed consent

True informed consent is a process—not merely an explanation and signing of documents. Informed consent requires that:

- All the treatments available to the child have been explained—not just the treatment available at your hospital or through your doctor, but all the treatments that could be beneficial, wherever they are given.

- The parents and, to the extent possible, the child, have discussed these options and decided they want to consider one of them.

- The option selected is thoroughly discussed, with all its benefits and risks clearly explained.

- Those aspects of the study that are considered experimental and those that are standard are clearly described.

- A fully informed medical decision is one that weighs the relative merits of a therapy after full disclosure of benefits, risks, and alternatives.

During the discussions between the doctor(s) and family, all questions should be answered in language that is clearly understood by the parents and child; and there should be no pressure on parents to enroll their child in a study. The objective of the informed consent process is that all family members are comfortable with their choice and can comply with it.

> We had many discussions with the staff prior to signing the informed consent to participate in the clinical trial. We asked innumerable questions, all of which were answered in a frank and honest manner. We felt that participating gave our child the best chance for a cure, and we felt good about increasing the knowledge that would help other children later.

Sometimes the informed consent process does not work as it should because of several factors, including the state of mind of the parents, the communication style of the doctor, and the system (if any) in place to discuss treatment options, Usually, this situation is the result of miscommunication arising from some combination of the following:

- No formal meeting time was established in advance to discuss treatment options, so parents do not understand the importance of the discussion they are having with the doctor.

- Parents, who are tired, confused, and mentally numb, may appear to understand things they are barely hearing.

- The doctor does not recognize that the parents are not following what he is saying and that they need more guidance and time to absorb the choices.

- The doctor is unconsciously promoting the choice she believes is the best one and she interprets the lack of questions as agreement.

- There is no one in the room except the doctor and the parents; therefore, there is no one to intervene if communication breaks down.

It is a good idea to ask the treatment team immediately after diagnosis when and how the treatment decision will be made and to ask for a specific meeting date and time to discuss treatment, even if it means a slight delay before starting treatment. Parents may also want to invite a trusted friend or their pediatrician to attend this meeting to ensure they understand the options before them.

> *Two days after my child was diagnosed, the oncologist told me it was time to begin treatment. I do remember him talking a lot, but I swear it actually sounded like "Wah, wah, wah, protocol, wah, wah, very successful, wah, DNA, wah, wah, wah, sign here." And I did. It was several days before it sank in that I had authorized an experimental treatment protocol and not the standard of care. The irony is that I worked in clinical research. I knew how this was supposed to go. But I was alone and tired and frightened and went along like a sheep. Did he railroad me? Maybe; but I don't think he meant to and in the end it was my responsibility to hold it together and ask what needed to be asked. But it just wasn't in me at the time. Later, I told the doctor this and he was astonished to learn that I hadn't heard a word he said. My child is cured now, so I am happy, but if I had it to do again, I might not have made the choice I did.*

The clinical trail consent form

The form parents sign will have language similar to the following: "The study described above has been explained to me, and I voluntarily agree to have my child participate in this study. I have had all of my questions answered, and understand that all future questions that I have about this research will be answered by the investigators listed above."

The study that our institution was participating in at the time of my daughter's diagnosis was attempting to lessen the treatment to reduce neurotoxicity yet still cure the disease. My family began a massive research effort on the issue, and we had several family friends who were physicians discuss the case with the heads of pediatric oncology at their institutions. The consensus was that since my daughter was at the high end of the high-risk description, it was advisable to choose the standard care, which was more aggressive.

By the time a study is published in the literature, doctors on the cutting edge of treatment are 2 to 4 years into improving that treatment or learning of its shortcomings. For this reason, it is best to make decisions in partnership with knowledgeable medical caregivers, rather than on your own.

No matter how comfortable you are with your child's treating oncologist, it may be helpful to have another medical caregiver help sort out your options. Often, that person will be the family's pediatrician or family doctor. Second opinions can be obtained from physicians at other institutions in your region, or any of the larger pediatric cancer centers. They will arrange to review the information (e.g., pathology, cytogenetics) and outline recommendations. It is most useful to get a second opinion from a center that treats significant numbers of patients with your child's diagnosis. Most pediatric oncologists are willing to facilitate this process for you.

Assent

Children under the age of 18 do not have the right to refuse standard treatment for their cancer. They do, however, have the right to accept or reject experimental treatments. All clinical trials are considered to be experimental treatments. Regardless of whether children will receive the standard treatment or an experimental treatment, they have rights to have the disease, treatment, and procedures explained to them at an age-appropriate level.

Assent means that children and adolescents are involved in decisions about their treatment. Doctors and parents are required to allow children to provide input to the extent of the children's abilities. According to the American Academy of Pediatrics (AAP), assent means that the child:

- Is aware of the nature of his or her disease.

- Understands what to expect from tests and treatments.

- Has had his or her understanding assessed.

- Has had an opportunity to express willingness to accept or reject the proposed treatment.

Parents can read or download a copy of the AAP policy statement ("Informed Consent, Parental Permission, and Assent in Pediatric Practice") from the AAP website at *http:// aappolicy.aappublications.org*. In part, the policy states, "In situations in which the patient will have to receive medical care despite his or her objection, the patient should be told that fact and should not be deceived." This policy applies to standard treatment.

Clinical trials, however, are research. As such, assent is required from children who are able to give it. The U.S. Code of Federal Regulations (CFR) 46.402 (b) requires that children must agree to participate in research. A child's failure to object does not constitute assent.

In short, parents can legally make decisions about standard care, but both parents and children have decision-making rights about participating in research. Thus, for older children and teens, informed consent to participate in a clinical trial means that physicians need both parental permission and the written assent of the child.

Saying no to a clinical trial

Parents, older children, and teens have the legal right to decide whether or not to participate in a clinical trial. If the family chooses for the child not to participate in the proposed clinical trial, the child is given the best known treatment (standard arm) for his type of leukemia.

> *We just were not comfortable with the concept of a clinical trial. It seemed like gambling to us. We also felt totally overwhelmed about making decisions on important subjects that we didn't understand. Even though we asked many, many questions, we just couldn't come to grips with the whole idea in the 2 days after our daughter was diagnosed. So, we declined the trial and had the best known treatment. We were happy with our decision.*

The entire clinical trial document

If your child is enrolled in a clinical trial, the roadmap described earlier is actually a very small portion of an extensive document describing all aspects of the study. The entire document usually exceeds 100 pages and covers the following topics: study hypothesis, experimental design, scientific background and rationale with relevant references from the scientific literature, patient eligibility and randomization, therapy for each arm of the study, required observations, pathology guidelines, radiation therapy guidelines (if applicable), supportive care guidelines, specific information about each drug, relapse therapy guidelines, statistical considerations, study committee members, record-keeping requirements, reporting of adverse drug reactions, and a consent form.

The full protocol is intended for use by specialists in oncology medicine and nursing and is not written in lay language. It is highly technical and can be confusing or overwhelming for parents.

However, some parents throw themselves into research to better understand their child's illness. These parents may want to have a copy of the study document for several reasons. First, it provides a description of some of the clinical trials that preceded the present one and explains the reasons the investigators designed this particular study. Second, it provides detailed descriptions of drug reactions, which comfort many parents who worry that their child is the only one exhibiting extreme responses to some drugs. Third, motivated parents who have only one protocol to keep track of occasionally prevent errors in treatment. Finally, for parents who are adrift in the world of cancer treatment, it can return to them a bit of control over their child's life.

Other parents find that reading hundreds of pages of technical information is overwhelming or just not helpful. As with almost every topic discussed in this book, families need to make individual choices based on what works best for their unique needs.

If your child is enrolled in a clinical trial and you would like a copy of the entire document, ask your child's oncologist for one. If he or she will not provide it, call COG and ask for a copy (800-458-6223). Informed consent documents for COG trials specifically state that families will receive a copy of the full protocol upon request. After reading the protocol, it may be helpful to schedule an appointment with your physician, nurse practitioner, or research nurse to discuss any questions or concerns.

> Since knowledge is comfort for me, I really wanted to have the entire clinical trial document, despite its technical language. Whereas the brief protocol that I had listed day, drug, and dose, the expanded version listed the potential side effects for each drug, and what actions should be taken should any occur. I learned the parameters.

The protocol is not for general distribution, because it is unethical to use these protocols outside a controlled research setting. Parents who obtain a copy should not circulate it.

Removing a child from a clinical trial

Parents have the legal right to withdraw their child from a clinical trial at any time, for any reason. But before doing so, it's a good idea to discuss questions or concerns with your child's doctor. The decision to withdraw from a trial should not be held against the parent, and the child will still receive the best available care for her type of cancer. On the consent form signed by the parent, there will be language similar to this: "You are free not to have your child participate in this research or to withdraw your child at any time without penalty or jeopardizing future care."

Jesse was enrolled in a clinical trial to assess long-term neuropsychological conse-
quences of cranial radiation. The testing was free, and we were glad to participate.
Unfortunately, the billing department of the hospital continually billed us in error.
We tried to correct the problem, but it became such a hassle that we withdrew from
the study.

Making a decision

As soon as possible after diagnosis, parents sit down with the doctors to discuss treatment options. If the child is being treated at a research hospital, the first discussion is
usually about standard treatment and a clinical trial, if your child qualifies. Parents are
often very conflicted about choosing a treatment.

> *When my son was diagnosed, we were told we had two options: a clinical trial or*
> *standard treatment. We decided to get a second opinion before making our decision.*
> *Our pediatrician, my husband, and I met in the doctor's office for a telephone confer-*
> *ence with a pediatric oncologist from a major treatment center. We each presented*
> *our concerns. Our pediatrician thought of some issues neither my husband nor I had*
> *considered. I think we all came away better informed of our options.*

The choice to opt for standard treatment or a clinical trial is a strictly personal one, but
parents should only make it after they are certain they understand the implications of
each path. The doctor is legally and ethically bound to alert parents to the full range of
medically appropriate treatment options available to their child and to help the parents
understand what each option entails before asking them for written consent (and older
children and teens to provide assent) to begin a particular treatment plan; this system
is known as "informed consent." The physician may recommend a particular treatment
option that he believes to be in the best interest of the child, but he may not coerce or
deceive the parents into approving a treatment. Once the parents have consented to standard treatment or a clinical trial, the physician is obligated to abide by their decision.

Protocol changes

Many parents express anguish when their child's doses or schedules for chemotherapy
change during treatment. It is very common for doses to be lowered or treatment to be
delayed while a child recovers from low blood counts, infection, or toxic reactions to
the treatment. An important point to remember is that the protocol is a guideline that
is frequently modified, depending on each child's response to treatment.

> *I didn't know what a protocol was when Preston was diagnosed, and I understood*
> *from the doctors that this was the "exact" regime that must be followed to cure*
> *Preston. It frightened me whenever changes were made in the protocol. After several*

years, I came to view the protocol as merely a guideline that is individualized for each patient according to his tolerance and reaction to the drugs. We ended up deleting whole sections of Preston's protocol due to extreme side effects. He has been off therapy for 15 years now with no relapse.

• • • • •

It took me a long time to get over my hang-up that things needed to go exactly as per protocol. Any deviations on dose or days were a major stress for me. It took talking to many parents, as well as doctors and nurses, to realize and feel comfortable with the fact that no one ever goes along perfectly and that the protocol is meant as the broad guideline. There will always be times when your child will be off drugs or on half dose because of illness or low counts or whatever. It took a long time to realize that this is not going to ruin the effectiveness, that the child gets what she can handle without causing undue harm.

• • • • •

I sobbed every night for an entire week when Christine was first taken off chemotherapy for low counts. I was convinced that the immunosuppression was due to a relapse. That was 2 years ago, and we have changed her dosages almost every 2 weeks due to erratic counts. I wish I had known how normal it is to go off protocol.

In some cases, the treatment plan changes when cytogenetics and/or MRD results are available. Changing the treatment plan several weeks after diagnosis can be very difficult for family members. Sometimes oncologists disagree and may need to gather additional opinions before deciding how to proceed.

Matthew has T-cell ALL, and we received the cytogenetics info close to the end of induction. His translocation is t(10;12). At that time, t(10;12) was not a recurrent anomaly associated with ALL, the prognostic significance was not known. About 5 months later, a new study came out about this type of translocation. At that point, we were nearing the end of interim maintenance. The study findings suggested that children with t(10;12) have a "very poor" prognosis. It was the decision of our oncology team to go forward with a BMT (bone marrow transplant). Our oncologist was not in agreement with the team's recommendation and he sought a second opinion. It was their recommendation not to proceed with a frontline BMT. That decision was based on the fact that, first, these study findings were from children in treatment at least 5 years ago and protocols have changed in that time. Second, Matthew had an MRD of .2 percent at the end of induction and it was brought down to virtually undetectable at the end of consolidation. He also received cranial radiation during consolidation as well as escalating methotrexate during interim maintenance, which are both thought to increase his chances of remaining in remission. There was some talk about integrating pulses of thioguanine into his maintenance cycle, but in the end there was no evidence of whether or not that treatment would cause more harm than good. So we have stayed the course despite the cytogenetic findings.

When my daughter was diagnosed in 2006, her oncologist told us that the study she would normally follow, ALL0331, had been suspended due to problems with avascular necrosis. However, we would still follow the standard arm of the study protocol. He explained in great detail how great the survival rates were (80–90%) and how the treatment would be "bad at first but get much better." He mentioned that we would do cytogenetic testing and unless something showed up, we could expect a relatively standard course of treatment.

Sometime between weeks 2 and 3, he called and told me that the cytogenetics report had come back. He said that she had the t(4:11) translocation (MLL gene rearrangement), which is normally seen in infants. My daughter was 12 at time of diagnosis. Because of the translocation, we would need to follow the augmented arm of 0331 and the rates of survival were lower, 60–70%.

I have to say that hearing the news was like a physical blow. To have it all change in midstream was devastating. There was very little information about t(4:11) and its outcomes. However, it was clear from what little was out there that chances of relapse were much higher. Our oncologist had had only one other patient with a t(4:11) translocation.

Because of her translocation and the fact that we weren't "on study," my daughter's oncologist made modifications in her treatment. She received more and higher doses of IT methotrexate and other study drugs. He also tested her bone marrow at the end of each course of treatment. Having this information and a doctor who was willing to use it made a great deal of difference in determining our next steps.

My daughter Allison has been off treatment since January 2009. So far so good. We're still figuring out all the damage that was done to her body from treatment, but she is alive and beautiful and we live one day at a time.

Chapter 5

Coping with Procedures

Mommy, I didn't cry but my eyes got bright.

— A 4-year-old with leukemia

THE PURPOSE OF THIS CHAPTER IS TO PREPARE both child and parent for several common procedures by providing detailed descriptions of each. Because almost all procedures are repeated frequently during the long treatment for childhood leukemia, it is important to establish a routine that is comfortable for you and your child. The procedure itself may cause discomfort, but a well-prepared, calm child fares far better than a frightened one.

Planning for procedures

Procedures are needed to make diagnoses, check for spread of disease, give treatments, and monitor responses to treatment. Some procedures are pain-free and easy to tolerate once both the parent and child understand what to expect. Other procedures can cause both physical and psychological distress in the child, which can be amplified if the child sees that the parent is also traumatized. The best way to prepare the child is for the parents to prepare themselves, intellectually and emotionally, to provide the support and comfort their child will need to endure the procedures to come. In most cases, although the procedure itself is non-negotiable, options are available to lessen the pain or stress. Parents need to know what these choices are to be effective advocates for their children.

A family-centered approach works best when planning and implementing procedures. The procedures are often as frightening, or more so, for parents than for children; memories of the procedures can be long lasting. For this reason, children, parents, and staff should work together to plan for and cope with procedures.

Many hospitals have a child life program. These programs exist to minimize psychological trauma, promote optimal development, and maintain, as much as possible, normal living patterns for hospitalized children. The American Academy of Pediatrics considers child life programs the standard of care for hospitalized children. As soon as possible after admission, find out if your hospital has a child life program or an equivalent support team.

> Matthew was in sixth grade when he was diagnosed, and he was worried about the surgery for implanting the port. He didn't know what the scar would look like and he was concerned about AIDS, because it had been in the news a lot that year. The child life worker came in and really helped. She showed him what a port looked like; then they explored the pre-op area, the actual surgery room, and post-op. She showed him on a cloth doll exactly where the incision would be and how the scar would look. Then she introduced him to "Fred," the IV pump. She said that Fred would be going places with him, and that Fred would keep him from getting so many pokes. She told Matthew that he could bring something from home to hang on Fred. Of course, he brought in a really ugly stuffed animal. Throughout treatment, she really helped his fears and my feelings about losing control over my child's daily life.

Child life specialists or other team members may accompany children to and provide support during procedures. They establish relationships with children based on warmth, respect, empathy, and understanding of developmental stages. They also communicate with the other members of the healthcare team about the psychosocial needs of children and their families.

One way to help the child life specialists do their job is to communicate openly with them from the beginning. In particular, it is helpful to share insights about your child's temperament and history to help the specialist understand how to approach your child. Discuss with the child life professional or social worker when and how to prepare for upcoming procedures. Usually, parents need to experiment with how much advance notice to give younger children about procedures. Some children do better with several days to prepare, while others worry themselves sick if they are informed too far in advance. Sometimes, needs change over the years of treatment, so good communication and flexibility are essential.

> I started giving my 4-year-old daughter 2 days' notice before procedures. But she began to wake up every day worried that "something bad was going to happen soon." So we talked it over and decided to look at the calendar together every Sunday to review what would happen that week. We put stickers on "procedure days" so she knew what to expect. She was a much happier child after that.

Although it may not always be possible, try to schedule procedures so the same person does the same procedure each time. Call ahead to check for unexpected changes to prevent any surprises for your child. Repetition can provide comfort and reassurance to children. Ritual can also be important. A child may prefer a precise sequence of steps or the use of certain cue words to signal the start of the procedure. If the staff knows the child and complies with her wishes, the child is usually calmer and more compliant.

> Katy and I wrote down her requests for each procedure that first week in the hospital. For example, during spinal taps she wanted me (not a nurse) to hold her in position; she wanted xylocaine to be given with a needle, not with the pneumatic gun; and she had a rigid sequence of songs that I sang.

Parents can ask for the medical professional with the most experience to perform procedures. The most-experienced person is not always the senior one. Nurses, for example, are often better than doctors at drawing blood. In the case of procedures that must be performed by a physician, the nurses or technicians usually know which doctor is best at which procedure. Don't hesitate to ask.

Parents should have a choice whether to be present or not during a medical procedure. If your child does better if you are not in the room, ask the child life specialist or another member of the healthcare team to be present solely to comfort your child. Teens often want to handle the procedure on their own and it is normally best to respect their wishes.

During procedures, a parent's role is to be supportive and loving. In most cases, the best place to position yourself is at your child's head, at eye level. Speak calmly and positively to your child. You can tell stories, sing songs, or read a favorite book. It helps to praise your child for good behavior, but don't reprimand or demean your child if problems occur.

> We decided from the very beginning that, even though it's no fun to have a bone marrow aspiration or a spinal tap, we were going to make something positive out of it. So we made it a party. We'd bring pizza, popcorn, or ice cream to the hospital. We helped Kristin think of the nurses as her friends. We'd celebrate after a procedure by going out to eat at one of the neat little restaurants near the hospital.

Oncology clinics usually have a special box full of toys or a selection of rewards for children who have had a procedure. It sometimes helps for the child to have a treat to look forward to afterward. Some parents bring a special gift to sneak into the box for their child to find.

Children have definite opinions about how they like things to go at the clinic and, to the extent feasible, their wishes should be respected. For instance, *Having Leukemia Isn't So Bad. Of Course It Wouldn't Be My First Choice* describes a list of rules for clinic staff written by then 7-year-old Catherine Krumme in the car on the way to the hospital:

1. *Must have a good sense of humor.*
2. *Must always do a good lumbar puncture (LP) and bone marrow.*

3. *Must always remember the toy box.*

4. *Must tell the truth.*

5. *Must like people.*

6. *Must like junk food.*

7. *Must know a lot about chemotherapy.*

8. *Must not mind the sight of blood.*

9. *Must like bald heads.*

10. *Must never be grumpy.*

Pain management

The goal of pediatric pain management should be to minimize discomfort during procedures. The two methods to achieve this goal are psychological (using the mind) and pharmacological (using prescription drugs). These two methods can be used together to provide an integrated approach.

Psychological methods

It is essential to prepare for every procedure. Unexpected stress is more difficult to cope with than anticipated stress. If parents and children understand what is going to happen, where it will happen, who will be there, and what it will feel like, they will be less anxious and better able to cope. Here are some ways to prepare your child:

- Verbally explain each step in the procedure.

- Meet the person who will perform the procedure, if possible.

- Tour the room where the procedure will take place.

- Let small children use dolls to play-act the procedure.

- Let older children observe a demonstration on a doll.

- Have adolescents watch a video that describes the procedure.

- Encourage discussion and answer all questions.

> *For my child, playing about procedures helped release many feelings. Parents can buy medical kits at the store or simply stock their own from clinic castoffs and the pharmacy. We had IV bottles made from empty shampoo containers, complete with tubing and plastic needles. Several dolls had accessed ports, and many stuffed animals in our house fell apart after being speared by the pen during countless spinal taps. Katy's younger sister even ran around sometimes with her own pretend port taped onto her chest. Some suggestions for the child's medical kit are: gauze pads,*

tape, tubing, stethoscope, reflex hammer, pretend needles, syringes, medical chart, and toy box. Of course, lots of dolls or stuffed animal patients are required.

· · · · ·

My daughter (3 years old) took an old stuffed animal to the clinic with her. Having the nurse and doctor perform the procedure first on "Bear" helped her immensely.

Hypnosis, imagery, and distraction are three techniques widely used to help children cope with painful procedures. Following are descriptions of each.

Hypnosis is a well-documented method for reducing discomfort during painful procedures. If performed by a qualified healthcare professional (e.g., psychologist, physician, nurse, social worker, or child life specialist), hypnosis can help your child control painful sensations, release anxiety, and diminish pain. The professional guides the child into an altered state of consciousness that helps to focus or narrow attention. To locate a qualified practitioner, visit the American Society of Clinical Hypnosis' website at *www. asch.net* or call (630) 980-4740.

Imagery is a way to create a mental image of pleasurable sights, sounds, tastes, smells, and feelings. It is an active process that helps people feel as if they are actually entering the imagined place. Focusing on pleasant images allows the child to shift attention from the pain. The child can actually alter the experience of pain, which simultaneously gives the child control while diminishing pain. Ask if the hospital has someone who can teach your child this very effective technique.

The following description of using imagery was written by Jennifer Rohloff when she was 17 years old and is reprinted with permission from the *Free to Be Yourself* newsletter of Cancer Services of Allen County, Indiana.

My Special Place

Many people had a special place when they were young—a special place that they still remember. This place could be an area that has a special meaning for them, or a place where they used to go when they wanted to be alone. My special place location is over the rainbow.

I discovered this place when I was 12 years old, during a relaxation session. These sessions were designed to reduce pain and stress brought on by chemotherapy. This was a place that I could visualize in my mind so that I could go there anytime that I wanted to—not only for pain, but when I was happy, mad, or sad.

It is surrounded by sand and tall, fanning palm trees everywhere. The blue sky is always clear, and the bright sun shines every day. It is usually quiet because I am alone, but often I can hear the sounds of birds flying by.

Every time I come to this place I like to lie down in the sand. As I lie there, I can feel the gritty sand beneath me. Once in a while I get up and go looking for seashells. I usually find some different shapes and sizes. The ones I like the best are the ones that you can hear the sound of the ocean in. After a while I get up and start to walk around. As I walk, I can feel the breeze going right through me, and I can smell the salt water. It reminds me of being at a beach in Florida. Whenever I start to feel sad or alone or if I am in pain, I usually go jump in the water because it is a soothing place for me. I like to float around in the water because it gives me a refreshing feeling that nobody can hurt me here. I could stay in this place all day because I do not worry about anything while I am here.

To me this place is like a home away from home. It is like heaven because you can do anything you want to do here. Even though this place may seem imaginary or like a fantasy world to some people, it is not to me. I think it is real because it is a place where I can go and be myself.

Distraction can be used successfully with all age groups, but it should never be used as a substitute for preparation. Babies can be distracted by colorful, moving objects. Parents can help distract preschoolers by showing them picture books or videos, telling stories, singing songs, or blowing bubbles. Many youngsters are comforted and distracted from the pain by hugging a favorite stuffed animal. School-age children can watch videos or TV, or listen to music. Several institutions use interactive videos to help distract older children or teens.

My daughter went through her therapy prior to the days when kids were given any pain medications for procedures. She and I would make up a schedule of songs for me to sing during the spinal tap or bone marrow. I would stroke her skin and sing softly to her. She visibly relaxed, and the staff found it soothing, as well. I'll never forget the time that the oncologist, nurse, and I were all quietly singing "Somewhere Over the Rainbow" during a spinal tap.

Relaxation, biofeedback, massage, acupuncture, Reiki (Japanese energy healing), and accupressure are all also used successfully to manage pain. Ask the hospital's child life specialist, psychologist, or nurse to discuss and practice different methods of pain management with you and your child.

Pharmacological methods

Most pediatric oncology clinics offer to sedate or anesthetize children for procedures that are painful or that require them to lie completely still. If your clinic does not offer this option, strongly advocate for it. Sedation and anesthesia have the advantage of calming the child, reducing pain, and, in many cases, obliterating all memory of the procedure. Four classes of drugs are used:

- **Sedatives,** which depress the central nervous system and result in relaxation. The child or teen may fall asleep, but will remain conscious.

- **General anesthetics,** which induce a loss of consciousness to prevent the child or teen from experiencing pain or remembering a procedure.

- **Local anesthetics,** which temporarily interrupt nerve transmission at a specific site on the body to lessen pain.

- **Analgesics,** which relieve pain. Narcotics are a subclass of analgesics that induce sleep and are potent pain relievers. Many commonly prescribed pain relievers combine narcotic and non-narcotic drugs to achieve greater pain relief with less drowsiness.

One father, a doctor just completing his anesthesia residency, explained:

> That first bone marrow was horrible. To have my little 3-year-old look up at me with tears in her eyes and ask, "What else are you going to let them do to me, Daddy?" was just too much. It was the worst day of my life.

His wife, a nurse, said:

> We really made waves by insisting that Meagan be sedated for her spinal taps and bone marrows. It was mostly a logistical problem, but we held firm, and now it has become much more routine at our children's hospital for many other kids as well.

The ideal pain relief drug for children should be easy to administer, have a predictable effect, provide adequate pain relief, have a short duration, and have minimal side effects. Sedatives and general anesthetics are given intravenously. Some facilities take the child into the operating room (OR) for the procedure; others use a preoperating area or clinic sedation room and allow the parent to be present the entire time. Certain drugs must be administered by an anesthesiologist (a physician specializing in anesthesia) in a hospital setting. Drugs commonly used during procedures include:

- **Valium® or Versed®, plus morphine or fentanyl.** Valium® and Versed® are sedatives that are used with pain relievers such as morphine or fentanyl. These drugs can be given in the clinic, but the possibility of slowed breathing requires expert monitoring and the availability of emergency equipment. The combination of a sedative and a pain reliever will result in your child being awake but sedated. The child may move or cry, but he will not remember the procedure. Often, EMLA® or lidocaine are also used to ensure the procedure is pain-free.

*Joel was treated from ages 14 to 17. During his spinal taps he would get Versed®
once he was positioned on the table. I would always sit at his head and keep his
shoulders forward while his head rested on my arm. (Kind of a hug.) As the Versed®
took effect, he would look up at me with huge eyes and give me a grin a mile wide,
then he would say something off the wall. He had to spend an hour flat after the LP.
He'd be groggy the whole time, constantly asking me what time it was and how soon
we could leave. He'd forget he asked and ask me again 5 minutes later. This continued for the whole hour. Later, we'd laugh about it. He never remembered anything
from the LPs.*

- **Propofol.** Propofol is a general anesthetic and will cause your child to lose consciousness. It must be administered in a hospital by an anesthesiologist. It is given intravenously and has the benefit of acting almost immediately with little recovery time.
At low doses, propofol prevents memory of the procedure but may not relieve all the
pain; thus, it is often used with EMLA® or lidocaine.

    *Patrick (12 years old) hates the lack of control involved when having a procedure
and getting propofol. He attempts to regain some control by verbally explaining to
the doctors just exactly how he wants it done each time. He has his own little routine—tells them jokes, sings "I Want to Be Sedated" (you know, the Ramones song),
etc. Patrick's biggest problem is the taste from the propofol. We have tried so many
different things when he wakes up to mask the taste—Skittles®, gum, Gatorade®. We
now have a supply of Atomic Fireballs®. I give him one as soon as they bring him
out, and he says that really helps cover the taste.*

- **Ketamine.** Ketamine is no longer in common use, but it is sometimes given to children who have had reactions to other drugs. It is a potent anesthetic that needs expert
monitoring. It has a much longer recovery time than the drugs listed above and can
cause hallucinations or confusion.

There are many types of drugs and several methods used to administer them, from very
temporary (10 minutes) mild sedation to full general anesthesia in the operating room.
Discuss with your oncologist and anesthesiologist which method will work best for
your child.

*Let's face it, kids don't care about blasts, lab work, or protocols, they just want to
know if they are going to be hurt again. I think that one of our most important jobs
is to advocate, strongly if necessary, for adequate pain control. If the dose doesn't
work and the doctor just shrugs her shoulders, say you want a different dosage or
drug used. If you encounter resistance, ask that an anesthesiologist be consulted.
Remember that good pain control and/or amnesia will make a big difference in your
child's state of mind during and after treatment.*

Emotions may run high after a difficult procedure. Rather than engage in a lengthy dissection about what went wrong, schedule an appointment with your physician well in advance of the next scheduled procedure to air your concerns and problem-solve.

Because children with leukemia are treated for years, some children build up a tolerance for sedatives and pain relievers. Over time, doses may need to be increased or drugs changed. If your child remembers the procedure, advocate for a change in the drugs or dosage. It is reasonable to request the services of an anesthesiologist to ensure the best outcome for your child.

> My job as an oral surgery assistant required me to be very familiar with different types of sedation. From the first day of Stephan's diagnosis, I quietly insisted on Versed® for bone marrows and spinal taps. We have been in treatment for 2 years, and they still fight me every time, saying that it's just not necessary. When I make the appointment I tell them we want Stephan sedated, and then I call and remind them so that all will go smoothly.

Your child will not be allowed to eat or drink for several hours prior to a procedure that requires sedation or anesthesia. After the procedure, your child may eat or drink when she is alert and able to swallow.

Procedures

Knowing what to expect will lay the foundation for years of tolerable tests. Because each hospital and practitioner has their own preferences and guidelines, the descriptions of procedures in the rest of this chapter may not exactly mirror your experience; but the fundamentals are the same everywhere. Reading the rest of this chapter may lessen your fears and help you to calm and prepare your child.

Questions to ask before procedures

You need information prior to procedures to prepare yourself and your child. Some suggested questions to ask the physician are:

- Why is this procedure necessary and how will it affect my child's treatment?
- What information will the procedure provide?
- Who will perform the procedure?
- Will it be an inpatient or outpatient procedure?
- Please explain the procedure in detail.
- Is there any literature available that describes it?

- Is there a child life specialist on staff who will help prepare my child for the procedure?

- If not, are there nurses, social workers, or parents who can talk to me about how to prepare my child?

- Is the procedure painful?

- How long will it take?

- What type of anesthetic or sedation is used?

- What are the risks, if any?

- What are the common and rare side effects?

- When will we get the results?

Blood draws

Frequent blood samples are a part of life during leukemia treatment. Blood specimens are primarily used for three purposes: to obtain a complete blood count (CBC), to evaluate blood chemistries, or to culture the blood to check for infection. A CBC measures the types and numbers of cells in the blood. Blood chemistries measure substances contained in the blood plasma to determine if the liver and kidneys are functioning properly. Blood cultures help evaluate whether the child is developing a bacterial or fungal infection. (For a list of normal blood counts, see Appendix A, "Blood Counts and What They Mean.")

A finger poke provides enough blood for a CBC. Blood chemistries or cultures require one or more vials of blood. Children with catheters usually have blood drawn from the catheter rather than the arm or finger. These procedures are described in Chapter 8, "Venous Catheters." If the child does not have a catheter, blood is usually drawn from the large vein on the inside of the elbow. The procedures for a blood draw are similar to those for placing an IV, which are described later in the chapter. The only difference is that with a draw, the needle is removed as soon as the blood is obtained.

Finger pokes

During the course of treatment, your child will have hundreds of finger pokes. Many children cooperate better with this procedure if the finger is first anesthetized with a topical numbing agent to reduce pain. The four topical anesthetics in wide use for pediatric procedures are as follows.

EMLA® cream is a combination of two topical anesthetics, lidocaine and prilocaine. It is available by prescription only. Parents must remember to apply the EMLA® cream at least 1 hour before the scheduled poke. Children with darker skin may need to leave it on longer for the full effect.

Put a blob of EMLA® on the tip of the middle finger, then cover it so the cream doesn't get wiped off. Tegaderm® is a special bandage designed for this purpose, but you can also cover the fingertip with plastic wrap, then tape it on the finger. Another method is to buy long, thin balloons with a diameter a bit wider than the child's finger. Cut off the open end, leaving only enough balloon to cover the finger up to the first knuckle. Fill the tip of the balloon with EMLA® and slide it on the fingertip. Before the finger poke, remove the plastic wrap or balloon, wipe off the EMLA®, and ask the technician for a warm pack. Wrapping this heated pack around the finger for a few minutes opens the capillaries and allows blood to flow out more readily. The finger then should be washed or wiped with disinfectant. Now your child is ready for a pain-free finger poke.

LMX4® is a 4-percent solution of lidocaine in a cream form. It works much like EMLA®, but it is available over the counter. It is important not to wash the child's finger prior to applying LMX4®, because it works best when it mixes with the natural oils on the skin. LMX4® works more quickly than EMLA®, so in most cases it should not be applied until you arrive at the laboratory or treatment center. Also, because of its quick action, the parent should wear gloves before rubbing it onto the child's skin.

The procedure for applying LMX4® is slightly different than it is for EMLA®. A small amount should be rubbed onto the finger first and left for about 30 seconds, then a thick blob should be applied on top. Cover the finger loosely with tape, a balloon, or Tegaderm®. Remove the wrapping after 30 minutes, clean the site, and proceed with the poke.

Numby Stuff® is also cream anesthetic, but a mild electrical current is used to help it penetrate the skin. It works in just a few minutes, so it is applied at the clinic.

Ethyl chloride ("freezy spray") is sprayed on the skin immediately before the procedure. This medication requires a prescription.

After the skin is numbed by one of the above methods, the technician will hold the finger and quickly stick it with a small, sharp instrument. Blood will be collected in narrow tubes or a small container. It is usually necessary for the technician to squeeze the fingertip to get enough blood. If you have not used a topical anesthetic, the squeezing part is uncomfortable and the finger can ache for quite a while.

> *Even though we use EMLA®, Katy (5 years old) still becomes angry when she has to have a finger poke. I asked her why it was upsetting if there was no pain, and she replied, "It doesn't hurt my body anymore, but it still hurts my feelings."*

Not all treatment centers recommend a topical anesthetic for finger pokes; you may have to advocate for it.

Starting an intravenous drip (IV)

Most pediatric hospitals have teams of technicians who specialize in starting IVs and drawing blood. The IV technician will generally use a vein in the lower arm or hand. First, a constricting band is put above the site to make the veins larger and easier to see and feel. The technician feels for the vein, cleans the area, and inserts the needle. Sometimes she leaves the needle in place and sometimes she withdraws it, leaving only a thin plastic tube in the vein. The technician will make sure the needle (or tube) is in the proper place, then will cover the site with a clear dressing and secure it with tape.

Methods that help when starting an IV include:

- **Stay calm.** The body reacts to fear by constricting the blood vessels near the skin surface. Small children are usually more calm with a parent present; teenagers may or may not desire privacy. Listening to music, visualizing a tranquil scene (mountains covered with snow, floating in a pool), or using the same technician each time can help.

- **Use a topical anesthetic.** Use EMLA® cream, LMX4®, Numby Stuff®, or ethyl chloride, as described earlier in the chapter. Topical anesthetics are not recommended when giving medications (for example, vincristine) that can burn the skin if leakage occurs.

- **Keep warm.** Cold temperatures cause the surface blood vessels to constrict. Wrapping the child in a blanket and putting a hot water bottle on the arm can enlarge the veins.

- **Drink lots of fluids.** Dehydration decreases the fluid in the veins, making them harder to find, so encourage lots of drinking.

- **Let gravity help.** If your child is lying in bed, have her hang her arm down over the side to increase the size of the vessels in the arm and hand.

- **Let your child have control as appropriate.** If your child has a preference, let him pick the arm to be stuck. If he is a veteran of many IVs, let him point out the best vein. Good technicians know that patients are quite aware of their best bet for a good vein.

- **Stop if problems develop.** The art of treating children requires spending lots of time on preparation and not much time on procedures. If a conflict arises, take a time-out and regroup. Children can be remarkably cooperative if they feel you are respecting their needs and if they are given some control over the situation.

> *You'll think I'm crazy, but I'll tell you this story anyway. After getting stuck constantly for a year, my daughter (5 years old) just lost it one day when she needed an IV. She started screaming and crying, just flew into a rage. I told the tech, "Let's just let her calm down. Why don't you stick me for a change?" She was a sport and started a line in my arm. I told my daughter that I had forgotten how much it hurt and I could understand why she was upset. I told her to let us know when she was ready. She just walked over and held out her arm.*

Traditionally, infants and young children have been restrained on their backs to insert the IV, a technique that minimizes the risk of misplacing the IV, but which causes significant fear and distress. Many treatment centers are now allowing a parent to hold their child upright in his or her lap to minimize stress.

Blood transfusions

Leukemia treatment can cause severe anemia (a low number of oxygen-carrying red cells). The normal life of a red cell is 3 to 4 months, and as old cells die the diseased or chemo-stressed marrow cannot replace them. Many children require transfusions of red cells when first admitted and periodically throughout treatment.

> *Whenever my son needed a transfusion, I brought along bags of coloring books, food, and toys. The number of VCRs at the clinic was limited, so I tried to make arrangements for one ahead of time. When anemic (hematocrit below 20 percent), he didn't have much energy, but by the end of the transfusion, his cheeks were rosy and he had tremendous vitality. It was hard to keep him still. After one unit (bag) of red cells, his hematocrit usually jumped up to around 30.*

One bag (called a "unit") of red cells takes 2 to 4 hours to administer and is given through an IV or catheter. Mild allergic reactions are common. If your child is prone to allergies or experiences an allergic reaction, it may be necessary to premedicate her with an antihistamine such as Benadryl®. Acute allergic reactions are rare, but they do happen. If your child develops chills and/or fever or any difficulty breathing during a transfusion, notify the nurse immediately so she can stop the transfusion.

There are some risks of infection from red cell transfusions. Since tests have been devised and used to detect the AIDS virus in donated blood, the risk of exposure is minuscule. Although there are excellent tests for the various types of hepatitis, exposure to this disease is still possible (the risk is less than 1 in 4,000). Exposure to cytomegalovirus is also a concern. These risks are the reason transfusions are given only when absolutely necessary.

> *My daughter received several transfusions at the clinic in Children's Hospital with no problems. After we traveled back to our home, she needed her first transfusion at the local hospital. Our pediatrician said to expect to be in the hospital at least 8 hours. I asked why it would take so long when it only took 4 hours at Children's. He said he had worked out a formula and determined that she needed two units of packed cells. I mentioned that she only was given one unit each time at Children's. He called the oncologist, who said it was better to give the smaller amount. We went to the hospital, where a unit of red cells was given. Then a nurse came in with another unit. I questioned why he was doing that and he said, "Doctor's orders." I asked him to verify that order, as we had already discussed it with the doctor. He went into another room to call the doctor, and came back and said the pediatrician thought my daughter needed 30 cc more packed cells. I called Children's and they said she didn't*

need more, so I refused to let them administer any more blood. It just wasn't worth the risk of hepatitis to get 30 cc of blood. Even though I was pleasant, the nurses were angry at me for questioning the doctor.

During transfusions, sometimes the nurse will strap the child's arm to a board for the duration of the procedure. This method of restraint prevents the child from accidentally bending his arm, which can be very painful and can reposition the needle, but the board can be cumbersome.

Platelet transfusions

Platelets are an important component of the blood. They help form clots and stop bleeding by repairing breaks in the walls of blood vessels. A normal platelet count for a healthy child is 160,000 to 380,000/mm^3. Chemotherapy can severely depress the platelet count. If a child's counts are very low, it may be necessary to transfuse platelets so uncontrollable bleeding does not occur. Many centers require a transfusion when the child's platelet count goes below 10,000 to 20,000/mm^3, and sometimes repeat transfusions are required every 2 or 3 days until the marrow recovers. Platelet transfusions usually take less than an hour.

As with other blood products, an allergic reaction is possible and platelets are capable of transmitting infections such as hepatitis, cytomegalovirus, and HIV. Even though the chance of contracting these viruses is extremely low, platelets are transfused only when necessary.

Platelet transfusions are a snap! Platelets are short-lived and boosted Matt's counts for only a few days, just long enough to get over the danger levels during chemo. He often needed them two to three times every cycle. He had a reaction of hives on one occasion, cured with Benadryl®. Ironically, that was one of the last times he needed platelets.

· · · · ·

Three-year-old Matthew had countless platelet transfusions, and only once did he have a reaction. It was an awful thing to watch, but the nurse who was monitoring him was very calm and professional, which helped both of us. Matthew was always premedicated for his platelet transfusions with Benadryl®, which made him very drowsy. Most often he would sleep through the entire transfusion.

Bone marrow aspiration

Protocols for children with leukemia require bone marrow aspirations, a process by which bone marrow is removed with a large-bore needle. The purpose of the first, or diagnostic, bone marrow aspiration is to see what percentage of the cells in the marrow are abnormal blasts. Then these cells are analyzed microscopically to determine which type of leukemia is present. For children or teens with ALL, the next bone marrow aspiration usually is done on day 8 and then on day 29 of treatment to determine how many blasts are still present. This information, along with other test results such as the amount of minimal residual disease (MRD), is used by oncologists to determine how intensive treatment should be. For instance, if the marrow still contains too many blasts, the child might be described as a "slow responder," who would require a more intensive course of treatment.

> *Since the doctors knew my daughter had leukemia from the blood work, they did her first bone marrow while she was under anesthesia to implant her PORT-A-CATH®. This was a blessing, as her marrow was packed tight with blasts.*

Most centers require additional bone marrow aspirations at the end of each phase of treatment and at the end of maintenance (or at the end of postremission treatment, if your child does not require the maintenance phase).

Doctors usually take a sample of the marrow from the iliac crest of the hip (the top of the hip bone in back or front). This bone is right under the skin and contains a large amount of marrow. The child lies face down on a table, sometimes on a pillow to elevate the hip. The doctor puts on sterile gloves, finds the site, then wipes it several times with an antiseptic to eliminate any germs. The nurse places sterile paper around the site, then an anesthetic (usually xylocaine) may be injected into the skin and a small area of bone. This causes a burning and stinging sensation that passes quickly. The physician usually rubs the area to distribute the anesthetic around the site. When she is convinced that the insertion site is numb, the doctor pushes a hollow needle (with a plug inside) through the skin into the bone, withdraws the plug, and attaches a syringe. She then aspirates (sucks out) the liquid marrow through the syringe. Finally, she removes the needle and bandages the area.

Without sedation, bone marrow aspiration is very painful, so most centers anethetize children for this procedure. Do not hesitate to advocate for this at your center. Here are some descriptions from children and adult survivors who have experienced it:

> *It was the worst thing of all. It felt really, really bad.*

> • • • • •

> *It hurts a lot. It feels like they are pulling something out and then it aches. You know, it hurts so much that now they put the kids to sleep. Boy, am I glad about that. It feels like they are trying to suck thick Jell-O® from inside the bone. Brief but incredible pain.*

> • • • • •

> *I would become very anxious when they were cleaning my skin and laying the towels down. Putting the needle in was a sharp, pressure kind of pain. Drawing the marrow*

feels tingly, like they hit a nerve. I always asked a nurse to hold my legs because I felt like my legs were going to jump up off the table.

Echocardiograms and electrocardiograms

Several drugs used to treat leukemia can damage the muscle of the heart, decreasing its ability to contract effectively. Many protocols require a baseline echocardiogram to measure the heart's ability to pump before any chemotherapy drugs are given. Echocardiograms are then given periodically during and after treatment to check for heart muscle damage.

An echocardiogram uses ultrasound waves to measure the amount of blood that leaves the heart each time it contracts. This percentage (blood ejected during a contraction compared to blood in the heart when it is relaxed) is called the ejection fraction.

The child or adolescent lies on a table and a technician, nurse, or doctor applies conductive jelly to the chest. Then the technician puts a transducer (which emits the ultrasound waves) on the jelly and moves the device around on the chest to obtain different views of the heart. He applies pressure on the transducer to obtain clear images; this pressure can be uncomfortable. The test results are videotaped for the technician to see the results as he works and so the radiologist can interpret the findings later.

> *Meagan used to watch a video during the echocardiogram. Sometimes she would eat a sucker or a Popsicle®. She found it to be boring, not painful.*

An electrocardiogram (EKG) measures the electrical impulses that the heart generates during the cardiac cycle. An EKG can be performed at an office, a lab, or your child's bedside. Before placing the electrodes, the technician cleans the area with alcohol and applies a cool gel under the electrodes. Your child must lie quietly during the test. You can remain with him throughout the procedure, which generally takes less than 10 minutes. Your child will feel nothing during the procedure other than the gel on the electrodes.

MUGA scan

A multiple-gated acquisition (MUGA) scan tests cardiac function. It is more sensitive than an echocardiogram. Children are sometimes sedated for the procedure to help them relax and stay perfectly still for the 15- to 20-minute test. The technician injects red cells or proteins tagged with a mildly radioactive substance, called technetium, into an IV while the child lies on a table with a large movable camera overhead. This special camera records sequential images of the technetium as it moves through the heart. These pictures of the heart's function allow doctors to determine how efficiently the heart muscle is pumping and if any damage to the heart has occurred.

My 3-year-old daughter had a MUGA scan before she started chemotherapy. They gave her an injection, and she fell asleep. They laid her on her back on a big table and moved a huge contraption around her to take pictures of her heart beating. We watched on a screen, and they printed out a copy on paper for the doctors.

If either the echocardiogram or MUGA scan shows heart damage, the oncologist may reduce the dosage or remove the drug that is causing the damage from your child's protocol.

Spinal tap (lumbar puncture or LP)

The body has a structure, called the blood–brain barrier, to protect the brain from poisons that may be circulating in the blood. Due to this barrier, systemic chemotherapy usually cannot destroy any blasts in the central nervous system (brain and spinal cord). Chemotherapy drugs must be directly injected into the cerebrospinal fluid to kill any blasts present and prevent a possible central nervous system relapse; this is called intrathecal administration. The drugs most commonly used are methotrexate, ARA-C (cytarabine), and hydrocortisone. The number of spinal taps required and when they are done varies depending on the child's risk level, the clinical study involved, and whether radiation is used.

Some hospitals routinely sedate children for spinal taps, and others do not. If the child is not sedated, EMLA® cream is usually prescribed to lessen the pain. Even with sedation, sometimes EMLA® is applied to minimize the sting of the topical anesthetic. To perform a spinal tap, the physician or nurse practitioner first ask the child to lie on her side with her head tucked close to the chest and knees drawn up. A nurse usually helps hold the child in this position. The doctor, wearing sterile gloves, finds the designated spot in the lower back and swabs it with antiseptic several times. The antiseptic feels very cold on the skin. The nurse then drapes the area with a sterile sheet. The doctor will administer one or two shots of an anesthetic (usually xylocaine) into the skin and deeper tissues. This causes a painful stinging or burning sensation that lasts about a minute. If EMLA® was used, the doctor may still inject anesthetic into the deep tissues. It is necessary to wait a few moments to ensure the area is fully anesthetized.

My 4-year-old daughter had finished 18 months of her treatment for ALL when EMLA® was first prescribed. She had been terrified of going to the clinic. After using EMLA® for her next LP, a dramatic change occurred. She was no longer frightened to go for treatment, and her behavior at home improved unbelievably. We use it for everything now: finger pokes, accessing port, bone marrows, even flu shots.

The child must hold very still for the rest of the procedure. The doctor will push a needle between two vertebrae and into the space where cerebrospinal fluid (CSF) is found. The CSF will begin to drip out of the hollow needle into a container. After collecting a small amount of CSF, the doctor attaches a syringe to the needle and slowly injects the medicine. This causes a sensation of coldness or pressure down the legs. He removes the needle and bandages the spot. The CSF is sent to the laboratory to see if any cancer cells are present and to measure glucose and protein.

> *During spinals, Brent listens to rock and roll on his Walkman®, but he keeps the volume low enough so that he can still hear what is going on. He likes me to lift up the earpiece and tell him when each part of the procedure is finished and what's coming next.*

It is important to lie extremely flat for at least 30 minutes after an LP to reduce pressure changes in the CSF. Sitting or standing up too soon can cause severe headaches. If your child or teen develops a persistent severe headache following the procedure that lessens while he lies flat, but throbs when he sits up, notify your physician or nurse.

The nurse will most probably tell you child or teen to lie flat and will offer high-caffeine beverages (such as Mountain Dew®) to drink. If these measures fail to give your child relief from the headache, an anesthesiologist sometimes does a procedure called a "blood patch." Your child lies in the same position as for the spinal tap. The anesthesiologist will draw a small amount of blood from your child's arm or central line. She will then inject it at the site of the prior spinal tap where CSF may be slowly leaking from the canal into the tissues. If this is the cause of the headache, the relief is immediate. This procedure is generally performed in the recovery room, emergency room, clinic, or inpatient unit. You can stay with your child during the procedure.

Subcutaneous and intramuscular injections

Some medications are given by injection, either under the skin (subcutaneous, or subQ, injection) or into a large muscle (intramuscular, or IM, injection). One drug commonly administered subcutaneously is Neupogen® (G-CSF), a medication that is often used to boost the white blood cell count. Methotrexate is given by IM injection, usually into the thigh.

> *We found that giving 4-year-old Joseph as much power in the process as possible really helped. The shots themselves are non-negotiable, but there are many parts of the process where the child can have some control (where to put the EMLA® cream, where to be sitting for the cream and/or the shot, who holds him, what Beanie Baby® to hold during the procedure, etc.). We also made sure to have a consistent little treat available afterwards, although this became unnecessary after a while. Even at 4, Joseph loved money, so for a long time he kept a pint jar, which would travel to the hospital and back home again, and he'd get to drop in a nickel for each pill successfully swallowed (a huge chore for him) and a quarter for each shot. Of course, adults would look very surprised when we told them we gave Joseph "quarter shots."*

Something tells me the bar scene will be very confusing to him when he gets to college.

To minimize pain caused by injections, apply EMLA® cream 1 to 2 hours before administration. Parents can also reduce pain by rubbing ice over the site to numb the area prior to injection. Other ideas are on the Internet at *http://webpages.charter.net/drshrink/gcsftips.htm.*

My two boys had ALL. Brian and Kevin both received IM methotrexate as part of their protocols. Brian, because of his age (12), was very macho about it, used "freezy" spray to numb the thigh, then giggled or made funny faces while the methotrexate was pushed. He had no aftereffects. Kevin, only 4 when they began, still doesn't like them. There were 3 or 4 months of overlap, when both boys got shots at the same time every week. This made it easier for Kevin, but he still insisted on an ice pack and freezy spray. Now, he uses the spray only.

Oral medication

As the parents of a child with leukemia, one of your most important jobs is to administer every dose of every oral medication on time every day. Research has proven that children who do not comply completely with the dosing regimen have a lower survival rate than others. Your child will need thousands of pills or liquid doses throughout treatment. To accomplish this, it is essential to get off to a good start and establish cooperation with your child early in the process.

To teach Brent (6 years old) to swallow pills, when we were eating corn for dinner I encouraged him to swallow one kernel whole. Luckily, it went right down and he got over his fear of pills.

· · · · ·

I wanted Katy (3 years old) to feel like we were a team right from the first night. So I made a big deal out of tasting each of her medications and pronouncing it good. Thank goodness I tasted the prednisone first. It was nauseating—bitter, metallic, with a lingering aftertaste. I asked the nurse for some small gel caps, and packed them with the pills which I had broken in half. I gave Katy her choice of drinks to take her pills with and taught her to swallow gel caps with a large sip of liquid. Since I gave her over 3,000 pills and 1,100 teaspoons of liquid medication during treatment, I'm very glad we got off to such a good start.

Gel caps come in many sizes. Number 4s are small enough for a 3- or 4-year-old child to swallow. Many pills can be chewed or swallowed whole without taste problems. Steroid medications (prednisone, dexamethasone, etc.) should not be chewed, because they have a bitter aftertaste and may cause your child to develop an aversion to all oral medications.

Just remember that different children develop different taste preferences and aversions to medications, and gel caps are useful for any medication that bothers them.

Very young children are often given liquid doses of medication, which can taste terrible. Gel caps can be used to help take unpleasant-tasting liquid medication as well. Using a syringe and needle, draw the correct dose and inject it into the gel cap so the child can swallow it.

> After much trial and error with medications, Meagan's method became chewing up pills with chocolate chips. She's kept this up for the long haul.

· · · · ·

> I always give choices such as, "Do you want the white pill or the six yellow pills first?" It gives him a little control in his chaotic world.

For younger children, many parents crush the pills into a small amount of pudding, applesauce, jam, frozen juice concentrate, or other favorite food. However, your child may develop a lifelong aversion to these foods after treatment is over.

> Jeremy was 4 when he was diagnosed, and we used to crush up the pills and mix them with ice cream. This worked well for us.

· · · · ·

> We used the liquid form of prednisone for my son, mixed it with a chocolate drink, and followed this with M&Ms®. The chocolate seemed to mask the taste.

· · · · ·

> Our son was 2½ years old when diagnosed. We put the med in an oral syringe and put very hot water in a tiny glass. Then we would draw a wee bit of the hot water into the oral syringe and then we would cap it. Then you gently shake the syringe and turn it back and forth while the med completely dissolves. Then we would take off the cap and fill it the rest of the way with nice cold Kool-Aid®. Alexander would get to choose the flavor of Kool-Aid® each day and we would just mix up a couple different batches of flavors and keep them in the fridge. He felt like he was in control because he chose the flavor, and it covered up the lousy taste of the medication. We asked our oncologist about this at the very beginning, and he said it was a great way to do it because neither the water nor the Kool-Aid® had any unwanted effects on the medication. Anyway, we never once had any problem with this method.

· · · · ·

> The method we used for getting Garrett to take his foul-tasting chemo/meds was the mixing agent Syrpalta®. This is a grape-flavored syrup available from the pharmacy. It doesn't react with most meds and the flavor can hide almost anything.

We used quite a bit of the stuff. First, we crushed Garrett's pills with a pill crusher/cutter, then we mixed them in a cup before putting them in a syringe to squirt in his mouth. (Keep in mind he was only about 15 months old when he got sick.) We had to make sure he got every drop though, since some of the pills were really small and a little bit of syrup could hide a significant portion of the dose.

You should make sure that any med you do this with is safe to crush or mix with Syrpalta® (or chocolate, or anything else for that matter). This particular mixing agent is designed to be "inert," but you can't be too careful. Meds with time-release or slow-release agents should never be crushed. Some meds should never be mixed with milk, for example.

Most children on maintenance take SMZ-TMP (sulfamethoxazole and trimethoprim), Bactrim®, or Septra® two to three times a week to prevent a specific type of pneumonia that can develop in children whose immune systems are suppressed. These drugs come in either liquid or pill form and are produced by several different manufacturers. Ask your pharmacist for a kid taste test. Letting your child choose a medicine that appeals to him encourages compliance.

Whenever my son had to take a liquid medicine, such as antibiotics, he enjoyed taking it from a syringe. I would draw up the proper amount, then he would put it in his mouth and push the plunger.

Because children associate taking medicine with being sick, it is helpful to explain why they must continue taking pills for years after they feel well. Some parents use the Pac-Man® analogy, "We need these pills to gobble up the last few bad cells." Others explain that the leukemia can return, and the medicine prevents it from growing again.

Teens and medication

Issues for teenagers about taking pills are completely different from those for young children. The problems with teens revolve around autonomy, control, and feelings of invulnerability. It is normal for teenagers to be noncompliant, and they cannot be forced to take pills if they choose not to cooperate. Trying to coerce teens fuels conflict and frustrates everyone. If you need help, ask for an assessment by the psychosocial team at the hospital to work out a plan for treatment adherence. Everyone will need to be flexible to reach a favorable outcome.

I think the main problem with teens is making sure that they take the meds. Joel (15 years old) has been very responsible about taking his nightly pills. I've tried to make it easy for him by having an index card for the week, and he marks off the med as he takes it. I also put a list of the meds on a dry erase board on the fridge as a reminder. As he takes the med, he erases it. That way it's easy for him (and me) to see at a glance if he's taken his stuff. The index card alone wasn't working because he couldn't find a pen or forgot to mark it off.

• • • • •

One of the biggest concerns with teens and maintenance is noncompliance. I think it's a delicate balancing act to allow the teen to be responsible for taking his own meds and yet have some supervision of the process. Our meds are kept in a small plastic basket on the kitchen counter. All meds are taken there. I'd never want him to keep his meds in his room where I would have no idea if he had taken them or not.

On Friday nights when he is to take his weekly methotrexate—a 16-pill dose—I will count it out and put it in a medicine cup on the counter. I am not always an awake and alert person when he comes home at midnight on Friday night. When I get up Saturday morning, I know immediately if he's taken his meds.

If he had shown any resistance to taking the meds, or any sign of telling me that he had taken them when he had not, I'd be doing this differently. But he's aware of the importance of each dose and the importance of his participation in the team beating the leukemia.

My only other advice is to be sure and ask the doctors what to do about a missed dose for each med. In 3-plus years of treatment, you are going to have a missed dose, and it helps to know how to handle it.

Taking a temperature

Fever is the enemy during treatment because it signals infection, and children on chemotherapy cannot fight infection effectively, especially when their white counts are depressed. Parents take hundreds of temperatures, especially when their child is not feeling well. Temperatures can be taken under the tongue, under the arm, or in the ear using a special type of thermometer. Rectal temperatures are not recommended due to the risk of tears and infection. Here are a few suggestions that might help.

• Use a glass thermometer under the tongue.

• Use a digital thermometer under the tongue or arm. Some have an alarm that beeps when it is time to remove the thermometer.

> *We bought a digital thermometer that we only use under his arm. It has worked well for us.*

• Tympanic (ear) thermometers measure infrared waves and are very easy to use.

> *When my in-laws asked at diagnosis if there was anything that we needed, I asked them to try to buy a tympanic thermometer. The device cost over 100 dollars then, but it worked beautifully. It takes only 1 second to obtain a temperature. I can even*

use it when she is asleep without waking her. They are now sold at pharmacies and drug stores, and cost much less.

Before you leave the hospital, you should know when to call the clinic because of fever. Usually, parents are told not to give any medication for fever and to call if the fever goes above 101° F (38.5° C). It is especially important for parents of children with implanted catheters to know when to call the clinic, as an untreated infection can be life-threatening. It is also really helpful to have a copy of your child's most recent blood counts when you call to notify your physician about fever issues.

Urine collections

Certain chemotherapy drugs can cause damage to the kidneys, so it is sometimes necessary to perform timed urine collections to evaluate your child's kidney function. Also, by measuring certain substances in the kidneys, doctors can tell how well the chemo drugs are working. If your child is toilet trained, the collection is done by saving all the urine your child produces in a defined period of hours.

Urine specimens

Chemotherapy requires frequent urine specimens. One way to help obtain a sample is to encourage drinking lots of liquids the hour before. If your child has an IV, you can also ask the nurse to increase the drip rate. Explain to the child why the test is necessary. Ask the nurse to show how the dip sticks work. (They change color, so they are quite popular with preschoolers.) Use a "hat" under the toilet seat. This is a shallow plastic bucket that fits under the seat and catches the urine.

Turn on the water while the child sits on the toilet. I don't know why it works, but it does.

As all parents learn, eating and elimination are functions that the child controls. If she just can't or won't urinate in the hat, go out, buy her the largest drink you can find, and wait.

It may be necessary to obtain a sterile specimen, or "clean catch," if infection is suspected. You or your child will need to cleanse the perineal area with soap or an antiseptic towelette, and she will need to urinate in a small sterile container.

If your child is not yet toilet trained, if a clean catch is impossible, or if your child is unable to urinate, it may be necessary to insert a Foley catheter. This procedure can be quite stressful because it involves placing a sterile rubber tube up the urethra and into the bladder. It is definitely appropriate to ask for your child to be given a mild sedative or muscle relaxant before the procedure if he is anxious, and to request that the most skilled person available perform the procedure. In skilled nursing hands, the procedure takes less than 5 minutes to perform.

X-rays

X-rays, a type of electromagnetic radiation, provide the doctor with a quick and simple method of viewing organs and structures inside your child's body. X-rays are performed for many reasons during a child's treatment for leukemia. Although large and repeated doses of x-ray radiation pose health risks, the number of x-rays your child is likely to need will not significantly impact his health. X-rays are:

• Needed before operations.

• Needed after your child's central venous catheter is placed to confirm it is in the proper location.

• Used as part of a workup for fever to determine whether your child may have pneumonia.

The technician positions your child in a manner that will make it easiest to get the images she needs. For chest x-rays, your child may be asked to breathe in, hold her breath, and remain perfectly still for a few seconds. The technician leaves the room during the time the x-rays are taken. If you are planning to stay with your child, you need to wear a lead apron to protect yourself from radiation. Your child may also have to wear a lead apron or lead shield to protect specific areas of her body. Pregnant women should not be present in the room when x-rays are taken.

Meagan is scheduled to go off therapy this May. She's doing well and is very happy. A father at our support group was advising a new set of parents to remember to view life from the child's perspective. He said that, especially with the little ones, parents sometimes agonized more than the child. He told us that at the end of the first year of treatment, he and his wife were reflecting on how much misery their child had endured, and then she piped up and said, "This has been a great year for me!" Meagan is the same. When I have bad days and get preoccupied with the uncertain future, I see Meagan skipping along and saying as she frequently does, "I'm such a happy girl!"

Chapter 6

Forming a Partnership with the Medical Team

It is our duty as physicians to estimate probabilities and to discipline expectations; but leading away from probabilities there are paths of possibilities, toward which it is our duty to hold aloft the light, and the name of that light is hope.

— Karl Menninger
The Vital Balance

IT IS VITALLY IMPORTANT that parents and the healthcare team establish and maintain a relationship based on excellent medical care, good communication, and caring. In this partnership, trust is paramount. Unlike children with some other diseases, children with leukemia spend years being treated primarily on an outpatient basis. Physicians rely on parents to make and keep appointments, give the proper medicines at the appropriate times, prepare the child for procedures, and monitor the child for signs of illness or side effects. Parents rely on physicians for medical knowledge, expertise in performing procedures, good judgment, caring, and clear communication. It is a delicate dance that spans years of trauma and emotional upheaval.

A climate of cooperation and respect between the healthcare team and parents allows children to thrive. This chapter explores ways to create and maintain that environment.

The hospital

Your child will probably be treated in a teaching hospital: a hospital that is affiliated with a medical school that serves as a training ground for young doctors and medical students. After admission to the hospital, a steady parade of anonymous faces enters the life of a child with leukemia, and it is not always clear to parents who is responsible for their child's treatment. The various specialty units in a hospital, such as pediatric oncology, cardiology, or neurology, are called "services." Within each service, the pecking order is roughly the same.

The doctors

A *medical student* is a college graduate who is attending medical school. Medical students often wear white coats, but they do not have M.D. after the name on their name tags. They are not doctors.

An *intern* (also called a first-year resident) is a graduate of medical school who is in her first year of postgraduate training. Interns are doctors who are just beginning their clinical training.

A *resident* is a graduate of medical school in his second or third year of postgraduate training. Most of the residents at pediatric hospitals will be pediatricians upon completion of their residencies. Residents are temporary: they rotate into different services every 4 weeks.

A *fellow* is a doctor pursuing post-residency study in a particular specialty. Most of the fellows you will encounter will be specializing in pediatric oncology. Not all teaching hospitals have fellowship programs.

Attending physicians (or simply, *attendings*) are highly trained doctors hired by the hospital to provide and oversee medical care and to train interns, residents, and fellows. Many of them also teach at a medical school.

Consulting physicians are doctors from other services who are brought in to provide advice or treatment to a child in the oncology unit. The attending may ask for consults with other specialists, who may appear in your child's hospital room unexpectedly. If questions arise about who these doctors are and what role they play, you should ask the fellow or attending assigned to your child.

Each child in a teaching hospital is assigned an attending, who is responsible for the child's care. This doctor should be "board-certified" or have equivalent medical credentials. This means that he has taken rigorous written and oral tests by a board of examiners in his specialty and meets a high standard of competence. You can call the American Board of Medical Specialties at (866) ASK-ABMS (275-2267) or visit *www.abms.org/Contact_Us* to find out if your child's physician is board-certified.

> *Our medical team was wonderful. They always answered our questions and spent the time with us that we needed. We had a group of doctors who were all working together for the patients. I always felt that we were known by each doctor, and that they were on top of Paige's treatment.*

If your family is insured by a health maintenance organization (HMO), you probably will be sent to the affiliated hospital, which will have one or more pediatric oncologist on staff. If this hospital is not a regional pediatric hospital or is not affiliated with the Children's Oncology Group, you can go elsewhere to get state-of-the-art care.

The nurses

An essential part of the hospital hierarchy is the nursing staff. The following explanations will help you understand which type of nurse is caring for your child.

An *RN* is a registered nurse who obtained an associate or higher degree in nursing, and then passed a licensing examination. RNs supervise all other nursing and patient care staff, give medicines, take vital signs (heart rate, breathing rate, blood pressure), monitor IV machines, change bandages, and care for patients in hospitals, clinics, and doctors' offices. Many RNs in the pediatric oncology service have received specialized training in pediatric oncology nursing.

A *nurse practitioner* or *clinical nurse specialist* is a registered nurse who has completed an educational program (generally a master's or doctoral degree) that has taught him advanced skills. For example, in some hospitals and clinics, nurse practitioners perform procedures such as spinal taps. Nurse practitioners or clinical nurse specialists are often the liaison between the medical teams and patients and families. They help parents keep all the different multidisciplinary team "players" straight and help interpret medical jargon.

> At our hospital, each of our nurses is different, but each is wonderful. They simply love the kids. They throw parties, set up dream trips, act as counselors, best friends, stern parents. They hug moms and dads. They cry. I have come to respect them so much because they have such a hard job to do, and they do it so well.

An *LPN* is a licensed practical nurse. LPNs complete certificate training and must pass a licensing exam. In some medical facilities LPNs are allowed to perform most nursing functions except those involving administration of medications. Many pediatric oncology services limit the involvement of LPNs to personal care, such as patient hygiene and monitoring fluid input and output.

The *head* or *charge nurse* is an RN who supervises all the nurses on the floor for one shift. If you have any problems with a nurse, your first step in resolving the issue should be to talk to the nurse involved. If this does not resolve the problem, a discussion with the charge nurse is necessary.

The *clinical nurse manager* is the administrator for an entire unit, such as a surgical or medical floor or outpatient clinic. She is in charge of all of the nurses on the unit.

Finding an oncologist

Usually, parents do not have the luxury of time in choosing a pediatric oncologist. At diagnosis, the family is usually referred to the nearest regional pediatric hospital. The young patient may be assigned the fellow or attending who happens to be on call at the time of diagnosis.

During induction and consolidation, it may not be clear which of the many doctors who see your child is in charge. Before your child is released to outpatient treatment, his case will be assigned to an oncologist, who will probably supervise the rest of your child's treatment. If you are not comfortable with the oncologist assigned, following are several traits to look for in the physician you request to supervise your child's care:

- Board-certified in the field of pediatric oncology.

- Establishes a good rapport with your child.

- Communicates clearly and compassionately.

- Skillful in performing procedures.

- Answers all questions in language that you understand.

- Consults with other doctors on complex problems.

- Makes available the results of all tests.

- Acknowledges parents' right to make decisions.

- Respects parents' values.

- Delivers the truth with hope.

If you don't develop a good rapport with the physician assigned to your child, ask to be assigned to a different physician you may have met on rounds or during clinic visits. Most parents are accommodated, for hospitals realize the importance of good communication between families and physicians. You will, however, still see different physicians, because many institutions have rotating physicians on call.

> I've been very lucky that our doctors have been very open with us. When Samantha was first diagnosed, our doctor spent 2 hours explaining and answering our questions, and it has never stopped. Even if we haven't asked, but the doctors notice concern in our faces, they sit and take the time to find out our worries. They've all been great—the nurses, hospital, and support staff.

Types of relationships

Three types of relationships tend to develop between physicians and parents:

- **Paternal.** In a paternal relationship, the parent is submissive, and the doctor assumes a parental role. This dynamic may seem desirable to parents who are uncomfortable or inexperienced in dealing with medical issues, but it places all responsibility for decisions and monitoring on the doctor. Doctors are human. If your child's doctor makes a mistake and you are not monitoring drugs and treatments, these mistakes may go unnoticed. You are the expert on your child and you know best how to gauge his reactions to drugs and treatments.

    After we left Children's and returned home for outpatient treatment, the local pediatrician's nurse called and said, "Doctor wanted me to tell you that the blood results were normal." I thought that unlikely since she was on high-dose chemotherapy, so I politely asked for the actual numbers for my records. She read them off and my daughter's ANC (absolute neutrophil count—see Appendix A, "Blood Counts and What They Mean") had dropped far below 500. I said, "Would you tell the doctor that her counts have dropped dramatically from last week?" She said in a frosty voice, "Doctor said they were fine." So I called Children's, and they told me to keep her at home, take her off all medications for a week, and then have her blood retested. I was glad that I paid attention to the counts.

Some parents are intimidated by doctors and express the fear that if they question the doctors their child will suffer. This type of behavior robs the child of an adult advocate who speaks up when something seems wrong.

- **Adversarial.** Some parents adopt an "us against them" attitude that is counterproductive. They seem to feel that the disease and treatment are the fault of the medical staff, and they blame staff for any setbacks that occur. This attitude undermines the child's confidence in his doctor, which is a crucial component for healing.

    I knew one family who just hated the Children's Hospital. They called it the "House of Horrors" or the "torture chamber" in front of their children. Small wonder that their children were terrified.

- **Collegial.** This is a true partnership in which parents and doctors are all on the same footing and they respect each other's domains and expertise. The doctor recognizes that the parents are the experts on their own child and are essential in ensuring that the protocol is followed. The parents respect the physician's expertise and feel comfortable discussing various treatment options or concerns that arise. Honest communication is necessary for this partnership to work, but the effort is well worth it. The child has confidence in his doctor, the parents have lessened their stress by creating a supportive relationship with the physician, and the physician feels comfortable that the family will comply with the treatment plan, thus giving the child the best chance for a cure.

> *We had a wonderful relationship with the oncologist assigned to us. He blended perfectly the science and the art of medicine. His manner with our daughter was warm, he was extremely well-qualified professionally, and he was very easy to talk to. I could bring in articles to discuss with him, and he welcomed the discussion. Although he was busy, he never rushed us. I laughed when I saw that he had written in the chart, "Mother asks innumerable appropriate questions."*

· · · · ·

> *Justin's oncologist had remarkable interpersonal skills. At our first meeting he said, "Justin has leukemia. There are two kinds of leukemia, and both of them are treatable." So right away he emphasized the positive. He then wrote on his notepad what all of Justin's blood counts were; he told us what normal counts were and explained clearly what we needed to do next. He was very reassuring. It has been years since that day, and he has always been very caring. He still frequently calls us on the phone.*

Another mother relates a different experience:

> *We tried very hard to form a partnership with the medical team but failed. The staff seemed very guarded and distant, almost wary of a parent wanting to participate in the decisions made for the child. I learned to use the medical library and took research reports in to them to get some help for side effects and get some drug dosages reduced. Things improved, but I was never considered a partner in the healthcare team; I was viewed as a problem.*

A pediatric oncologist shares her perspective:

> *All parents are different and have different coping styles. Some deal best with a lot of information (lab results, meds, study options) up front, while others are overwhelmed and want the information a little bit at a time. There is no way for the doctor to know the parents' coping styles at the beginning. (Even the parents may not yet know!) So if they let the doctor know how much information they want or don't want, it is very helpful.*

Communication

Clear and frequent communication is the lifeblood of a positive doctor/parent relationship. Doctors need to be able to explain clearly and listen well, and parents need to feel comfortable asking questions and expressing concerns before they grow into grievances. Nurses and doctors cannot read a parent's mind, nor can a parent prepare her child for a procedure unless it has been explained well. The following are parent suggestions about how to establish and maintain good communication with their child's healthcare team:

- Tell the staff how much you want to know.

  I told them the first day to treat me like a medical student. I asked them to share all information, current studies, lab results, everything, with me. I told them, in advance, that I hoped they wouldn't be offended by lots of questions, because knowledge was comfort to me.

  · · · · ·

  If the doctors at Children's told me to do something, I didn't question it because I trusted them.

- Inform the staff of your child's temperament, likes, and dislikes. You know your child better than anyone, so don't hesitate to tell the clinic staff about what works best.

  Whenever my daughter was hospitalized, I made a point of kindly reminding doctors and nurses that she was extremely sensitive, and would benefit from quiet voices and soothing explanations of anything that was about to occur, such as taking temperatures, vital signs, or adjustments to her IV.

- Encourage a close relationship between doctor, nurse, and child. Insist that all medical personnel respect the young person's dignity. Do not let anyone talk in front of your child as if she is not there. If a problem persists, you have the right to ask the offending person to leave. Marina Rozen observes in *Advice to Doctors and Other Big People*:

  The best part about the doctor is when he gives me bubble gum. The worst part is when he's in the room with me and my mom and he only talks to my mom. I've told him I don't like that, but he doesn't listen.

- Most children's hospitals assign each patient a primary nurse who will oversee all care. Try to form a close relationship with your child's nurse. Nurses usually possess vast knowledge and experience about both medical and practical aspects of cancer treatment. Often, the nurse can rectify misunderstandings between doctors and parents.

  The nurses at Children's were splendid. They were gentle with both kids and parents. Once, when I asked to have Christine's spinal done by the fellow rather than the resident, the fellow said in a nasty voice, "Well, we'll see about that!" and he disappeared. He didn't come in for 2 hours; my child was crying, we missed an appointment with radiation, and everyone was upset. The nurse ran back and forth between the fellow and us trying to get it resolved. In the end—after the resident had done

*the spinal—she hugged me, and told me that she was going to talk with the fellow
because his actions were unacceptable.*

- Children and teenagers should be included as part of the team. They should be consulted about treatments and procedures and be given age-appropriate choices.

- Cooperate. If your hometown pediatrician will handle all of your child's outpatient treatments, find ways to facilitate communication between the oncologist and pediatrician.

  *Before we left Children's, I called our pediatrician to ask what paperwork he had
  received and what he needed. He had received nothing, so he gave me a list of what
  he needed, which I was able to get from the primary nurse and carry home with me.
  When maintenance started, I asked if there was anything that he thought might help
  keep his staff aware of the cycles of blood work and chemotherapy orders. He asked
  me to write a letter at the beginning of every 3-month cycle listing what needed to be
  done and when. They put this in the front of her chart, and it helped keep the orders
  and communication flowing smoothly.*

- Go to all appointments with a written list of questions. This prevents you from forgetting something important and saves the staff from numerous follow-up phone calls.

- Ask for definitions of unfamiliar terms. Repeat back the information to ensure it was understood correctly. Writing down answers or tape recording conferences are both common practices.

  *We found that sitting down and talking things over with the nurses helped immensely. They were very familiar with each drug and its side effects. They told us many
  stories about children who had been through the same thing and were doing well
  years later. They always seemed to have time to give encouragement, a smile, or
  a hug.*

- Some parents want to read their child's medical chart to obtain more details about their child's condition and to help in formulating questions for the medical team. Often, the doctor or nurse will let the parents read it in the child's hospital room or in the waiting room at the clinic. Most states and provinces have laws that allow patient access to all records. You may have to write to the doctor asking to review the chart and pay any photocopy costs.

- If you have questions or concerns, discuss them with the resident. If she is unable to provide a satisfactory answer, ask the fellow or attending physician assigned to your child.

- The medical team includes many specialists: doctors, nurses, physical therapists, nutritionists, x-ray technicians, radiation therapists, and more. At training hospitals, many of these people will be in the early stages of their training. If a procedure is not going well, the parent has the right to tell the person to stop, and to request a more skilled person to do the job.

> *At our hospital, family practice residents rotate through, and are often assigned to do the spinal taps. My son was on a high-dose methotrexate protocol, which required a rescue drug to be administered at a certain time. Once, the resident tried for an hour to do the tap, and just couldn't do it. My son was very late getting the rescue drug, and I was worried. Later, I requested a conference with the oncologist and asked him to perform the spinal taps in the future to prevent the residents from practicing on my child. He agreed, but I didn't intervene that first time and I felt very guilty.*

• • • • •

> *While I truly supported the teaching hospital concept, it was difficult to deal with a first-year resident who couldn't do a spinal tap or insert an IV. We had a tendency to lose patience rather quickly when our child was screaming and the doctor was getting impatient. More than once we requested a replacement and had someone else do the test.*

• Know your rights—and the hospital's. Legally, your child cannot be treated without your permission. If the doctor suggests a procedure that you do not feel comfortable with, keep asking questions until you feel fully informed. You have the legal right to refuse the procedure if you do not think it is necessary.

> *One day in the hospital, a group of fellows came in and announced that they were going to do a lung biopsy on Jesse. I told them that I hadn't heard anything about it from her attending, and I just didn't think it was the right thing to do. They said, "We have to do it," and I repeated that I just didn't think it needed to be done until we talked to the attending. They seemed angry, but we stood our ground. When the attending came later, he said that they were not supposed to do a biopsy because the surgeon said it was too risky of an area in the lung to get to.*

However, if the hospital feels you are endangering the health of your child by withholding permission for treatment, they can take you to court. All parties must remember that the most important person in this circumstance is the child. Don't let problems turn into grievances.

> *We had a problem with the pediatrician's office not calling me with the results of my daughter's blood work in time for me to call the clinic. This would result in worry for me and a delay in changes to her chemotherapy doses. I told the pediatrician's nurse that I knew how busy they were and I hated having to keep calling to get the results. I asked her if it was possible for them to give the lab authorization to call me with the results. They thought it was a great idea, and it worked for 3 years. The lab would fax the doctor the results, but call me. Then I would call the clinic and get the dose changes. The clinic would then fax that information to the pediatrician's office.*

It was a win/win situation: the doctor's office received no interruptions, they got copies of everything in writing, and I got quick responses from the clinic on how to adjust her meds to her wildly swinging blood counts.

- Use "I" statements. For example, "I feel upset when you won't answer my questions," rather than, "You never listen to me."

- If it helps you feel more comfortable, keep track of your child's treatments to check for mistakes.

  A nurse thought Arielle had a double-lumen catheter and put two incompatible drugs through her single lumen line. It immediately turned to concrete. Arielle had to have the line removed. When they took it out, we saw the drugs had precipitated and formed what looked like little tablets. If this had become dislodged into her blood-stream (a very real possibility) it could have been fatal. Scary!

- Be specific and diplomatic when describing problems. Allow room for the staff to save face. For example, "My daughter feels very comfortable with Dr. Smith, so I would really appreciate it if we could wait for him," rather than, "I'm not going to let that intern near my daughter again." Another example is, "My son gets very nervous if we must wait a long time for our appointment, which makes him less compliant with the doctor. Could we call ahead next time to see if the doctor is on schedule?" rather than, "Do you think your time is more valuable than mine?"

- If you have something to discuss with the doctor that will take some time, request a conference. These are routinely scheduled between parents and physicians, and should be scheduled to allow enough time for a thorough discussion. Grabbing a busy doctor in the hallway is not fair to her and may not result in a satisfactory answer for you.

- Do not be afraid to make waves if you are right or to apologize if you are wrong.

  When Meagan was in the hospital during induction, the nurse came in with two syringes. I asked what they were, and she said immunizations. I said that it must be a mistake, and the nurse said that the orders were in the chart. So I checked Meagan's chart, and the orders were there, but they had another child's name on them.

- Show appreciation.

  I sent thank-you notes to three residents after my daughter's first hospitalization. The notes were short but sweet. I wanted them to know how much we appreciated their many kindnesses.

I always try to thank the nurse or doctor when they apologize for being late and give the reason. I don't mind waiting if it is for a good cause, and I feel they show respect when they apologize.

. . . . .

Erica's doctor would sometimes call up just to say, "How's my little chickadee?" He really cared. It touched me that he took the time to call, and I told him that I appreciated it.

. . . . .

Early in my daughter's treatment, we changed pediatricians. The first was aloof and patronizing, and the second was smart, warm, funny, and caring. He was a constant bright spot in our lives through some dark times. So every year during my daughter's treatment, she and her younger sister put on their Santa hats and brought home-made cookies to her pediatrician and nurse. This year was the first time she was able to walk in, and she looked them in the eye and sang, "We Wish You a Merry Christmas." Her nurse went in the back room and cried, and her doctor got misty-eyed. I'll always be thankful for their care.

The National Coalition for Cancer Survivorship (NCCS) has developed an excellent resource for communicating with healthcare providers. This audio resource program, called the *Cancer Survival Toolbox*, is available free by request. Its goal is to "help develop practical tools in daily life" to deal with a cancer diagnosis and treatment. The CDs in the Toolbox include the topics: Communicating, Finding Information, Making Decisions, Solving Problems, Negotiating, Standing Up for Your Rights, and Finding Ways to Pay for Care. Call the NCCS at: (877) NCCS-YES (622-7937), or e-mail your request to *info@canceradvocacy.org*. If you have Internet access, you can read, listen to, or download the Toolbox materials at: *www.canceradvocacy.org/toolbox*.

Getting a second opinion

There are times during your child's treatment when a second opinion may be advisable. Parents are sometimes reluctant to request a second opinion because they are afraid of offending their child's doctor or creating antagonism. Conscientious doctors will not resent a parent seeking a second opinion. If your child's doctor does resist, ask why. Second opinions are a common and accepted practice, and they are sometimes required by insurance companies.

The two ways to get a second opinion are: see another specialist or ask your child's physician to arrange a multidisciplinary second opinion. If you choose to see another specialist, do not do it in secret. Explain your concerns to your child's oncologist and ask for his recommendation or simply tell him that you are obtaining a second opinion.

Multidisciplinary second opinions incorporate the views of several different specialists. Parents who would like to get various viewpoints can ask to have their child's case discussed at a tumor board, which usually meets weekly at major medical centers. These boards include medical, surgical, and radiation oncologists, as well as fellows and residents. Your child's oncologist will present the facts of your child's case for discussion. Ask him to tell you what was said at the meeting.

Doctors informally seek second opinions all the time. Residents confer with their fellow for complicated situations; fellows might confer with the attending when unusual drug reactions or responses to treatment occur. Attendings call colleagues at other institutions. Parents should feel free to ask their child's physician if he has conferred with other staff members to gain additional viewpoints.

> Brent developed a seizure disorder after a rare drug reaction, so he was on anticonvulsants as well as chemotherapy for 2 years. We worried about the interaction of all the drugs, as well as the advisability of his continuing on the more aggressive arm of the protocol. We asked the fellow to arrange a care conference, and she met with the clinic director as well as Brent's neurologist to discuss how best to manage his case.

Conflict resolution

Conflict is a part of life. In a situation where a child's life is threatened, such as childhood leukemia, the heightened emotions and constant involvement with the medical bureaucracy guarantee conflict. Because clashes are inevitable, resolving them is of paramount importance. A speedy resolution may result if you adopt Henry Ford's motto, "Don't find fault; find a remedy."

Following are some suggestions from parents about how to resolve problems:

• Treat the doctors with respect, and expect respect from them.

> I always wanted to be treated as an intelligent adult, not someone of lesser status. So I would ask each medical person what they wished to be called. We would either both go by first names or both go by titles. I did not want to be called 'Mom.'

• Expect a reasonable amount of sensitivity from the staff.

> Soon after my daughter began treatment, I was walking by the open door of the residents' room, which was directly across from the nurses' station. Written in large letters on the blackboard were the words "Have a blast of a day!" with a picture of a smiling leukemia blast drawn below. I felt like I had been punched in the stomach. I was too upset to say anything, but I always regretted not complaining.

- Treat the staff with sensitivity. Recognize that you are under enormous stress, and so are the doctors and nurses. Do not blame them for the disease or explode in anger. Be an advocate, not an adversary.

- If a problem develops, state the issue clearly, without accusations, and then suggest a solution.

> *I found out late in my daughter's treatment that short-acting, safe sedatives were being used for many children at the clinic to prevent pain and anxiety during treatments. Only parents who knew about it and requested it received this service. I felt that my daughter's life would have been incredibly improved if we had been able to remove the trauma of procedures. I was angry. But I also realized that although I thought that they were wrong not to offer the service, I was partially at fault for not expressing more clearly how much difficulty she had the week before and after a procedure. I called the director of the clinic and carefully explained that I thought that poor staff/parent communication was creating hardships for the children. I suggested that the entire staff meet with a panel of parents to try to improve communication and to educate the doctors on the impact of pain on the children's daily lives. They were very supportive and scheduled the conference. From then on, children were sedated for painful procedures. This is a classic example of how something good can come out of a disagreement, if both parties are receptive to solving the problem.*

- Recognize that it is hard to speak up, especially if you are not naturally assertive; but it is very important to solve the problem before it grows and poisons the relationship.

- Most large medical centers have social workers and psychologists on staff to help families. One of their major duties is to serve as mediators between staff and parents. Ask for their advice about problem solving.

- Monitor your own feelings of anger and fear. Be careful not to dump on staff inappropriately. On the other hand, do not let a physician or nurse behave unprofessionally toward you or your child. Parents and staff members all have bad days, but they should not take it out on each other.

- Do not fear reprisal for speaking up. It is possible to be assertive without being aggressive or arguing.

- There are times when no resolution is possible; but expressing one's feelings can be a great release.

> *My son and I waited in an exam room for over an hour for a painful procedure. When I went out to ask the receptionist what had caused the delay, she said that a parent had brought in a child without an appointment. This parent frequently failed to bring in her child for treatment, and consequently, whenever she appeared, the doctors dropped everything to take care of the child. When the doctor finally came in, an hour and a half later, my son was in tears. The doctor did not explain the delay or apologize, he just silently started the procedure. After it was finished, I went out*

of the room, found the doctor, and said, "This makes me so angry. You just left us in here for hours and traumatized my son. Our time is valuable, too." He told me that I should have more compassion for the other mother because her life was very difficult. I replied that he encouraged her to not make appointments by dropping everything whenever she appeared. I added that it wasn't fair to those parents who played by the rules; she was being rewarded for her irresponsibility. After we had each stated our position, we left without resolution.

Changing doctors

Facing cancer is one of life's greatest struggles. With a skilled physician you trust, who communicates easily and honestly with you, the struggle is greatly eased. If the doctor adds to your family's discomfort rather than reduces it, you may have to change doctors. Changing doctors is not a step to be taken lightly, but it can be a great relief if the relationship has deteriorated beyond repair. It is a good policy to exhaust all possible remedies prior to separating and to examine your own role in the relationship, or the same problems may arise with the new doctor. Mediation by social service staff and improved communication can often resolve the issues and prevent the disruption of changing doctors.

Although there are many valid reasons for changing doctors, some of the most common are:

- Lack of qualifications.

- Grave medical errors being made.

- Poor communication skills or refusal to answer questions.

- Serious clash of philosophy or personality; for example, a paternalistic doctor and a parent who wishes to be informed and share in decision-making.

Do not change doctors because you're searching for a better diagnosis. If two reputable physicians, or a tumor board, have agreed on the diagnosis and treatment, it is best for the child to begin treatment immediately.

Many parents, fearing reprisals, choose to continue with a physician in whom they have no confidence. Such reprisals rarely happen at large, regional children's hospitals. While there may be lingering bitterness or anger between parents and doctors, the child will continue to benefit from the best-known treatment. Children may actually suffer more from the additional family stress caused by a poor doctor/parent relationship than from changing doctors.

In a small treatment center like Group Health, there are only two pediatric oncologists. When parents change doctors, the situation becomes very tense because the terminated doctor still cares for their child nights, weekends, and when he is on call. I would not recommend changing doctors if there are only two doctors in the clinic. It's probably better to change treatment centers if possible.

Once the decision to change doctors is made, parents must be candid. Either verbally or in writing, they should give an explanation for the change and make a formal request to transfer records to the new physician. Physicians are legally required to transfer all records upon written request.

We've had wonderful docs, mediocre docs, and one who made a terrible mistake. We've had warm, compassionate docs, ho-hum docs (on a good day they're nice, on a bad day they're neutral), and we've met some world-class jerks. Sounds pretty much like a slice of humanity, right?

Parents hold doctors to a different standard since the stakes are so high—our kids' lives. But the reality is they are usually overworked, exhausted, and deal with newly diagnosed families on an almost daily basis, day after day, week after week, year after year. I can't even begin to imagine the emotional toll that must take.

I tell my kids all human relationships are like a goodwill bank. If you make lots of deposits, an occasional withdrawal won't be so noticeable. I tell my docs and my kids' docs whenever things go right. I like to write, so I send many thank-you notes. When our pediatrician went on sabbatical, he took me into his office and showed me every mushy Christmas card I'd sent him lined up on the back of his messy desk.

I also have been known to bring in brownies for the office staff. We did this on my daughter's last day of radiation and several people broke down and cried when they saw the thank-you note she drew—a picture of herself holding a Snow White and the seven dwarves audiotape. She listened to that during every radiation session because I'd promised that day's radiation treatment would be over before the dwarves appeared.

I recently asked one of my favorite doctors (a pediatric oncologist who has incredible compassion) how many thank-you notes she had received from parents over the years. She said she could count them on two hands. I asked how many complaints, and she said, "You wouldn't want to know."

So, while I think docs should be called out for bad behavior and bad medicine, I also think we should acknowledge good medicine and good behavior. I'd like to encourage the good ones to stick around—new little innocents keep getting cancer every day.

Chapter 7

Hospitalization

Every day is a journey, and the journey itself is home.
— Matsuo Basho

THERE ARE FEW THINGS in life more uncomfortable than rising from a lumpy pullout couch to face another day of your child's hospitalization for leukemia. Hospitals are noisy bureaucracies that run on a time schedule all their own. For a child, being hospitalized means being separated from parents, brothers, sisters, friends, pets, and the comfort and familiarity of home. A child's hospitalization can rob both parent and child of a sense of control, leaving them feeling helpless. With a little ingenuity, however, you can make the most of the facilities, liven up the atmosphere, and even have some fun.

The room

Because kids on chemotherapy are at increased risk of infection, many hospitals give them private rooms. This means more space for the child, the parents, and visitors; it also means much more freedom to personalize and decorate the room. Covering the walls with big, bright posters of interest to your child can liven up the room immensely.

> *The first thing we put up in Meagan's room was a huge poster of The Little Engine That Could saying, "I think I can, I think I can."*

Cards can be displayed on the walls, hanging from strings like a mobile, or taped around the windowsills. Put up pictures of your child engaged in her favorite activity, and add photos of her friends. Most hospitals don't allow flowers on oncology floors because they can grow a fungus that can make children sick; but it's fun to have bouquets of balloons bobbing in the corners. Younger children derive great comfort from having a favorite stuffed animal, blanket, or quilt on their bed. If it doesn't bother your child, make the room smell good with potpourri or aromatherapy oils.

> *I went and bought a travel bag on wheels. It is so much easier than trying to carry several handle bags when Zach is admitted. It has several pockets to carry stuff. I love it and wished I had done it 2 years ago when we started this!*

I take these things to the hospital: flavored creamer for my coffee (a little treat for me); a book for us to read together so I don't go crazy from Cartoon Network (we are reading the Narnia series, and Zach begs me to read to him. I snuggle up with him in his bed while we read); his favorite pillow from home; little airplanes and parachuters to drop from the third floor at night when the lobby is empty (if he's feeling well enough); my thermometer so I can check his temp anytime I want to; lots of Legos®; phone numbers of friends; canned ravioli; toaster strudels; story tapes (Adventures in Odyssey®); and music CDs with earphones.

To personalize visits, some parents bring a guestbook for people to sign. Others put up a medical staff sign-in poster, which must be signed before examinations begin or vital signs are taken. Another variation of the sign-in poster is to have each staff member or visitor outline his or her hand and write her name within the handprint. If your budget allows, a digital camera can help identify the many staff members involved in your child's care and can provide a fun activity for your child.

In my position as a parent consultant, I suggest that a journal (possible titles are Book of Hope, Book of Sharing, My Cancer Experience, and Friends Indeed) be kept in the child's room for any visitor, family member, or medical caregiver to write in at any time. Leaving a message if the child is sleeping or out of the room for procedures can be a nice surprise. Later, a surviving child and her family, or the family of a child who has died, have a memory book of those who have touched their lives.

Bringing music will help block out some of the hospital noise, as well as help everyone relax. An iPod® or other portable device with headphones makes the time pass more quickly.

My daughter's preschool teacher sent a care package. She made a felt board with dozens of cutout characters and designs that provided hours of quiet entertainment. She also included games, drawings from each classmate, coloring books, markers, get well cards, and a child's tape player with earphones. Because we had run out of our house with just the clothes on our backs, all of these toys were very, very welcome.

The floor

As soon as possible after admission, ask for a "floor tour." Find out if a microwave and refrigerator are available, learn what the approved parent sleeping arrangements are, and ask about showers and bathtubs for both patients and parents. Obtain a hospital handbook if one is available. These booklets often include information about billing, parking, discounts, and other helpful items.

Either my husband or I stayed with Delaney the entire time she was in the hospital (with AML, that is not a small number of nights). To improve the comfort of the fold-out chair that the hospital provides for the sleep-in parent, we used a self-inflating camping mat. When it is rolled out, it self-inflates with a one-way valve. The straps can be used to secure it to the vinyl chair. It makes the chair much more comfortable and allows your muscles to relax. When it is not in use, it can be rolled up with straps and set in the corner.

Many children's hospitals have in-room or portable VCRs or DVD players available. Sign up for a convenient time and bring in or rent a favorite funny movie or TV show. Ask if the floor has a sign-out media library and review the list for your child's favorite movies or cartoons. Bring in age-appropriate games, puzzles, and books. Humor helps, so joke books and things that make kids laugh (such as silly string) are great items to pack.

A friend brought in a bag from the local dime store. He included a water pistol (good for unwelcome visitors or unfriendly interns), play dough, a Slinky®, checkers, dominos, bubbles, a book of corny jokes, and puzzles.

Although many hospitals provide brightly colored smocks for young patients, most children and teens prefer to wear their own clothing if at all possible. This can pose a laundry problem, so find out if the hospital has washers families can use.

Food

Buying meals day after day in the hospital cafeteria is expensive. Check with the hospital social worker to find out if the hospital has food discount cards or free meal trays for parents. Many of the food items available in the cafeteria deserve the notorious reputation of "hospital food." Check to see if the floor has a refrigerator for parents' food and stock it with your favorite items from home. Remember to put your name in a prominent place on your containers.

Our hospital provides vouchers for the cafeteria that can be used instead of ordering food for the room. For us, they have been a godsend. The food on the tray is much worse than what is in the cafeteria. Also, oncology patients have no spending cap on the vouchers, so we can get a few extras. When our son is not able to go to the cafeteria, we go down and bring the food back to his room.

Many hospitals have cooking facilities for families where they can cook or microwave favorite meals brought from home. Ask family and friends to bring food in when they visit, and consider ordering extra items to come up on your child's tray. Ordering out for dinner can also be a nice change of pace for you and your child. As long as there are no medical restrictions, there's no reason why pizza can't be delivered to the hospital. Ask the nurses if they have menus from local restaurants.

Just the smell of food nauseated my daughter. I'll never forget taking the tray out in the hall and gobbling the food down myself. I always felt so guilty, and thought that the staff viewed me as that parent who ate her kid's food. But it saved money and prevented her meals from going to waste. I also did not want to leave her side for the few minutes it took to go to the cafeteria although, in hindsight, the walk would have done me some good.

Parking

Many parents of children with cancer have unpleasant memories of driving around in endless loops looking for a parking space while their child is throwing up in a bucket in the back seat (or even worse when the bucket was left at home). Learn about both long-term and short-term parking arrangements. Ask the nurses and other parents if parking passes are available or where the cheapest parking is located. Some hospitals have valet parking, which may be as inexpensive as self-parking for an appointment of an hour or two.

I had no idea that the hospital gave out free parking passes to their frequent customers. Now I tell every new parent to check as soon as possible to see if they can get a parking pass. It will save them lots of money that they would have spent on meters and parking tickets, and time that they would have spent running out to move the car out of the emergency parking spot.

The endless waiting

Everything seems to take forever in the hospital, so parents must learn the art of waiting patiently or they will go nuts. For example, the nurse might tell you not to go to the playroom because someone will be "right up" to take your child for an echocardiogram. "Right up" can easily mean 2 hours or more. Many parents find themselves getting nervous or angry while waiting for the doctors to appear during "rounds" each morning (when the attending physicians, residents, and interns move from room to room in a large group), then feeling let down when the visit lasts only a few moments. If you have questions to ask the doctors, write them down and tell the doctors when they come in that you would like a moment to discuss concerns or ask questions.

Our emergency bag had two sides. The most important was mine, because our hospital provided nothing for parents. I would pack deodorant (plus an extra set of clothes), a book I had not read (I survived on romance novels that I bought at the used bookstore, four for a dollar), decent lighting, a soft sweatshirt top and bottom to wear at night, paper and pen for taking notes, and clean socks. You might laugh, but I can deal with a scared, irritable kid for a L-O-N-G time as long as I have clean soft socks!

On the kids' side was an art kit with play dough, crayons, pencils, markers, scissors, glue, finger paints, clay, and reams of paper. It also had plastic cutlery, and some cookie cutters for the play dough. I always brought the game Trouble®, since it's self-contained and the dice are enclosed in the little bubble. The pieces fit nicely in a plastic sandwich bag (or medication bag). The lifesaver was a Game Boy®, games, and batteries. They provided hours of enjoyment. We also brought a Lego® table with blocks. Since Matthew is usually neutropenic, or in isolation for some mysterious complication, we bring our own games. Monopoly® and Battleship® are both long games that can take an entire morning to play.

We also made it a habit to always bring Matthew's special blanket on any clinic or ER visits. We left it in the car, or I snuck it in the trunk of the car. I cannot imagine trying to have him in the hospital without it. He does not carry it around, but it is always there at bedtime.

I also kept a box of stuff for me to do in case of incarceration at Club Children's. In particular, the box had pictures and photo albums. One nurse remarked how organized I was, but I pointed out that the album I was putting together was of Matthew's first birthday. (He was almost 6 at the time.)

It helps for both caregiver and child to come prepared for long waits each time they go to the hospital. Some progressive or well-supported institutions have VCRs or DVDs, video games, toys, and games available, but usually you need to bring your own entertainment. Have your child pick out favorite card games, board games, computer games, drawing materials, and books. Remember to bring food and drinks. Some children will take comfort from having a favorite blanket or pillow along with them for a day in the clinic or during a lengthy hospitalization. If your child is scheduled for surgery, you can bring a good book, a model airplane project, a jigsaw puzzle that several people can work on together, your holiday card list, or a recipe file that needs revision.

You don't have to go too crazy. Make sure you watch the videos or eat the popcorn or flirt with the nurses or taunt the residents or leave notes for the cleaning lady or chat with the security guard or make coffee for all the parents or pretend you like puking or show the nurses how to hack into the hospital mainframe or paint your face with Butt Paste. Or, all of the above, if you like. Just do something.

Working with the staff

There are wonderful and not-so-wonderful people employed by hospitals, but it helps to remember that working in the pediatric oncology service is extremely stressful and that most of the staff are working hard on behalf of the children. Even the tiniest effort on your part to ease their burden or empathize with their circumstances will go a very long way toward establishing a cooperative and friendly relationship. For example, if a parent helps change soiled bedding, takes out food trays, and gives their child baths, it can free up overworked nurses to take care of medicines and IVs. If you are making a run to the coffee shop, ask if you can bring them something, too. Simply remembering to thank them every day will make a big difference. Chapter 6, "Forming a Partnership with the Medical Team," contains additional suggestions to enhance your relationship with the staff.

As soon as possible, learn about the shift changes on the oncology floor. If you need to leave during the day or night, don't leave a request with one nurse if another will be coming on duty soon. If you have a request or reminder, you can post it on your child's door, on the wall above the bed, or on the chart.

> I always made a point of introducing myself to my daughter's nurse and resident for each shift. I told them my child's name and which room we were in. I told them that I would be there the whole time and that I would help as much as I could. I tried to talk to them about non-hospital matters to give them a break from their routine, as well as to get to know them. I thanked them for any kindnesses and told them I appreciated how hard their jobs were. Although I wasn't angling for favors, I found that they soon came to like me and helped me out whenever any difficulty arose. Although there were a few that I didn't care for, on the whole I found the staff members to be warm, caring, dedicated people.

In addition, parents and staff can help children regain some control by encouraging choices whenever possible. Older children should be involved in discussions about their treatments, while younger children can decide when to take a bath, which arm to use for an IV, what to order for meals, what position their body will be in for procedures, what clothes to wear, and how to decorate the room. Some children request a hug or a handshake after all treatments or procedures.

Find out if there are support groups for teens. Visiting restrictions vary from institution to institution, but most are liberal regarding adolescent visitation. You might also try to bend the rules a bit to allow your teen to have friends in as much as possible.

Being an advocate for your child

Hospitals can be frightening places for children. Parents need to provide comfort, protection, and advocacy for their vulnerable child. To fulfill these needs, parents need to be present.

Most pediatric hospitals are quite aware of how much better children do if a parent is allowed to sleep in the room. Sometimes small couches convert into beds, or parents can use a cot provided by the hospital. If hospital policy requires the parent to leave, insist on staying. Geralyn Gaes tells a story in *You Don't Have to Die* about a confrontation at her local hospital.

One night a nurse came into Jason's room and curtly informed me that I would have to leave, since it was past visiting hours. With my son pale and retching from chemotherapy, I was not about to go anywhere. Looking her in the eye, I said, "You can send security after me if you like, but I'm not leaving here." No one disturbed me again.

Of course, sometimes it isn't possible to stay with your child if you are a single parent or if both parents work full time. Many families have grandparents or close friends who stay with the hospitalized child when the parents cannot be present. Older children and teenagers may not want a parent in the room at night, but they may need an advocate there during the day just as much as the preschoolers.

Whenever my husband couldn't be at the hospital at bedtime, he would bring in homemade tapes of him reading bedtime stories. Our son would drift off to sleep hearing his daddy's voice.

· · · · ·

We were always there with her in the hospital, and one of us was always with her for treatments. However, she did not want us going back with her into the examining room, so we respected those wishes. Her doctor was very kind in always coming out and talking to us. He showed her complete respect as a 15-year-old and also took time to meet our needs. She has always kept up with her own medical reports and concerns. Although her father and I have always been there with her and for her in the background, she has been much more knowledgeable about the whole cancer experience than we have in her treatments, medications, etc. She loves being in charge of her medical needs.

· · · · ·

Brian was 12 and could have stayed alone, but we never left him for more than 5 minutes to run down the hall for coffee, bathroom, etc. Someone—my husband, me, a grandparent, an aunt or uncle—was always there. If we had needed them, church members and friends had also volunteered, as Kevin (the younger brother) was only 2 at the time. With my husband rotating days at work and the hospital, and me rotating home and hospital, somehow we managed. The shift usually changed mid-day, so we each got a half day at both. A caring employer is essential.

Also, Brian became very familiar with all his drugs, allergies, reactions, and doses. Several times he corrected the staff even before I could. We also had errors and near-errors, as I'm sure everyone does, but many fewer, I'm sure, because of the constant presence and watchful eyes. Operating room doctors and nurses accessed his line without first swabbing with alcohol. Someone wanted to give ibuprofen for fever. Non-oncology nurses were working the pediatric oncology floor and knew less than we did. Our hospital is now greatly improved, but things like this happen everywhere.

Other families find staying at the hospital day and night to be too stressful. An oncologist made the following suggestion:

> *When people are subject to stress, some people cope by focusing on all the details. For these people, being there all the time reduces their stress level. In other words, they would be more stressed if they were at home or work because they would be worrying all the time. Other people cope with stress by blocking out the details and trying to make life normal. I think that you need to think about how your family can best cope with this process and make your decisions based on that. Have a family meeting to sort out these issues, and don't feel bad if you decide what is best for your family is different from what other people say you should do.*

Whenever a family member is not present, children who are old enough should be taught to use the telephone. Tape a phone number nearby where a parent can be reached and have the child call if anyone tries to do procedures that are unexpected. The hospital staff should be informed that any changes in treatment (except emergencies) need to be authorized by a parent.

Having cancer strips children of control over their bodies. To help reverse this process, parents can take over most nursing care. Children may prefer to have their parents help them to the bathroom or clean up their diarrhea or vomit. Making the bed, keeping the room tidy, changing dressings, and giving back rubs helps your child feel more comfortable and lightens the burden on the nurses. However, some children and teens may feel better if the nurses provide these services. Parents should respect the child's preferences, even if it feels like rejection.

> *I was embarrassed to have the nurse change the sheets when I had an accident in the bed. I couldn't help it when I was taking the cytoxan, but I was still embarrassed.*

Everyone makes mistakes and hospital workers are no exception. Parents can help out by checking for mistakes. It is useful to have a written copy of the protocol that should be followed; if you weren't given one, you can ask the hospital staff for a copy. If your child is enrolled in a clinical trial, you may have the short roadmap that describes dates, drugs, and tests, which you may find sufficient. However, you also have a right to get a copy of the full trial protocol if you would like one. For more information, see Chapter 4, "Choosing a Treatment." Parents can be the last line of defense against mistakes.

> *Know every drug your child takes. Write down the name of the drug and the dosage. Watch that the name on the drug matches what YOU are expecting them to get, and ask if it isn't something you recognize. Watch that the name on the blood matches up with the child's name band. Watch everything.*

If the pill or liquid looks different or you don't recognize the label on the IV, do NOT let them give it to your child without confirming that it is correct. My kid nearly died the one time I allowed myself—uncharacteristically—to be bullied by a nurse who assured me that the strange-looking pill was just a different generic version of a drug we were supposed to get. In fact, it was the same drug at 10 times the normal dose. The staff care, but they have dozens of patients to look after over long 12-hour shifts. You may be tired, too, but you have only one patient, who is dear to you, so never lose vigilance.

Playing

Children need to play, especially when hospitalized. Ask whether the hospital has a recreation therapy department. Often, a large room is devoted to toys, books, dolls, and crafts, and is staffed by specialists who really know how to play with children. These rooms provide many therapeutic activities such as medical play with dolls, which helps children express fears or concerns about what is happening to them. By encouraging contact with other children in similar circumstances, recreation therapy helps children feel less alone and less different from other children.

The fun-filled activities and smiling staff people in the recreation therapy rooms are a cheerful change from lying in a hospital bed. If the child is too ill or if her counts are too low to go to the play area, arrangements can be made for a recreational therapist to bring a bundle of toys, games, and books to the room. This can give the parent time to go out to eat or take a walk.

When I wanted to have a conference with the oncologist about Katy's protocol, I called recreation therapy and they sent two wonderful ladies to the clinic. The doctor and I were able to talk privately for an hour, and Katy had a great time making herself a gold crown and decorating her wheelchair with streamers and jewels.

Exercise is important, too. For kids strong enough to walk, exploring the hospital can be fun. Even if they can't walk, you can wheel them around or pull them in a wagon if they feel up to it. (This is also a great workout for you.) Plan a daily excursion to the gift shop or the cafeteria. Go outside and walk the entire perimeter of the hospital if weather and the neighborhood permit. Don't feel limited by an IV pole; it can be pushed or pulled and will feel normal after a while. Many children stand on the base of the IV pole with a parent pushing them down the hall at a good clip.

Check to see if the hospital has a swimming pool (for you to swim in; your child probably can't use it) or gym. Ask if there is an outdoor playground for patients and parents and make use of it whenever your child feels well enough to go outside. Your child will probably sleep much better at night in the hospital if he can get some daily fresh air and exercise. Also, the physical therapy department may have an exercise program in which you can participate.

> *In our hospital photos, I have several of a grinning 4-year-old, hooked up to an IV, in a hospital bed, with the head raised waaaaaaayyyy up, as she'd slide down to the bottom. Of course I was doing guard duty at the door, to alert the happy child when a nurse was coming and she needed to "cease this unsafe behavior immediately!" Sometimes you have to make memories while you can, wherever you are.*

· · · · ·

> *At Egleston, there was a large metal tricycle with a huge metal basket on the back. I would cap off Kenny's IV, toss him in the back, then we would pedal all over the hospital. There is one part of the hospital called "the tunnel," which connects the children's hospital with Emory Hospital. It is about a mile-long tunnel—all downhill. Man, we would fly—laughing and screaming. Of course, coming back up was pure hell.*

Many children and teens feel refreshed by going up on the roof just to feel the wind on their faces and have the sun warm their skin. Some hospitals even grant passes to young patients whose white counts are high enough so they can take trips away from the hospital. Before requesting a pass, be sure to check whether your insurance plan allows this. Over the last several years, third-party payers have begun to frown on this practice and may not pay for that day of hospitalization.

> *Preston left the hospital several times on passes. His IV was capped off and his arm was taped to a board resembling a cast. He attended a birthday party and went Christmas shopping on a pass.*

Any action that parents, family members, and friends take to support and advocate for the youngster with cancer buoys up the spirit. Courage is contagious.

> *Sometimes you can create your own fun with just a little imagination. On one particular occasion, Matthew was feeling especially bored. With a little ingenuity, we soon discovered that four unused IV poles and as many blankets as we could steal from the linen cart made for one pretty cool tent. We then used the mattress from a roll-away cot, and spent the night "camping" in his hospital room. He had a wonderful time.*

Chapter 8

Venous Catheters

Do what you can, with what you have, where you are.

— Theodore Roosevelt

MOST CHILDREN WITH LEUKEMIA require intensive treatment, including chemotherapy, intravenous (IV) fluids, IV antibiotics, blood and platelet transfusions, frequent blood sampling, and sometimes IV nutrition. Venous catheters provide a very effective method for allowing entry into the large veins for intensive therapy. Venous catheters eliminate the difficulty of finding veins for IVs and allow drugs to be put directly into the heart, where they are rapidly diluted and spread throughout the body. They also reduce stress and discomfort for the child by eliminating the need for hundreds of needle sticks.

The three types of venous catheters are: external catheters, subcutaneous ports, and peripherally inserted central catheters (PICC). Other names for a venous catheter include: venous access device, right atrial catheter, implanted catheter, indwelling catheter, central line, Hickman®, Broviac®, Port-a-cath®, Medi-port®, and PICC line.

External catheter

The external catheter is a long, flexible tube with one end in the right atrium of the heart and the other end outside the skin of the chest. The tube tunnels under the skin of the chest, enters a large vein near the collarbone, and threads inside the vein to the heart (see Figure 8-1). Because chemotherapy drugs, transfusions, and IV fluids are put in the end of the tube hanging outside the body, the child feels no pain. Blood for complete blood counts (CBC) or chemistry tests can also be drawn from the end of the catheter. With daily care, the external catheter can be left in place for years.

The tube that channels the fluid is called a lumen. Some external catheters have double lumens, in case two drugs need to be given at the same time. External catheters are usually put in under general anesthesia. Once the child is anesthetized, the surgeon makes two small incisions. One incision is near the collarbone over the spot where the catheter will enter the vein, the other is the area on the chest where the catheter exits the body.

To prevent the catheter from slipping out, it is stitched to the skin where it comes out of the chest (see Figure 8-1). There is a cuff around the catheter right above the exit site (under the skin) into which body tissue grows. This further anchors the catheter and helps prevent infection. After healing is complete, normal activities can resume.

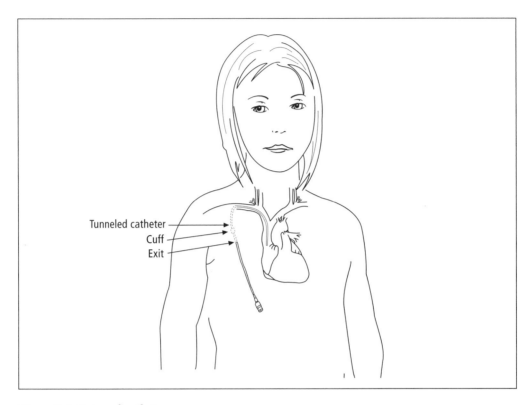

Figure 8-1: External catheter

Daily care

The external catheter requires careful maintenance to prevent infection or the formation of blood or drug clots. It is necessary to frequently clean and bandage the site where the catheter exits the body (schedules range from daily to weekly). Procedures and schedules for daily cleaning and bandaging vary from one institution to another. Some pediatric oncology centers also place a small antibiotic-impregnated disk around the catheter at the exit site. The site should be checked daily for redness, swelling, or drainage.

To prevent clots, parents or older children are taught to flush the line with a medication called heparin that prevents blood from clotting. Each institution uses its own flushing schedule. Nurses at the hospital instruct parents and children in catheter care.

Both parent and child should be given ample opportunity to practice the procedure with supervision and should not be discharged until they are comfortable with the entire procedure. At discharge, it may be desirable to arrange home nursing visits to provide further help.

> We were very grateful for Matthew's Hickman® line. Like a lot of children, he was terribly afraid of needles. The maintenance that was necessary to keep his line working properly became second nature to me. After his diagnosis, and again after his relapse, he had a Hickman® implanted. In total, he had his external catheter for more than 4 years.

Risks

The major complications of using the external catheter are infections—either in the blood or at the insertion site—and the formation of clots in the line or the blood vessel where the catheter is placed. Rare complications include kinking of the catheter, the catheter moving out of place, or breakage of the external segment of the catheter.

Infections. Even with the best care, infections are common in children with external lines. Children who have low blood counts for long periods of time are at risk for developing infections anyway, and each time the line is flushed or cleaned, there is a chance of contamination. Usually, it is a bacterium called staphylococcus epidermidis—which lives on the skin—that is the culprit, although a host of other organisms can cause infections in children receiving chemotherapy.

If your child develops a fever over 101° F (38.5° C), redness or swelling at the insertion site, or pain in the catheter area, you should suspect an infection. This is a life-threatening situation, so call the doctor immediately. To determine if bacteria are present, blood will be drawn from the catheter to culture (grow in a laboratory for 24–48 hours). Treatment will start whenever an infection is suspected and will end if the culture comes back negative. If the culture is positive, treatment usually continues for 10–14 days. Some physicians require that the child be hospitalized for antibiotic treatment, while others allow the child to receive treatment at home. Treatment with antibiotics is usually effective. However, if the infection does not respond to treatment, the catheter will need to be removed.

> When my daughter had a line infection, I wanted to use the antibiotic pump at home. It was hard, though. It took 2 hours per dose, three doses per day, for 14 days. I would get up at 5 a.m. to hook her up, so that she would sleep through the first dose. The second dose I would give while she watched a TV show in the early afternoon. Then I would hook her up at bedtime so she would sleep through it. I had to wait up to flush and disconnect, so I was very tired by the end of the 2 weeks.

. . . . .

We used the IV infusion ball when Joseph needed a 3-hour vancomycin infusion because he didn't have to sit chained to a pump. The IV infusion ball is cool because if you have a sweatshirt with front pockets, you can make a tiny hole in the back of the sweatshirt to put the tubing through and stash the ball in the pocket so you can go about your business while your IV is infusing and no one has to know a thing! It's handy for pain meds, too. He even used it at school, as long as I was there with him. An awesome invention—brilliantly simple. Here's the website that describes it: www. iflo.com/prod_homepump.php.

Clots. Even with excellent daily care, some external catheters develop blockages or clots. If the catheter becomes blocked with a blood clot, it will be flushed with a drug to dissolve the clot, such as activase, urokinase, and streptokinase. These agents are given in the clinic or hospital, and the child usually needs to remain nearby for 1–2 hours, depending on the institutional protocol. On rare occasions, the catheter becomes blocked by solidified medications, which can occur if two incompatible drugs are administered simultaneously. In this case, a diluted hydrochloric acid solution may be used to dissolve the blockage.

We had no choice of catheter in 1985, and Judd received the Hickman® line from Dr. Hickman himself. We had very little trouble with it until the last 6 months of the 3-year protocol. It was found that Judd had a very large blood clot on the end of the line in his heart, possibly due to being too slow in flushing the line. With only one treatment to go, we had the line removed.

. . . . .

Two months before the end of Kristin's treatment, her line plugged up. We tried several maneuvers at home unsuccessfully. We had to bring her in for the IV team to work on it. I think the bumpy ride to the hospital loosened it because at the hospital they were able to dislodge the clot just by flushing it with saline.

Kinks. Rarely, a kink develops in the catheter due to a sharp angle where the catheter enters the neck vein. In such cases, the fluids may go in the catheter but it is hard to get blood out. Parents and nurses are often able to work around this problem by experimenting with different positions for the child when the blood is drawn. The nurse may ask your child to bear down as if to have a bowel movement, take a deep breath, cough, stretch, or laugh.

Catheter breakage. Breaks in the line do happen, but they are extremely rare. If a break or rupture of the line inside the body occurs when the line is not in use, only heparin will leak into surrounding tissues (not a major problem). If the break occurs when corrosive chemotherapy drugs are flowing through the catheter, they may leak and cause damage to surrounding tissue. The risk of an internal line leaking is far lower than the chance of leakage from an IV in a vein of the hand or arm.

The external portion of the catheter can also break. If this occurs, clamp the line between the point of breakage and the chest wall, cover the break in the line with a sterile gauze pad, and notify the physician immediately. In most cases, the line can be repaired. Many institutions send a catheter repair kit home with parents.

> *I think it is important for parents to obtain clamps from the treating institution to carry with them. The preschool or school the child attends should also have one, in case something happens to the external line above the clamps that exist on the catheter. Younger children should wear a snug tank top that helps hold the catheter in place. Pinning it to the shirt is not the best solution for an active or younger child.*

Other factors to consider

The proper care and maintenance of an external catheter requires motivation and organization. The site needs to be cleaned and dressed frequently, and heparin must be injected using sterile techniques. The dressing must be taped to the skin. If your child's skin is quite sensitive, or if she cries when tape or Band-Aids® are removed from her skin, the external line may not be the best choice.

> *One of my most difficult times was learning to change the dressing for Ben's catheter. I am totally freaked out by syringes, and anything like that, and here we were given a 10-minute demonstration in the hospital and an instruction book and that was it. I was petrified of doing something wrong to hurt my son. My husband tried, but he does not have very good balance, and he could not get the sterile gloves on without contaminating them. I went into panic mode the first week home from the hospital. I felt like the most inadequate mother in the whole world. Since neither of us could do what had to be done, my husband called a home health agency and they sent a nurse.*

> *Kathy was the most wonderful person on earth. She told me that even though she had been a nurse for 20 years, she didn't think she could change the dressing on her own child, and she perfectly understood my fears. She had me watch her over and over again until I was comfortable enough to do it with her watching, and then finally on my own. She also talked to our insurance company numerous times to explain why she had to change the dressing instead of the family, and they ended up paying for her services! It was totally amazing. In addition, she helped my mental mood immensely, always telling me how good Ben was doing and sharing stories with me. I could tell her anything and she always understood. After I no longer needed her, she still stopped by about once a month to see how Ben was doing. She was my guardian angel.*

The external line is a constant reminder of cancer treatment and can cause changes in body image. Both parent and child need to be comfortable with the idea of seeing and handling a tube that emerges from the chest. It is noticeable under lightweight clothing and bathing suits, but not under heavier clothing like sweaters or coats. If a younger sibling might pull or yank on the catheter, the Hickman® or Broviac® might not be the appropriate choice.

On the other hand, the reason external lines are chosen so frequently is that there are no needles and no pain. This is a very important consideration for young children or for any person who is frightened of needles and/or pain. Some treatment protocols require double lumen access and the external catheter is the only option. For instance, children who need a bone marrow transplant use double-lumen external venous catheters. In most cases, however, families have a choice of which catheter to use.

> We didn't get a choice when Morgan needed a stem cell transplant. They needed to put in two Broviac® lines to accommodate all of the meds, fluids, and TPN (liquid nutrition) she needed for the procedure. I remember seeing six bags hanging up at once. I did the dressing changes, and we didn't have any trouble with the lines throughout the recuperation.

An external catheter may require restrictions regarding swimming, use of hot tubs, and sometimes bathing and showering, although care protocols vary by institution.

Subcutaneous port

Several types of subcutaneous (under the skin) ports are available. The subcutaneous port differs from the external catheter in that it is completely under the skin. A small metal chamber (1.5 inches in diameter) with a rubber top is implanted under the skin of the chest. A catheter threads from the metal chamber (portal) under the skin to a large vein near the collarbone, then inside the vein to the right atrium of the heart (see Figure 8-3). Whenever the catheter is needed for a blood draw or infusion of drugs or fluid, a needle is inserted by a nurse through the skin and into the rubber top of the portal.

How it's put in

The subcutaneous port is implanted under general anesthesia in the operating room in a procedure that generally takes less than an hour. Sometimes local anesthesia is used for older children or teens. The surgeon makes two small incisions: one in the chest where the portal will be placed, and the other near the collarbone where the catheter will enter a vein in the lower part of the neck. First, one end of the catheter is placed in the large blood vessel of the neck and threaded into the right atrium of the heart. The other end of the catheter is tunneled under the skin where it is attached to the portal. Fluid is injected into the portal to ensure that the device works properly. The portal is then placed under the skin in the right chest and stitched to the underlying muscle. Both incisions are then stitched closed. The only evidence that a catheter has been implanted are two small scars and a bump under the skin where the portal rests.

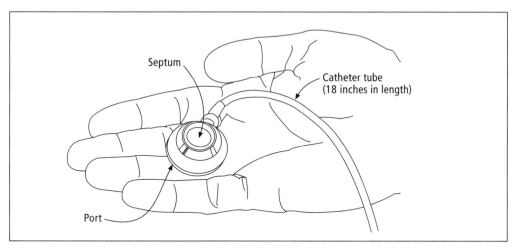

Figure 8-2: Parts of the subcutaneous port

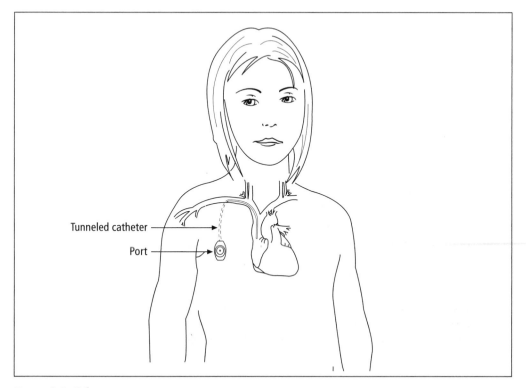

Figure 8-3: Subcutaneous port

Before my child's surgery to have a port implanted, I saw other children being wheeled into the operating room screaming and trying to climb off the gurney to return to the parents. It broke my heart. When it was Jennifer's turn, I asked them to give her enough premedication so that she was relaxed and happy to go. I also insisted that I be in the recovery room when she awoke.

• • • • •

Christine had her port surgery late at night. The resident gave her some premedication, then the chief resident ordered him to give her more. She felt so silly that she looked at me, giggled, and said "Mommy has a nose as long as an elephant's." I asked the surgeon if I could be in the recovery room before she awoke, and he said, "Sure." When I told the nurse that I had permission to go in recovery, she refused. When I persisted, she became angry. I told her that my child was expecting to wake up seeing my face, and I wanted to be there. I suggested that she go in and ask the surgeon to resolve the impasse. When she came out, she let me in the recovery room.

How it works

Because the entire subcutaneous port is under the skin, a needle is necessary to access it. The skin is thoroughly cleansed with antiseptic, then a special needle is inserted through the skin and the rubber top of the portal. The needle is attached to a short length of tubing that hangs down the front of the chest. A topical anesthetic cream (see Chapter 5, "Coping with Procedures") can be applied 1 hour before the needle poke to anesthetize the skin, or ethyl chloride ("freezy spray") can be sprayed on right before the poke. Subcutaneous ports have a rubber top (septum) that reseals after the needle is removed. It is designed to withstand years of needle insertions, as long as a special "non-coring" needle is used each time. Fluid will leak into the tissues if the wrong needle is used.

If the child is in a part of treatment that requires using the line every day, the nurse will attach the tubing to IV fluids or will close the end off with a sterile cap after flushing the line with saline solution. A transparent dressing will be put over the site where the needle enters the port. The port can remain accessed in this way for up to 7 days. After that time, to avoid the risk of infection, the needle should be removed and the port reaccessed when necessary. If the needle and tubing are to be left in place, it is important to tape them securely to the chest to avoid accidents.

At the end of delayed intensification while getting Cytoxan®, Meagan (3 years old) got a line infection. Because she hated tape removal, we did not secure the IV tubing to her stomach or chest. On one of her many trips to the potty, we accidentally tugged on the tubing and caused a very small tear in the skin around the needle. It became infected. We did home antibiotics on the pump and felt very fortunate that we were able to clear the line with antibiotics. We were glad our doctor was not too quick to remove the line, but it did require 2 weeks off chemotherapy.

If the port is only needed infrequently (e.g., during the maintenance phase), this will be the sequence of events: clean the site, put in the needle, rinse the line with saline, give the drug or draw blood, rinse the line with saline, add heparin to the line, withdraw the needle, and place an adhesive bandage over the site.

Care of the subcutaneous port

The entire port and catheter are under the skin and therefore require no daily care. The skin over the port can be washed just like the rest of the body. Frequent visual inspections are needed to check for swelling, redness, or drainage. Signs of infection include redness, swelling, pain, drainage, or warmth around the exit site. Fever, chills, tiredness, and dizziness may also indicate that the line has become infected. You should notify the doctor if any of these signs are present or if your child has a fever above 101° F (38.5° C).

The subcutaneous port must be accessed and flushed with saline and heparin at least once every 30 days, which usually coincides with the monthly clinic visit and blood checks. This procedure is done by a nurse or technician. The port system requires no maintenance by the parent or patient.

My son had a Port-a-cath® for 3 years, from ages 14 to 17. During that time, he played basketball, football, softball, and threw the shot in track. His port was placed on his left side just below his armpit. For football, I worked with the trainer, and we developed a special pad that went into a "custom" pocket I sewed into some T-shirts. That way the port had a little extra padding. We also found shoulder pads that had a side piece that covered the area. He never had any problems or soreness from the port.

Risks

The risks for a subcutaneous port are similar to those for the external catheter: infection, clots, and, rarely, kinks or rupture. If the needle is not properly inserted through the rubber septum, or if the wrong kind of needle is used, fluids can leak into the tissue around the portal.

Brent (8 years old) has had a Port-a-cath® for 33 months with absolutely no problems. He uses EMLA® to anesthetize it prior to accessing. He hates finger pokes so much that he has his port accessed every time he needs blood drawn.

We had a few unusual problems in the beginning with the catheter. It was a bit kinked where the catheter went under the clavicle (collarbone) and would not easily draw. This caused more stress than anything in the hospital, because their middle-of-the-night blood draws were always an ordeal for our daughter. They needed to wake her up and try multiple manipulations. Once we were familiar with its idiosyncrasies and were outpatient, we worked it out much better. Then about halfway through maintenance, her catheter broke at the kink and travelled into her heart. To make a long story short, it was retrieved by a cardiologist without major surgery, and she got a new one placed, this time with the catheter going down from her neck. It works like a dream.

Infection. Most studies show that the infection rate of subcutaneous ports is lower than that of external catheters. If the subcutaneous port does become infected, it is treated the same as an infected external catheter is treated.

Katy had two infections in her Port-a-cath® during the 27 months of her leukemia treatment. One occurred during reinduction when the tape loosened during a blood transfusion. She developed a fever the next day and required 14 days of vancomycin. Eighteen months later, we went in for her monthly vincristine, and she became ill in the car on the way home. Her skin became white and clammy, and she felt faint and nauseated. She spiked a 102° temperature which only lasted for 2 hours. The blood culture both times grew staphylococcus epi.

Kinks, clots, ruptures. These events rarely occur with the subcutaneous port. If they do occur, they are treated as described in the external catheter section.

My son had a very bad blood clot in his Port-a-cath®. In fact, he had two. He was put on Lovenox® (low molecular weight heparin for 3 months twice a day). We went for an ultrasound last week and it showed that the clots are mostly gone now.

Peripherally inserted central catheters

A peripherally inserted central catheter is also referred to as a PICC line. This type of catheter is placed in the antecubital vein (a large vein in the inner elbow area) and is threaded into a large vein above the right atrium of the heart (see Figure 8-4). Unlike other catheters, a PICC line can be inserted by an IV nurse, rather than by a surgeon.

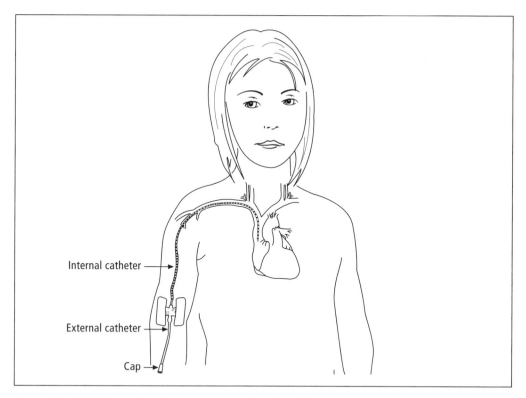

Internal catheter

External catheter

Cap

Figure 8-4: PICC (peripherally inserted central catheter) line

The PICC line can remain in place for many weeks or months, avoiding the need for a new IV every few days. PICC lines can be used to deliver chemotherapy, antibiotics, blood products, other medications, and IV nutrition. When the PICC line needs to be accessed, an IV line is connected to the end of the catheter. When it is not in use, the IV is disconnected and the catheter is flushed and capped.

How it's put in

The PICC line can be inserted in your child's hospital room by a nurse or physician. Your child will be positioned on a flat surface, and she will need to keep her arm straight and motionless during the procedure. An injection to numb the area is given to decrease discomfort during insertion. A special needle is used to place the PICC line into the arm vein. The catheter is then threaded through the needle. Once the line is in place, a chest x-ray is taken to ensure that it is positioned properly.

Brian had his Hickman® pulled when he started maintenance in February 1997, but 2 weeks later he developed pancreatitis and needed total parenteral nutrition. Since he was still on active treatment, he was given the choice of another Hickman® or a PICC, which he decided to try. It was inserted right in our room with no anesthetic other than the morphine pump he was already on for the pancreatitis pain. He pushed his PCA button (the control that allows patients to administer their own doses of pain medication) moments before it was inserted, because he was not sure what to expect. The procedure was uncomfortable, but not terribly painful. They did an x-ray to make sure that it was in the right place. It wasn't, but after some aerobics (moving him into different positions) and lots of flushing, they checked again, and it was.

Care of the peripherally inserted central catheter

The PICC line, like the external catheter, requires care to prevent problems. The nurses will teach you how to change the dressing, flush the line, change the injection cap, and inspect the site for possible signs of infection. The dressing covering the exit site is changed on a weekly basis, and is changed if it becomes wet or is exposed to the air. The line must be flushed after every use, or every day. You should get plenty of practice under the supervision of a nurse until both you and your child are comfortable with caring for the line. The care required for your child's PICC line may be slightly different from what has been described in this section because institutional preferences vary.

Kelsey had a PICC line in her right arm, and she would not straighten it out, but kept it a little bent. I definitely think she was protecting it, and also I think when she tried to straighten it, it pulled on the suture and on the dressing in an uncomfortable way that could have been painful, so she just wouldn't try. I had to do a heparin flush every day and change the dressing twice a week. She could not tolerate Tegaderm®, so we used another kind of porous adhesive bandage, and doused it with Detachol®, which dissolved the adhesive within a few minutes, allowing us to get the bandage off quite easily. The Detachol® was a godsend for her, as removing the adhesive was like pulling teeth and a source of unnecessary pain. [For more information on Detachol®, see the section "Adhesives" later in the chapter.]

Risks

The problems associated with a PICC line are similar to those with any external catheter. Veins may become irritated, infection can occur, or the line can be accidentally torn or moved.

Irritated veins. Within the first few days of insertion, the vein where the catheter is located may become irritated. Signs of irritation include swelling or pain in the area. Often, the discomfort can be alleviated by placing a warm, moist cloth or a carefully monitored heating pad on the vein. Elevating the arm on a pillow is also sometimes helpful.

Infection. Meticulous care using sterile techniques is extremely important to reduce the risk of infection. The dressing over the exit site should be changed every week, or if it becomes wet or exposed to the air. Injection caps must also be regularly changed using sterile techniques when the line is not in use, and the line must be flushed on a regular basis. Signs of infection include redness, swelling, pain, drainage, or warmth around the exit site. Fever, chills, tiredness, and dizziness may also indicate that the line has become infected. You should notify the doctor if any of these signs are present or if your child has a fever above 101° F (38.5° C).

Torn catheter. Accidents sometimes happen, and a hole or tear in the line can occur. Careful handling of the catheter can help prevent these accidents. You should suspect a torn catheter if fluid leaks out of the line, especially during an injection. If a tear is found, you should find the hole, fold the line above the tear, tape it together, and cover it with sterile gauze. You should immediately notify your child's doctor of the problem.

Displacement of the catheter. As with the external catheters discussed earlier in this chapter, it is important that the PICC line be securely taped to the exit site to prevent movement. Signs of a displaced catheter include chest pain, burning or swelling in the arm above the exit site or in the chest, fluid leaking around the catheter, or pain when fluid is injected into the line. If you suspect that the line has moved, you should tape the catheter in place and immediately notify your child's doctor.

Cost

The external catheter and the PICC line require supplies for cleaning, dressing, and irrigating the line, but the subcutaneous port does not. The port itself, however, is usually more costly than the external catheter. The external catheter and the subcutaneous port require operating room time and the services of a surgeon and an anesthesiologist to insert. PICC lines are usually inserted in the hospital room by a doctor or nurse. External catheters can be removed in the clinic with only IV sedation, but subcutaneous ports can only be removed in the operating room. A good rule of thumb to consider is that, if the lines stay in place at least 6 months, the overall costs are almost equal.

Most insurance plans will cover the placement of any central venous catheter and the services of the surgeon, anesthesiologist, and operating room facility. Many plans, however, will not cover the cost of the supplies to maintain the line, and this can be an additional financial hardship for families. You may want to consider this when making the final decision about the type of catheter that is best for your child.

Choosing not to use a catheter

Many physicians automatically schedule surgery for catheter implantation as soon as a child is diagnosed with leukemia. Others do not recommend using implanted catheters in their pediatric patients with leukemia, while some physicians only use catheters in high-risk patients. Ask the physician the reason for his recommendation, and discuss it thoroughly if you are uncomfortable with the options presented.

> *Stephan (6 years old) has no catheter. Sometimes I wish he had one. It seems like it would be easier. We were told he didn't need it. He is running out of usable veins and it is getting harder and harder.*

Some children and teens prefer IVs to an implanted catheter.

> *My son had a port for a very short time, and due to frequent fevers (with no evidence of infection) and because he had a blood clot form in his heart, they pulled the port. He had IVs for the remainder of treatment and was much happier with the IVs than with what he called "that foreign object in my chest."*

Some physicians recommend trying treatment without a catheter before making a decision.

> *Our physician gave us the option of using a catheter for our 6-year-old daughter with low-risk ALL, but he recommended against it. He said if she could stand the pokes it was better not to use it due to the chance of infection. She had several sessions with the staff psychologist to teach her visualization and imagery, which she used successfully to deal with the 2 years of IVs.*

To help you make the best decision for your particular situation, Table 8-1 outlines the pros and cons for each type of catheter. There is no right or wrong choice; different options are available because each child, each parent, and each family is unique.

Table 8-1: Comparison of Catheters

Things to Consider	External Catheter	Subcutaneous Port	Peripherally Inserted Central Catheter
Infection rate	Higher	Lower	Higher
Maintenance	Daily	Monthly	Daily
Body image	Changes: tube outside body	Minor: lump under skin	Changes: tube outside body
Pain	Dressing changes	Needle poke to access (use EMLA®)	Needle poke to insert the line; dressing changes
Anxiety	Low to high	Low to high	Low to high
Cost	Insertion cost moderate. Maintenance cost high.	Insertion cost highest. Maintenance cost low.	Insertion cost lowest. Maintenance cost high.
Risk of drugs leaking into tissues	Lowest	Low	Low

Making a decision

After reviewing the information, discuss with the doctor her opinion about the merits of each type of catheter. Talk about the pros and cons with your child if she is old enough. Then make the rounds of the cancer ward, asking both parents and children which type of catheter they chose and why. You will probably hear many opinions on the benefits and drawbacks for each catheter.

The nurses in the clinic and on the ward are another source of valuable information. They will have seen dozens (or hundreds) of children with catheters, and they will be able to give excellent advice, given your family situation. There is no right or wrong choice, just different options for each unique child.

> When we asked one of the young children on the ward which catheter she had, she pulled up her shirt with a big grin to show us her Hickman®. She had a coil of white tubing neatly taped to her chest. My husband's face turned as white as her tubing.

• • • • •

> My 4-year-old daughter loved ballet and was extremely interested in her appearance. Her younger sister was very physical, and we were worried that if we chose the Hickman® she would grab and pull on the tubing. We chose the Port-a-cath® so that she could wear her tutus without reminders of cancer, and so the children could play together without mishap.

· · · · ·

We chose the Hickman® for Shawn because we didn't want any needles coming at him. He spent almost the whole first year in the hospital, so it saved him from so many pokes. The line was a blessing. He went 3 years and 3 months with no infections. We thought it was just a beautiful thing.

Adhesives

Whether your child has a subcutaneous port, external catheter, or PICC line, dressing changes will be necessary. Some children don't mind having the Tegaderm® or tape pulled off. For others, it is traumatic every time. Parents have many suggestions for ways to make it easier for kids. These suggestions also work for removing tape used to hold plastic wrap over EMLA®:

- Don't use Tegaderm® if it bothers your child or reddens the skin. Try plastic wrap cut into a square and use paper tape or tape with perforations.

- Try Hypafix®. It's a dressing retention material that looks like gauze with a sticky side. Usually, several sterile 2x2 gauze pads are put over the needle entry site, then Hypafix® is applied to hold them in place.

  I like Hypafix® because when it's time to take it off, you can use the adhesive dissolver where it's stuck to the skin, and even without the dissolver, it comes off more easily and gently than the Tegaderm®. The nurses at our oncology clinic use this all the time. Our local clinic and hospital do not use Hypafix®, so I bought a roll and take it with me whenever we have to go locally for a port access so we don't have to use the Tegaderm®.

- When it's tape removal time, use an effective adhesive remover such as Detachol® (an orange-colored product made by Ferndale Laboratories, Ferndale, MI, *www. eloquesthealthcare.com/products/detachol.aspx*). If you douse the paper tape with adhesive dissolver and wait a couple of minutes, it will usually pull right off with no pain.

- Ask for expert advice.

  Apryl has had skin tears and reactions from the adhesives as a result of using Tegaderm®. We were using Primapore® dressings for a while, but after a year she started having the same reaction. When she had her line replaced, I asked for a consultation with the skincare nurse. She recommended All-Dress®. It is a waterproof dressing with non-stick gauze in the center surrounded by Hypafix® tape. Apryl changes hers once every 3 days, whether it gets wet or not. She also has this pink tape that has zinc oxide in the adhesive to protect the skin. These two have worked out great.

- Once you have found a routine that works well, negotiate with nursing staff to remove the tape yourself or to have them follow your system.

> *Using adhesive dissolver (or peeling off tape or Tegaderm® millimeter by millimeter) takes a bit of time—it's not just a swipe—and it works. It has to sort of soak in and takes some time to dissolve the sticky stuff. I know the nurses are really busy and under pressure to keep on time schedules, so it's probably a conflict for them. I deal with this by always being the one to get the Tegaderm® off. This took some "muscling in" with nurses who were used to doing it, but it works much, much better. I try to make a joke of it: "I have a deal with my kid that I'm taking off the Tegaderm®. It might take a while and I wouldn't want you to fall asleep waiting on us—how about if I holler out the door when it's off and we're ready?" That way they don't have to stand around and wait, and you don't feel like you need to hurry your child.*

Removal of catheters is explained in Chapter 19, "End of Treatment and Beyond."

> *When Scott (age 3) was diagnosed, his doctor gave us a choice of which central line we could use. He showed us a mannequin with a Broviac® and a Port-a-cath®. He also told us the pros and cons of each type, then asked us to decide. We chose the Broviac®, and feel it was the best decision for Scott. The day it was installed was the end of a lot of unnecessary pain (from needle sticks) for Scott.*

> *Scott finished all his treatments 3 months ago, and yesterday he had his Broviac® removed. It went extremely smoothly. He had only one cuff and it was halfway out already. And to think I fretted and worried about the removal all week!*

> *He has lots and lots of energy. His hair is coming back in and he actually has color in his face. He looks so healthy! I love it!*

Chapter 9

Chemotherapy

The first wealth is health.

— Ralph Waldo Emerson

THE WORD CHEMOTHERAPY IS DERIVED from a combination of the words "chemical" and "therapy" (meaning treatment). During chemotherapy, drugs are used individually or in combination to destroy or disrupt the growth of cancer cells without permanently damaging normal cells.

This chapter explains how chemotherapy drugs work, how they are given, and how dosages for children and teens are determined. It then describes the most common drugs used to destroy leukemia cells, as well as medications used to prevent nausea and treat pain. Numerous stories are included that show the range of responses to different chemotherapy drugs. A brief discussion of adjunctive and alternative treatments is also included.

Reading about chemotherapy's potential side effects can be disturbing. However, by learning what to expect from the various drugs, you may be able to recognize symptoms early and report them to the doctor so swift action can be taken to make your child more comfortable. On rare occasions, side effects may be life-threatening and some can persist throughout life. However, most are merely unpleasant and subside soon after treatment ends. Not all children respond to these drugs in the same way. Some may experience serious side effects from certain drugs while others appear to be completely unaffected. In most cases, it is impossible to predict how an individual child will tolerate chemotherapy.

How chemotherapy drugs work

Normal, healthy cells divide and grow in a well-established pattern. When these cells divide, an identical copy is produced. The body only makes the number of normal cells it needs at any given time. As each normal cell matures, it loses its ability to reproduce. Normal cells are also preprogrammed to die at a specific time.

In contrast, cancer cells reproduce uncontrollably and grow in unpredictable ways. They invade surrounding tissue and can travel in blood or lymph to lodge in other parts of the body.

All chemotherapy drugs work in some way to interfere with the cancer cells' ability to live, divide, and multiply. Some of the types of drugs used to treat leukemia are:

- **Alkaloids.** These drugs, derived from plants, interrupt cell division through a variety of mechanisms, including interfering with DNA and specific enzyme activities. They also disrupt the membrane (outer wall) of the cancer cell, causing cell damage or cell death.

- **Alkylating agents.** All cells contain DNA and RNA, which provide the instructions needed by the cells to make exact copies of themselves. Alkylating agents poison cancer cells by interacting with DNA or RNA to prevent cell reproduction.

- **Antibiotics.** This type of drug prevents cell growth by blocking reproduction, weakening the outer wall of the cell, or interfering with certain cell enzymes.

- **Antimetabolites.** These drugs starve cancer cells by replacing essential cell nutrients that are necessary during the synthesis (growth in preparation for cell division) phase of the cell cycle.

- **Hormones.** These drugs create a hostile environment that slows cell growth. They can also signal cancer cells that it is time to die.

- **Immunotherapeutic agents.** These substances, usually used in targeted therapies, either encourage the cancerous cells to die or help the body destroy them.

- **Protein inhibitors.** These drugs interfere with tumor cells' ability to reproduce by depriving the cells of specific proteins necessary for cell growth and division.

How chemotherapy drugs are given

The five most common methods for giving drugs during treatment for childhood leukemia are:

- **Intravenous (IV).** Medicine is delivered directly into the bloodstream through a venous catheter or IV in the arm or hand. IV medicines can be administered in a few minutes (IV injection or push) or as an infusion over a number of hours.

- **Oral (PO).** Drugs, taken by mouth in liquid, capsule, or tablet form, are absorbed into the blood through the lining of the stomach and intestines.

- **Intramuscular (IM).** Drugs that need to seep slowly into the bloodstream are injected into a large muscle such as the thigh or buttocks.

- **Intrathecal (IT).** Doctors perform a spinal tap and inject the drug directly into the cerebrospinal fluid (the fluid surrounding the brain and spinal cord), circumventing the barrier between the blood and brain.

- **Subcutaneous (Sub-Q).** Drugs that need to enter the bloodstream at a moderately rapid rate are injected into the soft tissues under the skin of the upper arm, thigh, or abdomen.

- **Sublingual (SL).** Several drugs are now available as lozenges that dissolve quickly when placed under the tongue.

Dosages

Dosages vary among protocols, but most are based on your child's weight or body surface area (BSA). BSA is calculated from your child's weight and height and is measured in meters squared (m^2). Doses of medications your child is scheduled to receive should be recalculated at the beginning of each new phase of treatment. Recalculating doses more frequently is necessary if your child has experienced significant weight gain or loss (more than 10 percent of his initial weight).

> My daughter's BSA ranged from .55 to .70 over the course of her treatment. During induction, the protocol required 60 mg/m² of prednisone on Days 0 to 27. To determine her dose, the doctor calculated .55 x 60 = 33. He then wrote a prescription that she take 33 mg of prednisone a day in three doses of 11 mg each. So I gave her one 10 mg tablet and one 1 mg tablet three times a day.

You do not need to do the calculations, but it is important to understand the dosage for each drug and how you should give it to your child. Most families write the dosages on a calendar and cross them out after each dose has been given to make sure they don't forget a drug or accidentally repeat a dose.

Variability in response to medications

Children's bodies have a wide range of responses to medications, some of which are due to their genes. Some children inherit genes that do not allow them to break down (metabolize) certain drugs, or that allow them to break the drugs down very slowly. If a child cannot metabolize a drug, it can build up in the blood stream and cause excessive toxicity.

Cancer cells also show dramatic variability in how they respond to different chemotherapy drugs. The leukemia cells in one child's body might be extraordinarily sensitive to a specific chemotherapy drug, while the cancer cells in another child's body might be very resistant to that same drug.

Therefore, the combination of variability in children's ability to metabolize drugs and variability in how sensitive cancer cells are to certain drugs causes a big range in effectiveness of standard doses of medications. How much of this variability is due to genetics is not well understood. However, researchers are identifying ways to test children's ability to metabolize certain drugs and are tailoring treatment based on that genetic information; this area of science is called pharmacogenetics. The following sections describe a few of the better-known genetic characteristics that help doctors tailor treatments to a child's unique genetic makeup.

Thiopurine methyltransferase (TPMT). Pharmacogenetics explores whether your genes allow your body to metabolize certain drugs, and if it can, how fast your body is able to do it. For instance, some children are not genetically coded to make a protein called thiopurine methyltransferase (TPMT), which metabolizes two common chemotherapy drugs used to treat leukemia—thioguanine (6-TG) and mercaptopurine (6-MP). Approximately 1 in 300 people cannot metabolize these drugs at all; when a child with this genetic makeup is given standard doses of these drugs, they quickly build up to toxic levels in the child's body. In these children, dramatic drops in the numbers of red cells, white cells, and platelets occur and the child is at risk for life-threatening infections.

Ten out of every 100 people are able to metabolize 6-TG and 6-MP, but very slowly; children with this genetic makeup need lower doses of 6-TG and 6-MP to prevent big drops in blood counts. The remainder of the population (approximately 90 percent) can break down these medications at the normal rate. Some treatment centers test all children with leukemia for their genetic ability to metabolize 6-TG and 6-MP before they give them either drug; other institutions test children if their blood counts drop dramatically after getting the first doses of these drugs. More information about this topic can be found at *www.candlelighters.org/Information/tpmt/tabid/331/Default.aspx*.

> *Josh has not been on full doses of 6-MP for over a year now. It did take the doctors a long time to realize that they needed to increase Josh's 6-MP slowly. For months they would drop the dose to 50%, and in 2 weeks his counts were okay. Not great, but high enough to increase the dose, so they would. Another 2 weeks at 75% and he would crash. Finally, they did the TPMT test and sure enough he does not metabolize the 6-MP. I remember them telling me that 0.03% of the population has this enzyme deficiency and you would never know unless you had to take 6-MP.*

CYP2D6. Another genetic variation currently being investigated concerns CYP2D6, which affects the metabolism of codeine. Approximately 10 percent of people do not get pain relief from codeine, because they are genetically not able to metabolize codeine into morphine. Because codeine products are often used for painful side effects of leukemia treatment (e.g., vincristine neuropathy), some institutions test all children with leukemia so appropriate pain medications can be prescribed.

Glucose 6 phosphate deficiency (G6PD). The drug rasburicase is increasingly used in the United States (it has been used in Europe for many years) to prevent tumor lysis syndrome in children with high white blood cell counts at diagnosis. When these children are first given chemotherapy, the destruction of the large number of cancer cells can cause tumor lysis syndrome. However, children with G6PD deficiency should not be given rasburicase because it increases the risk of destruction of red blood cells in such patients.

Methlyenetetrahydrofolate reductase (MTHFR). The chemotherapy drug methotrexate decreases the amount of folate in cells. Two common genetic variation—MTHFR C677T and A1298C—may increase some people's sensitivity to methotrexate. Children who cannot tolerate methotrexate are sometimes tested for these genetic variations, but how to tailor their treatment based on the results is not clear.

> *Our facility did not test for MTHFR or TPMT until after my daughter was in her second year of long-term maintenance. Her blood counts were continually bottoming out and she had elevated bilirubin. Her bilirubin has been as high as 6.5 and as low as 0.8 when she is not receiving her chemotherapy (at times up to 15 weeks). It was at my request that the tests were administered. The tests showed that she is homozygous (has two copies) of MTHFR C677T; however the tests show normal ability to process 6-MP and thioguanine. With that said, she has spent an enormous amount of time off chemo with elevated liver enzymes and/or counts that have bottomed out. She currently is off chemo again. This will be her fourth week with no 6-MP or methotrexate. As her doctor has said, "Her body really just doesn't like the stuff very well." When she is on chemo, she takes 25% of the standard amount of methotrexate and 50% of 6-MP dosing per protocol ALL0331.*
>
> *After MTHFR was confirmed (as it can be a positive indicator of clotting disorders), I conferred with her team and we agreed that because there is a history of clotting disorders in my family we would do further testing. Her doctor ordered a standard clotting panel and checked her homocysteine levels. We love and trust her team completely. This just goes to show how very different each child is, and why we must continue working toward protocols which are tailored to individuals and standardizing testing which helps to identify these types of anomalies at the beginning of treatment.*

Chemotherapy drugs and their possible side effects

The following section contains not only common and infrequent side effects of anticancer drugs, but also parent and survivor experiences and suggestions. You may be overwhelmed by reading about all the potential side effects of each drug. Please remember, each child is unique and will handle most drugs without major problems. Most side effects are unpleasant, not serious, and subside when the medication stops. The parent experiences included here may provide insight, comfort, and suggestions should your child have an unusual side effect. If you have any concerns after reading these descriptions, consult your child's oncologist. (Appendix C, "Books, Websites, and Videotapes" contains resources for obtaining information about drugs not covered here.)

Remember to keep all chemotherapy drugs in a locked cabinet away from children and pets.

If your child likes computer games, you might look at Captain Chemo, a free interactive online game designed by a teenaged cancer patient at the Royal Marsden Hospital in the United Kingdom. Captain Chemo, at *www.royalmarsden.org.uk/captchemo,* has several adventures that young cancer patients often enjoy.

Questions to ask the doctor

Before giving your child any drug, you should be given basic information, including answers to the following questions:

- What is the dosage? How many times a day should it be given?

- Should the drug be given at a particular time of day or under specific conditions (e.g., on an empty stomach or before bed)?

- What are the common and rare side effects?

- What should I do if my child experiences any of the side effects?

- Will the drug interact with any over-the-counter drugs (e.g., Tylenol®), foods, or vitamins?

- Will you give my teen detailed counseling about the risks associated with drinking alcohol, smoking cigarettes or marijuana, or getting pregnant while using this drug?

- What should I do if I forget to give my child a dose?

- What are both the trade and generic names of the drug?

- Should I buy the generic version?

Guidelines for calling the doctor

Sometimes parents are reluctant to call their child's physician with questions or concerns, so here are some general guidelines. Call the doctor when your child has:

- A temperature above 101° F (38.5° C)

- Shaking or chills

- Shortness of breath

- Severe nausea or vomiting

- Unusual bleeding, bruising, or cuts that won't heal

- Pain or swelling at a chemotherapy injection site

- Any severe pain that cannot be explained

- Exposure to chicken pox or measles

- Severe headache or blurred vision

- Constipation lasting more than 2 days

- Severe diarrhea

- Severe headaches

- Painful urination or bowel movements

- Blood in urine.

You can also call the doctor whenever your child appears sick and you are concerned.

Chemotherapy drug names

Drugs used to treat children with cancer are known by various names, which can get very confusing. You may hear the same drug referred to by its generic name, an abbreviation, or one of several brand names, depending on which doctor, nurse, or pharmacist you talk to. The list below provides the generic name of the most commonly used chemotherapy drugs and some of the most common brand names.

Drug name	Brand name(s)
Amsacrine	(No brand names)
Arsenic trioxide	Trisenox®
Asparaginase L-Asparaginase ASP PEG-asparaginase	Elspar® Oncaspar®
Azacytidine	Vidaza®
Cyclophosphamide	Cytoxan®, Cytoxan Lyophilized®, Neosar®
Cytarabine Cytosine arabinoside ARA-C	Cytosar-U®, Tarabine PFS®, Cytosar®
Daunorubicin Daunomycin	Cerubidine®
Dexamethasone DEX	Decadron®, Hexadrol®, and multiple other brand names
Doxorubicin	Adriamycin®

Drug name	Brand name(s)
Epirubicin	Ellence®, Pharmorubicin PFS®, Pharmorubicin RDF®
Etoposide VP-16	VePesid®, Toposar®
Fludarabine	Fludara®
Gemtuzumab	Mylotarg®
Hydrocortisone	Cortef®, Hydrocortone®, Hydrocortone Phosphate®, Solu-Cortef®, and multiple other brand names
Hydroxyurea	Droxia®, Hydrea®, Mylocel®
Idarubicin	Idamycin PFS®
Imatinib	Gleevec®
Interferon-alpha	Intron®
Isotretinoin 13-cis-retinoic acid	Accutane®, Amnesteem®, Claravis®, Sotret®
Mercaptopurine 6-MP	Purinethol®
Methotrexate MTX	Trexall®
Prednisone	Sterapred®
Thioguanine 6-TG	Tabloid®
Tretinoin Cis-retinoic acid All-trans retinoic acid ATRA	Vesanoid®
Vincristine	Oncovin®, Vincasar PFS®

Side effects terminology

Many of the side effects caused by the drugs described below have medical names that may be unfamiliar to you. This table defines those terms so you can understand what the members of your child's treatment team mean when they discuss side effects.

Medical Name	Description (most of these conditions are temporary)
Alopecia	Hair loss.
Amenorrhea	Absence of a menstrual period.
Anemia	Low red blood cell count, which causes weakness, fatigue, and paleness.
APL differentiation syndrome	Occasionally seen in children with acute promyelocytic leukemia (APL) who are treated with tretinoin or arsenic trioxide. This is a serious complication, characterized by breathing difficulties, lung and heart problems, fluid retention, and weight gain.

Medical Name	Description (most of these conditions are temporary)
Arrhythmia	Abnormal electrical rhythm in the heart; the term is usually used to describe an abnormal heartbeat.
Avascular necrosis	Death of bone tissue, caused by reduced blood supply.
Conjunctivitis	Inflammation or infection of the membrane that lines the eyelid (eyes can be red, irritated, crusty, and watery); vision may be blurry.
Dyspnea	Shortness of breath; breathing difficulties.
Dystonia	Muscle contractions that result in repetitive twisting or movement of a limb or other body part, which may be painful.
Dysuria	Painful urination.
Hematuria	Blood in the urine.
Hemorrhagic cystitis	Inflammation of the bladder; characterized by pus or blood in urine, pain with urination, and decreased urine flow.
Hyperglycemia	Increased blood sugar.
Hypoglycemia	Decreased blood sugar.
Hyperpigmentation	Darkening of the skin.
Hypertension	High blood pressure.
Hypotension	Low blood pressure.
Jaundice	Yellowish discoloration of the skin or eyes, caused by too much bilirubin in the blood. Jaundice may indicate liver toxicity.
Myelosuppression	Decreased bone marrow activity, resulting in lowered counts of all blood components (red blood cells, white blood cells, and platelets). Severe myelosuppression is called myeloablation.
Neutropenia	Not enough neutrophils (white blood cells that fight infection); this condition increases the risk of infection.
Pancreatitis	Inflammation of the pancreas, normally associated with abdominal pain, nausea, or vomiting.
Pancytopenia	Reduction in the number of all kinds of bloods cells: red blood cells, white blood cells, and platelets.
Peripheral neuropathy	Pain, numbness, tingling, swelling, or weakness, usually in the hands, feet, or lower legs. It is caused by damage to the nerves that transmit to the extremities; usually temporary, but occasionally permanent.
Petechiae	Small red spots under the skin caused by bleeding in tiny blood vessels.
Photosensitivity	Sensitivity to the sun; can cause sunburn, rash, skin discoloration, hives, and itching.
Somnolence	Sleepiness, drowsiness, and lethargy.
Stomatitis	Inflammation or irritation of the membranes of the mouth; mouth sores.
Thrombocytopenia	Not enough platelets, resulting in poor blood clotting, bleeding, bruising, and petechiae.
Veno-occlusive disease (VOD)	A blockage in the veins of the liver. Symptoms include weight gain, liver pain or swelling, and increased bilirubin levels in the blood.

Chemotherapy drug list

This section lists drugs commonly used to treat leukemia.

Amsacrine (AM-sah-creen)

How given: IV infusion over several hours.

How it works: Amsacrine interferes with the action of the enzyme topoisomerase II, breaking the strands of DNA in the cancerous cells and causing them to die.

Precaution: Amsacrine is a red-orange fluid. It may turn the urine orange, but this is normal and no reason for concern.

Common side effects:

- Nausea, vomiting, or diarrhea
- Low blood counts, which may increase risk of infection or bleeding and cause weakness, fatigue, and paleness.

Infrequent side effects:

- Hair loss
- Abdominal pain
- Mouth sores or ulcers
- Pain or swelling at the injection site
- Changes in heart rhythm.

Arsenic trioxide (AR-sen-ick try-OX-ide)

How given: IV injection or infusion over several hours.

How it works: Arsenic trioxide appears to work in several ways. It causes enzymes in a cell to signal that it is time to die. It also interferes with creation of DNA and other cellular processes.

Precaution: Arsenic trioxide is associated with a serious condition known as APL differentiation syndrome. This complication is characterized by breathing difficulties, lung and heart problems, fluid retention, and weight gain.

Common side effects:

- Fatigue
- Dizziness
- Headaches
- Swelling of arms, hands, feet, and lower legs
- Rash or itching
- Fever
- Swelling at the injection site
- Fluid retention
- Insomnia
- Numbness or tingling
- Constipation.

Infrequent side effects:

- Allergic reactions, including hives; swelling of the lips, tongue, and throat; and difficulty breathing
- Seizures
- Black, tarry stool
- Bloody vomit
- Bleeding or bruising
- Heart irregularities
- Decreased urination.

L-Asparaginase (L-a-SPARE-a-jin-ase)

How given: IM injection.

Types: The three types of L-asparaginase are E. coli asparaginase, Erwinia asparaginase, and pegylated asparaginase (also called PEG- or PEG-L-asparaginase).

How they work: These drugs are enzymes that block protein production in cancer cells to prevent them from reproducing.

Precaution: Occasionally a child will have a severe allergic reaction to L-asparaginase. It is important that the drug be given by trained medical personnel who have emergency equipment available. The child should be monitored at the clinic for 20 to 30 minutes after receiving the drug in case a reaction occurs. If a child has a reaction to E. coli asparaginase, Erwinia asparaginase or PEG-asparaginase may be tried. If the child reacts to all three drugs, L-asparaginase therapy is usually discontinued.

Common side effects:

- Loss of appetite and weight

- Fatigue

- Headaches

- Abdominal cramps

- Nausea and vomiting.

Infrequent side effects:

- Allergic reaction, including swelling, difficulty breathing, and rash

- Yellowish tint to skin or eyes (jaundice)

- Confusion or hallucinations

- Convulsions

- Swelling of feet or legs

- Unusually frequent urination

- High blood pressure

- Kidney or liver damage

- Stroke

- Inflammation of the pancreas

- Excessive bleeding

- Blood clots.

> *Meagan had no problem with the L-asparaginase other than that the shots in her thigh were painful. This was before EMLA® was available. I'd recommend that parents put EMLA® on 2 hours before the shot to reduce the pain.*

> • • • • •

> *A couple of hours after Preston's third dose of L-asparaginase his leg began to swell up around the injection site. His leg grew to three times its normal size. The doctors switched him to a different kind of L-asparaginase for all subsequent doses, and he had no further problems.*

. . . . .

A day after Brent received his last L-asparaginase dose, he began to have intense pain in his kidney area and began to pass blood in his urine. After his arrival at the hospital, his kidneys shut down and he stopped breathing. He was in the ICU (intensive care unit) on a ventilator and received kidney dialysis for a week. The doctors thought that he had a rare reaction to L-aparaginase which caused tiny blood clots in his kidneys. His kidneys function normally now, but he developed a seizure disorder as a result of the trauma to his brain.

Very few children have serious side effects from L-asparaginase; but for those who do, the effects can be both frightening and life-threatening.

Azacytidine (az-uh-SIGH-ti-deen)

How given: Subcutaneous injection, IV injection, or IV infusion.

How it works: Azacytidine disrupts RNA metabolism and inhibits protein synthesis within cells, which keeps diseased cells from multiplying.

Precaution: Children must be monitored closely for signs of liver or kidney toxicity.

Common side effects:

- Nausea, vomiting, or diarrhea

- Constipation

- Loss of appetite

- Low blood counts, which may increase risk of infection or bleeding and cause weakness, fatigue, and paleness

- Fever

- Shakiness

- Swelling or pain at the injection site

- Headaches

- Dizziness.

Infrequent side effects:

- Liver problems

- Kidney problems.

Cyclophosphamide (sye-kloe-FOSS-fa-mide)

How given: IV injection.

How it works: Cyclophosphamide is an alkylating agent that disrupts DNA in cancer cells, preventing reproduction.

Precaution: The child should drink lots of water or be given large amounts of IV fluids while taking cyclophosphamide to prevent bladder damage. A drug called Mesna® may be given to prevent bladder irritation. Antinausea drugs should be given before and for several hours after this drug is administered.

Common side effects:

- Low blood counts, which may increase risk of infection or bleeding, and cause weakness, fatigue, and paleness

- Nausea, vomiting, and diarrhea

- Loss of appetite

- Hair loss that is not permanent

- Mouth sores.

Infrequent side effects:

- Bleeding from the bladder

- Cough or shortness of breath

- Skin rash, dryness, and darkening of the skin

- Metallic taste during injection of the drug

- Blurred vision

- Irregular or absent menstrual periods in girls (temporary)

- Permanent sterility in post-pubertal boys (rare at routine doses, more common at doses given for high-risk or relapse treatment or for transplants).

> *Erica just could not tolerate the Cytoxan®. She had continuous vomiting. At one point she had lost more than one third of her body weight. Our HMO (health maintenance organization) wouldn't authorize using ondansetron (a very effective antinausea drug) because it was so expensive.*
>
> • • • • •
>
> *Christine breezed through the Cytoxan® infusions. She would go to Children's in the afternoon, they would give her lots of IV fluids, and then ondansetron a half hour*

before the Cytoxan®. She would sleep through the night with absolutely no nausea, because they were so good about giving her the ondansetron all night and the next morning. It was hard on me because I had to wake up every 2 hours to change her diaper so that the nurse could weigh it to make sure she was passing enough urine.

Cytarabine (sye-TARE-a-been)

How given: IV, IT, or subcutaneous injection.

How it works: Cytarabine kills cancer cells by disrupting DNA.

Common side effects:

- Low blood counts, which may increase risk of infection or bleeding and cause weakness, fatigue, and paleness
- Nausea, vomiting, and diarrhea
- Loss of appetite
- Hair loss that is not permanent
- Mouth sores
- Redness and irritation of the eyes.

Infrequent side effects:

- Fever with or without chills
- Yellow tint to skin or eyes (jaundice)
- Lethargy and excessive sleepiness
- Flu-like symptoms, including bone and joint pain
- Seizures
- Headaches
- Numbness or tingling of fingers and toes.

> *I told my daughter's oncologist how happy I was that she had not had any severe nausea after her first few doses of ARA-C (cytarabine). His only reply was, "It's cumulative." Within an hour, on the long drive home, she was vomiting constantly. We became ensnared in a 2-hour traffic jam. She ran out of clean clothes, so for 2 hours, I repeatedly carried her to the side of the road, a naked, bald, 25-pound 4-year-old with tubing hanging from her chest, and supported her as she dry-heaved. The people in the cars around us were in tears and kept asking if there was anything they could do to help. I just focused on comforting her, and getting her home to that vial of ondansetron in our fridge.*

Daunorubicin (daw-no-ROO-bi-sin)

How given: IV injection or infusion.

How it works: Daunorubicin is an antibiotic that prevents DNA from forming, thus preventing cancer cells from multiplying.

Precaution: Daunorubicin is a red color and may turn urine red for a day or two after each dose. This discoloration is normal.

Common side effects:

* Low blood counts, which may increase risk of infection or bleeding and cause weakness, fatigue, and paleness
* Nausea, vomiting, and diarrhea
* Hair loss
* Mouth sores.

Infrequent side effects:

* Burning pain and swelling if any drug leaks into skin
* Heart damage
* Shortness of breath
* Skin rash.

> My son didn't have any problems from daunorubicin, but I sure worried about heart damage. I went to a conference and learned that the cut-off dose was below what he had on the protocol. I requested an echocardiogram, and his heart function was normal, but I know we need to follow this for life.

Dexamethasone (dex-a-METH-a-zone)

See **Prednisone.**

Doxorubicin (dox-o-ROO-bi-sin)

How given: IV injection or infusion.

How it works: Doxorubicin is an antibiotic that prevents DNA from forming, thus preventing cancer cells from multiplying.

Precaution: It is a red color and may turn urine red for a day or two after each dose. This discoloration is normal.

Common side effects:

• Low blood counts, which may increase risk of infection or bleeding and cause weakness, fatigue, and paleness

• Nausea and vomiting

• Hair loss

• Mouth sores.

Infrequent side effects:

• Loss of appetite

• Diarrhea

• Burning pain and swelling if any drug leaks into skin

• Heart damage

• Shortness of breath

• Fever and chills

• Abdominal pains

• Dark or bloody stools

• Redness at the site of previous radiation ("radiation recall")

• Darkening or ridging of nails.

> The Adriamycin® (doxorubicin) just burned right through my son. He never got mouth sores, but he sure had problems at the other end. They had him lie on his stomach with the heat lamp on his bare bottom. His whole bottom was blistered so badly that it looked like he'd been in a fire. They used to mix up what they called "Magic Butt Paste," and I'll never forget the recipe: one tube Nystatin® cream, one tube Desitin®, and Nystatin® powder. It was like spackle that they would just slather on. He had a lot of gastrointestinal bleeding, too, so he was continuously getting platelets. That's when they decided that he wouldn't have the delayed intensification phase.

• • • • •

> Other than red urine and the expected low counts, hair loss, and nausea, Christine had no problems from her many doses of doxorubicin. She is now 21 and has an EKG (electrocardiogram) and echocardiogram every 2 years. So far, no problems.

Epirubicin (ep-ee-ROO-bi-sin)

How given: IV injection or infusion.

How it works: Epirubicin is an antibiotic that prevents DNA from forming, thus stopping cancer cells from multiplying.

Precautions: An uncommon but serious side effect is heart irregularities. Heart function must be tested before administering epirubicin and periodically during treatment. There is a lifetime maximum dose of this drug, which is dependent upon the health of the individual's heart. This drug can also cause infertility. And if the drug leaks into surrounding tissue, it can cause localized burning.

Common side effects:
- Hair loss
- Nausea and vomiting
- Low blood counts, which may increase risk of infection or bleeding and cause weakness, fatigue, and paleness
- Mouth sores
- Changes in taste or smell
- Rashes
- Discolored urine
- Temporary changes in menstrual cycle in girls.

Infrequent side effects:
- Changes in heart rhythm
- Diarrhea
- Discoloration of fingernails
- Inflammation or irritation of the eyelids
- Hot flashes.

Etoposide (e-TOE-poe-side)

How given: IV injection or infusion; pills by mouth.

How it works: Etoposide prevents DNA from reproducing and causes cells to die.

Precautions: No live vaccines should be given while taking etoposide. It also interacts with several common drugs and herbs, such as aspirin, cyclosporine, glucosomide, and St. John's wort. Etoposide may cause birth defects if taken during pregnancy. It can also irritate the vein where it is injected or damage nearby tissue if it leaks out of the vein.

Common side effects:

- Low blood counts, which may increase risk of infection or bleeding and cause weakness, fatigue, and paleness
- Loss of appetite
- Nausea and vomiting
- Hair loss that is not permanent
- Temporary changes in menstrual cycle in girls.

Infrequent side effects:

- Low blood pressure
- Shortness of breath
- Numbing of fingers and toes
- Fever with or without chills.

Fludarabine (flew-DARE-uh-bean)

How given: Pills by mouth, or by slow IV injection or infusion.

How it works: It causes cell death by interfering with the reproductive processes in the cell.

Precautions: This drug can cause infertility. Liver function may decrease while taking this drug, but this effect is usually temporary. If the child needs a blood transfusion while taking fludarabine, the blood must be irradiated to minimize the chance of an autoimmune reaction.

Common side effects:

- Low blood counts, which may increase risk of infection or bleeding and cause weakness, fatigue, and paleness
- Loss of appetite
- Fever, with or without chills
- Joint pain.

Infrequent side effects:

- Nausea, vomiting, and diarrhea
- Headaches
- Confusion or agitation
- Mouth sores
- Changes in taste
- Rash
- Bladder irritation
- Changes in lung function
- Vision changes
- Increased levels of uric acid in urine
- Infertility.

Gemtuzumab (jem-TOO-zah-mab)

How given: IV infusion.

How it works: Gemtuzumab is a monoclonal antibody that binds to and enters cancer cells, then delivers a substance that causes the cells' DNA to break, thus inhibiting growth. It is a targeted therapy that only affects cancer cells.

Precautions: Although few side effects have been reported, in very rare cases, patients suffer from veno-occusive disease (VOD), in which the small veins in the liver become blocked. This condition is a medical emergency. The signs of VOD include swelling or tenderness of the liver and increased bilirubin levels in the blood.

Common side effects:

- Low blood counts, which may increase risk of infection or bleeding and cause weakness, fatigue, and paleness
- Fever
- Chills.

Infrequent side effects:

- Liver toxicity
- Mouth sores
- Rashes

- Cold sores or fever blisters.

Hydroxyurea (hi-DROX-ee-yoo-REE-ah)

How given: Pills by mouth.

How it works: Hydroxyurea has an action that is not well understood, but it is thought to work by stopping DNA production.

Precaution: Taking this drug while pregnant can cause serious fetal abnormalities.

Common side effects:
- Low blood counts, which may increase risk of infection or bleeding, and cause weakness, fatigue, and paleness.

Infrequent side effects:
- Nausea, vomiting, and diarrhea
- Loss of appetite
- Fever, chills, and flu-like symptoms
- Headaches, drowsiness, dizziness
- Skin rash, itching, darkening of the skin
- Redness of the skin in areas of prior radiation ("radiation recall")
- Mouth sores
- Temporary discoloration or thickening of skin or nails
- Disorientation, hallucinations
- Seizures.

> *Drew has been on hydroxyurea for about 2 years. It is a pill that he can take long term. He is being weaned off it now because of sores (mouth and leg), which are very, very slow to heal.*

Idarubicin (EYE-dah-rue-buh-sin)

How given: Slow IV injection.

How it works: Idarubicin is an antibiotic that prevents cells from making DNA or RNA, thus preventing them from multiplying.

Precautions: Idarubicin causes urine to turn red; this discoloration is normal. This drug can injure the heart muscle, so heart function must be monitored before starting the drug and throughout treatment. If idarubicin leaks out into the tissue surrounding the injection site, it can cause localized tissue damage.

Common side effects:

- Low blood counts, which may increase risk of infection or bleeding and cause weakness, fatigue, and paleness
- Nausea and vomiting
- Temporary hair loss
- Abdominal pain
- Decreased appetite
- Mouth sores
- Rashes.

Infrequent side effects:

- Liver toxicity
- Darkening of nail beds
- Swelling, pain, itching, or numbness of hands or feet
- Heart damage.

Imatinib (im-AT-in-ib)

How given: Pills by mouth, which should be taken with food and water. Do not take with grapefruit juice, because the juice can interfere with the effectiveness of the drug.

How it works: This drug inhibits an enzyme (tyrosine kinase) produced in the cancer cells of most people with chronic myelogenous leukemia (CML) and in some with acute lymphoblastic leukemia (ALL).

Precautions: This drug causes birth defects if taken during pregnancy. It also interacts with numerous other compounds, which can increase or decrease the amount of imatinib in the system or interfere with the effectiveness of the other drugs. Some of the most common drug interactions are with dexamethasone, erythromycin, fentanyl, acetaminophen, cyclosporine, and some antibiotics, seizure medications, sedatives, and antidepressants.

Common side effects:

- Nausea or vomiting

- Fluid retention
- Low blood counts, which may increase risk of infection or bleeding and cause weakness, fatigue, and paleness
- Muscle cramps
- Rashes
- Birth defects if taken during pregnancy.

Infrequent side effects:
- Hemorrhage
- Liver damage
- Headaches
- Constipation
- Night sweats.

Interferon-alpha (in-ter-FEAR-on-AL-fah)

How given: Subcutaneous, IM, or IV injection.

How it works: Interferon-alpha boosts the body's immune system, enabling it to fight cancer cells. It may also directly interfere with the growth of malignant cells.

Precautions: In very rare cases, interferon-alpha can cause permanent vision loss or congestive heart failure. Patients using interferon should have regular thyroid tests. The drug interacts with theophylline, a drug used to treat respiratory diseases.

Common side effects:
- Fatigue
- Flu-like symptoms
- Low blood counts, which may increase risk of infection or bleeding and cause weakness, fatigue, and paleness.

Infrequent side effects:
- Dizziness or confusion
- Depression, anxiety, or irritation
- Swelling or irritation at the injection site
- Insomnia

- Abdominal pain, nausea, vomiting, and diarrhea

- Temporary hair loss

- Rashes, sweats, dry skin, or itching

- Allergic reaction

- Tingling in hands and feet

- Swelling of feet and ankles

- Changes in taste or smell

- Dry mouth

- Temporary liver or kidney toxicity

- Chest pain or irregular heartbeat.

Mercaptopurine (mer-kap-toe-PYOOR-een)

How given: Pills by mouth.

How it works: It is an antimetabolite that interferes with the growth and spread of cancer cells.

Precautions: Certain drugs, including allopurinol and the sulfa-based antibiotics, can worsen side effects of mercaptopurine or cause serious decreases in blood counts. Mercaptopurine can raise blood levels of uric acid, resulting in kidney damage.

Note: See earlier section in this chapter called "Variability in response to medications" to review the genetic tests that determine whether and how quickly your child might metabolize this drug.

Common side effects:

- Low blood counts, which may increase risk of infection or bleeding and cause weakness, fatigue, and paleness

- Loss of appetite.

Infrequent side effects:

- Nausea and vomiting

- Skin rashes

- Mouth sores

- Yellow tint to skin or eyes (jaundice)

- Liver damage (usually temporary)

- Kidney damage (usually temporary)

- Gout.

> *My son was diagnosed with Pre-B ALL. He is currently in long-term maintenance and doing very well. During interim maintenance he had a severe drop in all counts. This was labeled as pancytopenia. His marrow shut down. When this first happened all counts were at rock bottom, and they thought he had relapsed. He tested positive for a condition called thiopurine methyltransferase (TPMT). Basically, the full dosage of 6-MP was poisoning him. He is currently being treated at 50 percent of the drug and being monitored through bimonthly CBCs (complete blood counts). The doctor will slowly increase the dosage to maintain a desired ANC (absolute neutrophil count) if needed.*

Methotrexate (meth-o-TREX-ate)

How given: Pills by mouth, IV infusion, IT or IM injection.

How it works: Methotrexate is an antimetabolite that replaces nutrients in the cancer cells, causing cell death.

Precautions: Children should not be given extra folic acid in vitamins or the methotrexate will not be effective. Several drugs can cause methotrexate to stay in the system too long or worsen its side effects. Some of these drugs include aspirin, non-steroidal anti-inflammatory drugs, penicillin, Bactrim®, Septra®, and several anti-seizure drugs. Children taking methotrexate are very sensitive to the sun and should always wear protective clothing and sunblock.

Hints for parents: Most of the common side effects of this drug are temporary and reversible. Mouth sores can be quite painful, and your child may not eat or drink well when she has them. Always remember to have your child use sunscreen when playing outside (SPF 30 or higher). Minor skin rashes can be treated effectively with over-the-counter cortisone cream. When given as high-dose therapy, methotrexate requires administration of a reversing agent (antidote) called leucovorin. It is critical that your child begin the leucovorin at the correct time to prevent serious, possibly irreversible, side effects.

Common side effects:

- Low blood counts, which may increase risk of infection or bleeding and cause weakness, fatigue, and paleness

- Extreme sun sensitivity, including allergic reactions

- Diarrhea

- Skin rashes

- Headaches, tingling pain down legs, and spinal irritation (when given by IT injection).

Infrequent side effects:

- Mouth sores

- Temporary hair loss

- Nausea and vomiting

- Loss of appetite

- Fever with or without chills

- Liver damage (temporary)

- Kidney damage (temporary)

- Shortness of breath and dry cough

- Temporary or permanent nervous system damage

- Neurotoxicity that can cause learning disabilities

- Redness at the site of previous radiation ("radiation recall").

> *My daughter had serious problems with rashes during maintenance. The doctors thought she had developed an allergy to the weekly methotrexate. She often would be covered with rashes that looked like small, red circles with tan, flaky skin inside. They were extremely itchy and unattractive. We spent hundreds of dollars at the dermatologist trying various prescription remedies. None worked. In desperation, I went to our local herbalist and asked if she had anything totally nontoxic, which would help the rash but not affect her chemotherapy. She sold me a small tub of salve made from olive oil, vitamin E oil, and calendula flowers. We checked with my daughter's oncologist before using it. It totally cured the rash after 2 days and worked each time that the rash reappeared. What a relief!*

> • • • • •

> *Carl was on an experimental IV high-dose methotrexate protocol funded through the National Institutes of Health. Side effects ranged from nausea and vomiting to diarrhea, sore bones, mood swings, and disorientation.*

> • • • • •

> *My son developed learning disabilities from his high-dose methotrexate protocol. He received tutoring through high school and is doing extremely well in college.*

Prednisone (PRED-ni-zone) and dexamethasone (dex-a-METH-a-zone)

These two steroids are grouped together because they are closely related chemically and have similar action and side effects. The biggest difference in side effects appears to be the increased risk of avascular necrosis (death of bone due to decreased blood supply) from dexamethasone.

Dexamethasone is given in high doses as a chemotherapy drug and in low doses to prevent nausea. To see the side effects of dexamethasone when it is used as an antinausea drug, look under "Drugs given to prevent nausea" later in the chapter.

How given: Pills or liquid by mouth, IV or IM injection.

How they work: These drugs are hormones that kill lymphocytes.

Precautions: Every parent interviewed described problems that their child had while on prednisone or dexamethasone. The side effects ranged from mild to severe, but were universal. At high doses, steroids create major behavioral problems in children, which gradually subside after the drug is stopped.

Common side effects:

- Mood changes, from extreme irritability to rage
- Increased appetite and food obsessions
- Increased thirst
- Indigestion
- Weight gain
- Fluid retention
- Round face and protruding belly
- Sleeplessness
- Nightmares
- Nervousness, restlessness, hyperactivity
- Loss of potassium
- Loss of bone mass
- Hypersensitivy to lights, sound, and motion.

Infrequent side effects:

- Decreased or blurred vision

- Seeing halos around lights

- Increased sweating

- Weakness with loss of muscle mass

- Muscle cramps or pain

- Swelling of feet or lower legs

- High blood pressure

- High blood sugar

- Hallucinations.

Judson was a hyper, high-strung child who became extremely hyperactive when he was on prednisone. My recommendation for other parents dealing with this difficult side effect is to run—don't walk—to your nearest library or bookstore and get some books on hyperactive behavior in children. It is important that parents understand this problem and learn to deal with it in a loving way. Remember, too, that this side effect will go away when the prednisone is out of the child's system. Judd would be hyperactive for the entire 2 weeks, desiring to eat every 15 minutes or so, making noises constantly, itching all over, sleeping less, having a terrible temper, and losing his fine motor and concentration skills.

During this time he would develop bad behavior because we could not parent him the way we would normally. A few days after his prednisone ended, we would become very firm and structured in our parenting, and he would return to his normal behavior patterns. My son has been in remission 10 years, has never exhibited abnormal hyperactivity since ending chemotherapy, and is a well-adjusted teen and an excellent student.

· · · · ·

Meagan is very emotionally labile after only two doses of prednisone. She is very frustrated, quick to anger, hits, screams. For those 5 days we try to stay home, and this helps to decrease the stimulation. We plot it out on the calendar in advance so that we can plan accordingly. I think the kids deserve some tender, loving care while taking prednisone. Of course, I don't allow the hitting, but I do try hard not to aggravate the situation when she is on prednisone. I can see how she is uncomfortable being out of control, but she just can't help it.

· · · · ·

Prednisone sends Stephan into a whirlwind of emotions. Sometimes he seems especially happy, and the rest of the time he is in tears at the drop of a hat. We explained to Stephan that the pill can make him feel this way, and it's okay to tell us, "I'm grumpy and I need to be alone for awhile." He gets physical side effects, too. He takes prednisone 5 days a month, and, like clockwork, on Day 6 he gets itchy, on

Day 7 he aches all over, on Day 8 he has severe back, chest, arm, and leg pain, and on Day 9 he starts to feel better.

• • • • •

Preston didn't act out while on prednisone; instead he became depressed and too compliant. He spent most of his time moodily cooking himself food and eating. We bought a second wardrobe of sweat pants with elastic waists so that he would be comfortable.

• • • • •

Rachel had a dual personality on prednisone. She would be fine one minute and then fly into a rage. One time, she literally had an argument with herself. She asked to watch a tape, and then for 20 minutes she argued with herself over whether she should watch the tape. It was painful to watch.

• • • • •

Prednisone and dexamethasone were the worst drugs for Katy. When she was on steroids for a month straight, she hallucinated horrible things. She'd scream that boys were chasing her or that her heart had stopped beating. She'd sob that I was melting and would disappear. She'd dig her fingers into my arm begging me to help her. She sometimes did this all night, and nothing consoled her. She slept very little while taking steroids. She spent day after day and night after night in my arms while I rocked her in the rocking chair, only leaving my arms to eat huge amounts of food. She would eat an entire loaf of bread, and always asked to have "butter spread on it like icing on a cake." She has never once said that since ending treatment.

• • • • •

Elke is currently in long-term maintenance for ALL. After one particularly bad steroid pulse, I told her oncologist about how heart-rending it was to watch a 3-year-old repeatedly wail, "I'm so sad!" while lying despondently on the couch. Her doctor prescribed potassium supplements to counteract the severe depression and mood swings caused by the Decadron®. She starts the potassium a couple days before she begins the steroid pulse, and ends a couple of days after. Although she is by no means even-tempered during her pulses, she no longer seems despondent. The potassium has also greatly decreased the muscular pain she always suffered from the steroids.

• • • • •

Jeremy never slept well when he was on prednisone. He had nightmares of doctors chasing him through the hospital halls. He had a lot of night sweats and was hungry all night and day. He slept with a loaf of bread, and when we would go places, he always carried a can of Campbell's® chicken soup and a can opener. He desperately needed to make sure that he would never be without food.

• • • • •

When you add steroids to a teen boy's already hyped up emotional level, you get ignition. My son was ages 14 to 19 when taking steroids. It helped to talk to him about how it would change how he feels and thinks. After a while, he could describe how he was becoming more agitated and wanted to stay in his room alone. He really didn't like being crabby and angry and would voluntarily isolate himself. I suggested ways for him to control his environment while on the steroids so things wouldn't irritate him as much. He also knew that rules of behavior did not change just because he was on steroids.

· · · · ·

Jody just seemed a little high when on prednisone. He was crazy for food but didn't have any behavior problems. He had lots of energy.

Thioguanine (Thigh-oh-GWAN-neen)

How given: Pills taken by mouth on an empty stomach.

How it works: It is an antimetabolite that interferes with the growth and spread of cancer cells.

Note: See earlier section in this chapter called "Variability in response to medications" to review the genetic tests that determine whether and how quickly your child might metabolize this drug.

Precaution: In some cases, thioguanine (6-TG) has caused liver problems. If your child's abdomen rapidly enlarges, call your doctor immediately.

Common side effects:

• Low blood counts, which may increase risk of infection or bleeding and cause weakness, fatigue, and paleness

• Nausea and vomiting

• Headaches

• Darkening of the skin.

Infrequent side effects:

• Enlarged liver

• Yellow tint to skin or eyes (jaundice)

• Stomach pain

• Loss of appetite

• Mouth sores.

Tay's abdomen slowly began to enlarge and then it suddenly went from a little bloated to huge. He looked pregnant and his abdomen was rock hard. He gained 10 pounds in 1 day—from 55 to 65 pounds. It affected his white, red, and platelet counts. Tay was taken off all meds. He was given potassium by mouth, albumen by IV, and several blood and platelet transfusions. It was very scary! He also ran a fever off and on, and we were in the hospital for days. Once his abdomen shrank and his counts stayed steady we went home.

Tretinoin (tret-IN-oin) and isotretinoin (ICE-oh-tret-IN-oin)

How given: Capsules taken by mouth.

How they work: Tretinoin and isotretinoin are closely related and are used to treat APL. Although scientists don't know exactly why these drugs work, they cause the abnormal cells to mature into healthy white cells.

Precautions: Tretinoin interacts with the antifungal drug ketokozinaol and may also interact with several antibiotics and other classes of drugs. Patients using tretinoin should avoid taking vitamin A or any multivitamins containing it, as this vitamin can cause toxic levels of tretinoin to build up in the body. Children should not receive vaccinations while taking this drug. It can also cause birth defects if taken during pregnancy.

Common side effects:

- Low blood counts, which may increase risk of infection or bleeding and cause weakness, fatigue, and paleness
- Birth defects if taken during pregnancy
- Headaches
- Nausea or vomiting
- Bone pain
- Rashes
- Liver damage (usually temporary).

Infrequent side effects:

- APL differentiation syndrome (breathing difficulties, lung and heart problems, fluid retention, and weight gain)
- Mouth sores
- Increased sweating
- Sudden pain behind eyes with vision problems
- Hair loss

- Earaches
- Abdominal pain.

Vincristine (vin-CRIS-teen)

How given: IV injection or infusion.

How it works: Vincristine is an alkyloid derived from the periwinkle plant. It causes cells to stop dividing.

Precautions: Care should be taken to prevent leakage of vincristine from the IV site because it will damage tissue. Before taking the first dose of vincristine, your child should be started on a program to prevent constipation. Vincristine interacts with several other chemotherapy drugs, so care should be taken in planning the dosing schedule. Grapefruit or grapefruit juice may affect the functioning of this drug, so parents should check with the doctor about whether their child should avoid these while taking vincristine. Children on vincristine should be tested frequently for kidney or liver toxicity.

Note: The side effects of vincristine are most obvious during induction and consolidation, when it is given weekly. It is generally better tolerated during maintenance when it is given monthly.

Common side effects:
- Severe constipation
- Pain (may be severe) in jaw, face, back, joints, and/or bones
- Foot drop (child has trouble lifting front part of foot)
- Numbness, tingling, or pain (may be severe) in fingers and toes
- Extreme weakness and loss of muscle mass
- Drooping eyelids
- Temporary hair loss
- Pain, blisters, and skin loss if drug leaks during administration.

Infrequent side effects:
- Headaches
- Dizziness and light-headedness
- Seizures
- Inappropriate production of antidiuretic hormone
- Paralysis.

Hints for parents: This drug is given weekly for a number of weeks and then monthly. Start your child on a stool softener at the beginning of treatment with this drug and give it consistently. Jaw pain is an early and temporary side effect, but it is often severe enough to warrant an oral narcotic. Watch your child's gait and strength, especially going up and down stairs and performing fine-motor activities, such as coloring, writing, or buttoning clothes. Report problems in these areas to your physician promptly so your child's dose can be altered. Sometimes medications (e.g., Neurontin®) and physical therapy are necessary to counteract the neurological effects of the drug.

> Erica (diagnosed at age 1) once had a vincristine burn on her arm at the IV site. It was red when we went home from the clinic, but by the second day it was badly burned. She developed a blister as big as a half dollar, which left a bad scar. It hurt and was sensitive for a long time. She also developed severe foot drop (she could not lift up the front part of her foot) and fell a lot.

· · · · ·

> Preston (diagnosed age 10) had an awful time from vincristine. He would develop cramping in his lower legs, and would just curl up in bed, in great pain. It would start a couple of days after he received the vincristine, and would last a week. I would massage his legs, use hot packs, and give him Tylenol®. I would have to carry him into the clinic, because he couldn't walk. I did some research and discovered that when the bilirubin is high, the child can't excrete the vincristine and therefore the toxicity is increased. We lowered his vincristine dose and got him into physical therapy.

· · · · ·

> Vincristine incapacitated Katy. She couldn't walk, lift her head, or open one eyelid. She had trouble swallowing and stayed in bed for weeks during induction and consolidation. I read the package insert for vincristine and discovered that the manufacturer recommended that vincristine be given at least 12 to 24 hours before asparaginase to minimize toxicity. Katy's protocol required that both drugs be given at the same time. I negotiated with the doctors and had her schedule changed so that these two drugs were given on different days. She was soon back on her feet, but still, after a year off treatment, she has generalized muscle weakness and problems with balance.

· · · · ·

> My daughter Elke (age 2 ½ at diagnosis of ALL) is very sensitive to the neuropathic effects of vincristine. During induction she developed breathing and swallowing issues due to vocal cord paresis, had severe jaw and leg pain, and could not walk. Her doctors quickly started her on Neurontin® (generic name: gabapentin) to combat the neuropathy. She is currently in long-term maintenance and taking Elavil® for the same purpose. Although these are off-label uses of these medications, they are fairly

effective at alleviating some of the pain caused by the vincristine. Since the damage done by vincristine can be long-term and cumulative, it is important to be proactive in addressing its side effects. Elke may not be able to run yet but she can walk, thanks to the continuous use of these medications and the willingness of her doctors to withhold or reduce her dosages of vincristine when warranted.

· · · · ·

Soon after diagnosis at age 5 ½, Robby became so weak in the hospital that he stopped walking. He did not walk for at least a week, maybe more. When Robby did walk, he was up on his toes. I kept asking the doctors about it, and they poohpoohed it, saying it was just the vincristine. Finally, I took Robby to the pediatrician, who was horrified at how bad his feet had gotten. We immediately started daily physical therapy and major exercises and got traction boots to wear at night.

Prophylactic antibiotics

Children and teens on chemotherapy take antibiotics 2 to 3 days each week to prevent pneumocystis pneumonia (PCP). They usually continue taking the antibiotics a few months to a year after treatment ends. The antibiotic of choice for PCP prevention is a combination drug containing sulfamethoxazole and trimethoprim; it is sold under the brand names Bactrim® and Septra®. This antibiotic can cause gastrointestinal upset, skin rashes, sun sensitivity, and low blood counts. If a substitute is needed, one of the following is used:

- Pentamidine, administered as an aerosol or through a nebulizer (can be difficult for children because it takes 20 minutes to administer and it smells and tastes bad), or by IV once a month.

- Dapsone, pills given orally every day.

> *The oncologist explained it this way. Bactrim® is the best prophylactic antibiotic for PCP (pneumocystis), but it can affect counts. Pentamidine IV can affect counts, but nebulizer treatments (once a month) usually don't. Dapsone can be used, but it can cause anemia.*

> *We just started the dapsone because Katie was starting to buck the nebulizer treatment. (It smells and tastes horrible.) The Bactrim® costs about $3/month, the dapsone about $7/month, and the pentamidine nebulizer treatment is about $300/month!*

Colony-stimulating factors

Colony-stimulating factors (CSFs) are not generally used for children with ALL, unless they suffer persistent and drastically reduced blood counts. They are often used for children with acute myelogenous leukemia (AML) or for those who have stem cell transplants. High-dose chemotherapy reduces the number of white blood cells used by the body to fight infections. The administration of CSFs, such as granulocyte colony-stimulating factor (G-CSF) and granulocyte-macrophage colony-stimulating factor (GM-CSF), can reduce the severity and duration of low white blood counts, lessening the chance of infection. G-CSF may be administered by IV or by subcutaneous injection. GM-CSF must be administered as a subcutaneous injection.

> Kenny was only 2 years old when he was receiving G-CSF, so he was too young to understand why he needed the shots. He would cry and beg us not to hurt him—that he was sorry. My heart would break, but I would have to give him the shot. We finally developed a really good system. Right before being discharged after a round of chemo, we would put EMLA® on Kenny's arm and then have the nurse place an insuflon. It was a small catheter that Kenny didn't even notice was in his arm. It was good for 7 to 10 days, which was the duration of his G-CSF for the entire month. We would draw up the amount needed for injection, then place it in the insuflon and inject it very slowly. Kenny never felt it and no longer begged us not to do the G-CSF. Oh, how I wished we had done this from the beginning! Kenny's counts would usually start to decline about 4 days after his chemo. At about Day 10 the G-CSF would kick in, and his counts would skyrocket.

· · · · ·

> Katie had G-CSF (brand name is Neupogen®) after each high-dose cytarabine. But it is in her protocol to give it to her after her other chemotherapy if low counts caused a delay of over 7 days in treatment—and we were pretty close a few times.
>
> She's had no side effects from Neupogen® that I can recall. The worst thing about it for us was giving the shots at home. They're subcutaneous, so the needle is short, but Katie still said they hurt, even with EMLA®.

Antinausea drugs used during chemotherapy

Antinausea drugs, also referred to as antiemetics, make chemotherapy treatments more bearable, but they can potentially cause side effects. The following section lists some commonly used antinausea drugs.

There are many drugs used to prevent nausea that are not described here, including Marinol®, Reglan®, scopolamine patch, and Atarax®.

Antinausea drug list

As with chemotherapy drugs, several different names can be used to refer to each antinausea drug. The list below will help you find detailed information about each drug on the following pages:

Drug name	Brand name(s)
Aprepitant	Emend®
Dexamethasone	Decadron®
Diphenhydramine	Benadryl®
Granisetron	Granisol®, Kytril®, Sancuso®
Lorazepam	Ativan®
Ondansetron	Zofran®
Prochlorperazine	Compazine®
Promethazine	Phenergan®

Aprepitant (a-PREP-it-ant)

How given: It is given orally (capsule) 1 hour before chemotherapy or by IV injection over a 15-minute span, starting 30 minutes before chemotherapy. This drug interacts with many drugs, so make sure the pharmacist knows about every drug your child takes.

Common side effects:

- Fatigue
- Dizziness
- Constipation
- Diarrhea
- Hiccups
- Heartburn
- Itching
- Loss of appetite.

Dexamethasone (dex-a-METH-a-zone)

How given: IV injection, usually given in combination with other antinausea drugs, or by mouth.

Common side effects: Side effects are different than those experienced when it is given in high doses for long periods of time. When dexamethasone is used to treat nausea, side effects include:

- Euphoria
- Restlessness
- Confusion.

Diphenhydramine (die-fen-HIGH-dra-meen)

How given: Liquid, pills, or caplets by mouth, or IV injection.

When given: Usually given every 6 to 8 hours.

Common side effects:

- Drowsiness
- Dizziness
- Impaired coordination
- Dry mouth
- Excitability (in young children)
- Low blood pressure.

Granisetron (gran-ISS-eh-tron)

How given: IV injection, pills by mouth, or a patch on the skin (called Sancuso®).

When given: Granisetron is usually given 30 minutes prior to the start of chemotherapy infusion. Doses may be repeated every 12 to 24 hours.

Common side effects:

- Headaches
- Diarrhea
- Constipation.

Infrequent side effects:

- High blood pressure
- Fatigue
- Fever

- Allergic reaction
- Abnormal heart rhythms.

> *Sarah got Zofran® at first, then the clinic switched to liquid Kytril®. Sarah usually hates liquid meds (she much prefers pills), but she loves Kytril®. She thinks it's really yummy. And it works, too!*

Lorazepam (lor-AZ-a-pam)

How given: Pills or liquid by mouth, sublingually (pill dissolved under the tongue), or subcutaneous, IV, or IM injection.

When given: This tranquilizer is generally given in combination with other antinausea drugs.

Precaution: This drug interacts with several other drugs, so parents should tell the doctor about everything else their child is taking, including over-the-counter drugs.

Common side effects:
- Drowsiness and sleepiness
- Poor short-term memory
- Impaired coordination
- Low blood pressure
- Excitability (in young children).

Ondansetron (on-DAN-se-tron)

How given: IV injection, liquid by mouth, pills by mouth, or sublingual (pill dissolved under the tongue).

When given: Usually given 30 minutes prior to chemotherapy drugs, then every 4 to 8 hours until nausea ends or in a higher dose once a day.

Note: Ondansetron comes in flavored oral solutions; 1 teaspoon = 4 mg. You can mix the dose in a small amount of a drink your child prefers.

Common side effects:
- Headache with rapid IV administration
- Diarrhea

- Constipation.

Infrequent side effects:

- Serious allergic reaction
- Abnormal heart rhythm.

> *After Jeremy had his first inpatient treatment, he was allowed to go on an outpatient basis, wearing a cad pump at home. He felt fine, but every couple hours he would vomit for no reason. The next morning, when his oncologist asked him how it had gone, Jeremy was hesitant to tell him about the vomiting. When he did, the doctor asked us if the Zofran® hadn't helped. I gave him a confused look and asked him what a Zofran® was. I can laugh about it now, but it was an oversight. Everyone thought someone else had taken care of it! We rarely had any problems with nausea after that.*

Prochlorperazine (pro-chlor-PAIR-a-zeen)

How given: Pills, long-acting capsule, or liquid by mouth; rectal suppository; or IM or IV injection.

When given: Used alone if only mild nausea is expected.

Common side effects:

- Drowsiness
- Low blood pressure
- Nervousness and restlessness
- Uncontrollable muscle spasms, especially of jaw, face, and hands
- Blurred vision.

Promethazine (pro-METH-ah-zeen)

How given: Pills or liquid by mouth, rectal suppository, or IM or IV injection.

When given: Usually given every 4 to 6 hours.

Common side effects:

- Drowsiness
- Dizziness
- Impaired coordination

- Fatigue

- Blurred vision

- Euphoria

- Insomnia.

Drugs used to relieve pain

As with other medicines, drugs used for pain relief can be given by various methods and can cause side effects. The following section lists some drugs commonly used to relieve pain. Many other medications are used to relieve pain in children, including acetaminophen, nalbuphine, fentanyl, hydrocodone, and others.

Pain medication names

Several different names can be used to refer to each of the pain medications. You may hear the same drug referred to by its generic name, an abbreviation, or one of several brand names, depending on which doctor, nurse, or pharmacist you talk to. The list below provides the generic name of several commonly used pain medications and some of the most common brand names.

Drug name	Brand names
Codeine	Codrix®
Hydromorphone	Dilaudid®
Meperidine	Demerol®, Mepergan®
Methadone	Methadose®, Dolophine®
Morphine	Astramorph PF®, Avinza®, Duramorph®, Infumorph®, Kadian®, MS Contin®, Oramorph SR®, Roxanol®
Oxycodone	Percocet®, Percodan®, Oxycontin®, Roxicet®, Roxilox®, Roxycodone®, M-Oxy®, Oxyfast®, OxyIR®, ETH-Oxydose®, Tylox®

Codeine

How given: IM injection, IV injection or infusion, subcutaneous injection, or pills or liquid by mouth.

How it works: Codeine is an opiate that reduces pain.

Note: Codeine is added to numerous other non-narcotic pain relievers.

Common side effects:

- Light-headedness

- Dizziness

- Sedation

- Euphoria

- Constipation.

Infrequent side effects:

- Nausea

- Vomiting

- Allergic reaction

- Slowed heart rate.

Hydromorphone

How given: IV injection or infusion, pill by mouth, rectal suppository, or subcutaneous injection.

How it works: Hydromorphone is a narcotic pain reliever.

Precaution: Hydromorphone can cause respiratory depression (slowed breathing).

Common side effects:

- Dizziness and light-headedness

- Sedation

- Nausea and vomiting

- Excessive sweating

- Euphoria and other mood alterations

- Headaches

- Constipation

- Respiratory depression.

Infrequent side effects:

- Hallucination and disorientation

- Diminished circulation

- Shock

- Cardiac arrest.

Meperidine

How given: IV, IM, or subcutaneous injection; or liquid or pill by mouth. It is not as effective if taken by mouth.

How it works: Meperidine is a narcotic that works similarly to morphine.

Common side effects:

- Sedation

- Constipation

- Dizziness

- Nausea and vomiting

- Dry mouth

- Flushing or sweating.

Infrequent side effects:

- Respiratory depression

- Decreased blood pressure

- Seizures

- Headaches

- Visual disturbances

- Mood changes

- Slowed heart rate.

Methadone

How given: IV, IM, or subcutaneous injection; or liquid or pill by mouth.

How it works: Methadone is a narcotic pain reliever.

Common side effects:

- Light-headedness and dizziness

- Sedation

- Nausea and vomiting

- Excessive sweating

- Euphoria

- Constipation

- Loss of appetite.

Infrequent side effects:

- Respiratory depression

- Decreased circulation

- Depression or euphoria

- Confusion

- Shock.

Morphine

How given: IV injection or infusion, pill by mouth (long-acting or short-acting), liquid by mouth, or suppository.

How it works: Morphine is a narcotic derived from the opium plant.

Common side effects:

- Euphoria

- Nausea and vomiting

- Sedation

- Dry mouth

- Headaches

- Drowsiness

- Constipation.

Infrequent side effects:

- Reduction in body temperature

- Respiratory depression

- Allergic reactions, including hives

- Seizures.

Oxycodone

How given: Pills or liquid by mouth.

How it works: Oxycodone is a narcotic derived from opium.

Common side effects:

- Light-headedness

- Dizziness

- Sedation

- Constipation

- Nausea and vomiting.

Infrequent side effects:

- Respiratory depression

- Skin rash

- Mood changes

- Headaches

- Insomnia

- Low blood pressure

- Slowed heart rate

- Delayed digestion

- Allergic reactions.

Topical anesthetics to prevent pain

Several products are commonly used to prevent pain from injections, finger pricks, IV insertions, spinal taps, bone marrow aspirations, and blood transfusions. Most fall into three categories, which are described below. Use of these drugs is also discussed in Chapter 5, "Coping with Procedures."

Topical anesthetizing creams

Examples: EMLA®, ELA-Max®, and many other brand names.

How given: Each product has slightly different instructions. In general, they are applied to the skin between 30 to 90 minutes before a procedure. Some must be covered with an airtight dressing.

How they work: These are creams that contain the topical anesthetic lidocaine. ELA-Max® uses lidocaine alone; EMLA® uses lidocaine in combination with prilocaine.

Notes: It may take longer than an hour to achieve effective anesthesia in dark-skinned children. Sometimes, when using EMLA®, the blood vessels constrict making it harder to find a vein. To prevent this problem, it helps to apply a warm damp cloth immediately before the injection. For more information about use of these products, see Chapter 5.

> We use EMLA® for everything: finger pokes, accessing port, shots, spinal taps, and bone marrows. I even let her sister use it for shots because it lets her get a bit of attention, too. Both of my children have sensitive skin that turns red when they pull off tape, so I cover the EMLA® with plastic wrap held in place with paper tape. I also fold back the edge of each piece of tape to make a pull tab so the kids don't have to peel each edge back from their skin.

Numby Stuff®

How given: Numby Stuff® is a device that delivers pain medication through the skin without the use of needles.

How it works: A patch containing lidocaine and epinephrine is applied to the skin, then electrodes are attached. Low-level electric currents then deliver the medication deep into the skin layer. It takes 10 to 15 minutes for the drugs to take full effect.

Note: Numby Stuff® cannot be used on damaged skin, the temples, or the eyes. Some children and teens do not like the electrical sensation it causes.

Vapocoolant sprays

Examples: Fluori-Methane Spray® and Freezy Spray.

How given: An aerosol spray that is applied to the sterilized target area immediately before the procedure. It can also be applied by spraying the solution into a medicine cup for 10 seconds, then dipping a cotton ball into the solution and holding it on the site for 15 seconds immediately before performing the procedure.

How they work: Most vapocoolant sprays use the refrigerant ethyl chloride to numb the area before an injection or infusion.

Note: If the spray is applied too long, it can cause frostbite. Spray just until skin begins to turn white (3 to 10 seconds). The spray can should be held between 3 to 9 inches away from the skin.

Adjunctive treatments

In recent years increasing research has been done on mind-body medicine and its effect on coping with the side effects of illness. Adjunctive therapies are those that can be expected to add something beneficial to the treatment. For example, imagery and hypnosis are widely used to help children and teens prepare for or cope with medical procedures. Other helpful adjunctive therapies are relaxation, biofeedback, massage, visualization, acupuncture, meditation, music therapy, aromatherapy, Reiki, and prayer. Chapter 5 discusses adjunctive therapies and how to obtain information about them.

> My daughter was terrified of needles, and it was a nightmare every time we went in to get her port accessed or blood drawn. We went to a psychologist who specialized in methods to cope with pain. She taught my daughter visualization. They made an audiotape of an underwater snorkeling trip. It included watching all of the colorful fish and feeling the soothing warm water. She would listen to it in the clinic, or visualize the trip without the tape. It really helped my daughter develop a technique to cope with accessing the port.

Alternative treatments

Alternative treatments can be defined as either treatments that are used in place of conventional medical treatments or treatments that may have unknown or adverse effects when used in addition to conventional treatments. Sometimes alternative treatments are illegal or unavailable in the United States or Canada, and patients travel to other countries to obtain them. Alternative treatments are usually based on word-of-mouth endorsements, called anecdotal evidence. Medical therapy is based on scientific studies using large groups of patients. In treating cancer, these large clinical trials have resulted in increases in survival rates in the past 3 decades.

Many alternative treatments can help parents and children feel they are aiding the healing process. Even with a good prognosis for your child, it is difficult to ignore the advice of friends and relatives extolling the virtues of various alternative treatments. Parents just want to help their children in every way possible; they often feel helpless and agonize over the pain their child endures for many months or years while on conventional therapy. However, it is extremely important that any alternative therapy that involves ingestion or injection into the body (e.g., herbs, vitamins, special diets, enemas) only be given with the oncologist's knowledge. The oncologist's involvement is necessary to prevent you from giving something to your child that could lessen the effectiveness of the conventional chemotherapy or cause additional toxicity. For instance, folic acid (a type of B vitamin) replaces methotrexate in cells and reduces or eliminates its effectiveness, allowing cancer cells to flourish. The oncologist will be much more knowledgeable about these potential conflicts than a parent, herbalist, or health food store salesperson.

If you want to evaluate claims made about alternative treatments, here are several ways to collect enough information to make an educated judgment:

- Check the National Institutes of Health's National Center for Complementary and Alternative Medicine to see if any scientific evidence or warnings exist about the treatment that interests you. This information is available online at *http://nccam.nih.gov*.

- Contact your local American Cancer Society or Canadian Cancer Society's division office and ask for information about the therapy you are considering. These organizations have compiled information about many therapies describing the treatment, its known risks, side effects, opinions of the medical establishment, and any lawsuits that have been filed in relation to the therapy. The American Cancer Society has an online database at *www.cancer.org* with information about many alternative treatments.

- Ask specifically what this treatment is expected to do for your child, what is in it, and what tests will be done to determine whether your child needs it and whether your child is benefiting from it.

- Collect and study all available objective literature about the treatment. Ask the alternative treatment providers if they have treated other children with cancer, what results have been achieved, how these results have been documented, and where they have reported their results. Ask for the reports so your child's doctor can review them.

- Talk with other people who have gone through the treatment. Inquire about the training and experience of the person administering the treatment. Be sure to find out how much the therapy costs, because your insurance company may not pay for alternative treatments.

- Beware of any practitioner who will give your child the alternative therapy only if you stop taking the child in for conventional treatments.

- Never inject any alternative product into a central line. Children have developed life-threatening infections and have died from this method of treatment.

Take all the information you gather to your child's oncologist to discuss any positive or negative impacts the alternative treatment may have on your child's current medical treatment. Do not give any alternative treatment or over-the-counter drugs to your child in secret. Some treatments negate the effectiveness of chemotherapy, while other substances, such as those containing aspirin or related compounds, can cause uncontrollable bleeding in children with low platelet counts.

At one point, we decided to try some alternative therapies with our son. Our plan was to use it in conjunction with his conventional treatment. I scheduled a meeting with his oncologist and discussed the alternatives with him. I wouldn't dare attempt to start anything, not even vitamin supplements, without first talking it over with the doctor, because I was scared that I would cause my child more harm than good. I was grateful that the oncologist was willing to listen to what I had to say and offer his opinion.

We both agreed that the alternative therapy we had in mind wouldn't do any damage or interfere with the chemotherapy my son was receiving. Two months later, we decided that it was doing absolutely nothing for him, so we stopped. I figured the money would be better spent at the toy store than on a useless therapy. I learned a valuable lesson from that experience. I'm much more skeptical now than I used to be. My new motto is "show me the proof."

• • • • •

I gave my son echinacea when he received chemotherapy. I checked with his doctor first. He didn't think it would hurt but didn't think it would help, either. Still, all the nurses in emergency swore by the stuff. We got good results, too. We started the echinacea after lots of treatment, and it was the first time that he didn't have to be readmitted 3 days after chemo for febrile neutropenia. I'm convinced that it helped him during the recovery period when his counts would bottom out.

If, after thorough investigation, you feel strongly in favor of using an alternative treatment in addition to conventional treatment and your child's oncologist adamantly opposes it, listen to her reasoning. If you still disagree, get a second opinion from another oncology specialist. Remember, your child's health should be everyone's priority.

My daughter Meagan was diagnosed with average-risk ALL over 7 years ago. She had many chemotherapy-related side effects, including severe high blood pressure and ongoing liver problems. We were constantly adjusting her doses or taking her off chemo altogether. I was so obsessed about it that the doctor took me aside and told me that it's easier to treat leukemia than liver failure, and he just had to take her off her medications. He told me I had to stop worrying, but I couldn't.

When her hair fell out again during maintenance, I just worried more. I realized that every child seemed to have something that went wrong, but I was amazed at how many different "somethings" there were.

Now she has a head full of gorgeous hair. She was just chosen for the select soccer team and is quite an accomplished skier. She has no long-term effects and is healthy and happy.

Chapter 10

Common Side Effects
of Chemotherapy

*In the depths of winter I finally learned
there was in me an invincible summer.*

— Albert Camus

CHEMOTHERAPY DRUGS INTERFERE with cancer cells' ability to grow and reproduce. Because cancer cells are rapidly dividing cells, they are more susceptible to chemotherapy drugs than are most normal cells. Unfortunately, normal, healthy cells that multiply rapidly can also be damaged by chemotherapy. These normal cells include those of the brain, bone marrow, mouth, stomach, intestines, hair follicles, and skin.

This chapter explains the most common side effects of chemotherapy drugs, along with two uncommon but serious ones, and explores ways to deal with them effectively. It also covers questions about owning pets when your child is being treated for leukemia. Chemotherapy side effects that prevent good nutrition are discussed in Chapter 17, "Nutrition."

Hair loss

Because hair follicle cells reproduce quickly, chemotherapy causes some or all body hair to fall out. The hair on the scalp, eyebrows, eyelashes, underarms, and pubic area may slowly thin out or fall out in big clumps.

Hair regrowth usually starts 1 to 3 months after maintenance starts or intensive chemotherapy ends. The color and texture may be different from the original hair. Straight hair may regrow curly; blond hair may become brown. Sometimes during maintenance, some children's hair begins to thin or fall out again.

The following suggestions for dealing with hair loss come from parents:

• When hair is thin or breaking, use a brush with very soft bristles.

- Avoid bleaches, curlers, blow dryers, and hair gel, as these may cause additional damage.

- If hair is thin, use a mild shampoo specifically designed for overtreated or damaged hair.

- A flannel blanket placed on the pillow at night will help collect hair that is falling out.

- Recognize that hair loss is traumatic for almost all children; but it is especially hard on teenagers.

- Emphasize to your child that the hair loss is temporary and that it will grow back.

> *During the first year after Belle was diagnosed (and lost her hair), her brother and I found some Barbie® hats/bandanas with wigs attached at the local dollar store. So the Barbies® whose heads were shaved had something to wear while their hair grew out! Belle also made numerous outfits for "chemo Barbie®" out of supplies at the hospital: napkins, masks, various kinds of tape. She even made furniture out of straws and stuff!*

- Try to have your child meet children in maintenance or off therapy so they can see for themselves that hair will regrow soon.

- Allow your child to choose a collection of hats, scarves, or cotton turbans to wear. These are tax-deductible medical expenses and may be covered by insurance.

- To order several styles of reversible all cotton headwear for girls and teens, contact Just in Time™, in Philadelphia at (215) 247-8777, or online at *www.softhats.com*. Another company sells hats with human hair that are soft, comfortable, and fun to wear. Visit its website at *www.hatswithhair.com*.

- If your child expresses an interest in wearing a wig, take pictures of her hairstyle prior to hair loss. Also, cut snippets of hair to take in to allow a good match of original color and texture. The cost of the wig may be covered by insurance if the doctor writes a prescription for a "wig prosthesis" and includes the medical reason for the wig, such as "alopecia due to cancer chemotherapy."

To find a wig retailer, look in the phone book's yellow pages under "Hair Replacements, Goods, and Supplies" or do an online search. The American Cancer Society, (800) ACS-2345, and some local cancer service organizations offer free wigs in some areas.

- Advocate that school-age children be permitted to wear hats or other head coverings in school. (Use a 504 Plan, described in Chapter 15, "School," if necessary.)

• Separate your feelings about baldness from your child's feelings. Many parents rush out to buy wigs and hats without discussing with their child how he wants to deal with his baldness. Allow your child to choose whether to wear head coverings or not. Let it be okay to be bald. An oncologist comments:

> Consider whether hair loss bothers your child. If it bothers him, then you should pursue things to hide or resolve the problem. If it bothers you but not him, then focus your efforts on trying to deal with your concern and anxiety. Think of this as an opportunity to teach him that it is what is on the inside that counts. In today's culture that places so much emphasis on outward appearance and conformity, this is a valuable lesson. It has been my experience that kids who have visible late effects after cancer treatment can adjust quite well to external differences if they are given a lot of support at home. As a parent, if you let him know he is a great kid, he will believe it.

The amount of hair loss varies among children being treated for leukemia. Some only lose part of their hair, some have hair that thins out, and some quickly lose every hair on their head.

> Preston never completely lost his hair, but it became extremely thin and wispy. When he was first diagnosed, a friend bought him a fly-fishing tying kit, and he became very good at tying flies. He even began selling them at a local fishing shop. When his hair began to fall out, we would gather it up and put it in a plastic bag. He started tying flies out of his hair, and they were displayed in the shop window as "Preston's Human Hair Flies." He was only 11, but the shop owner hired him to help around the shop. He became very popular with the clientele, because everyone wanted to meet the boy who tied flies from his own hair. He really turned losing his hair into something positive.

• • • • •

> Three-year-old Christine's hair started to fall out within 3 weeks of starting chemo. She had beautiful curly hair, but she never talked about losing it, and I thought it didn't bother her. Occasionally she would wear a hat or the hood of a sweatshirt, but most of the time she went bald. One day, I learned how she really felt. We were talking about the different colors of hair in our family, and she began shouting, "I don't have brown hair! I'm bald, just like a baby."

• • • • •

> The chemo greatly affected Meagan's hair. During maintenance, it came back in lush and curly, then after a few months it began falling out again. This was very upsetting. She hasn't gone completely bald again, but it remains very thin and unhealthy hair, while others in the same stage of treatment have beautiful hair back again.

• • • • •

My daughter, Katie (age 11), cut and dyed her hair bright fuchsia as soon as she realized she had cancer. It made her hair seem less hers than something to play with. Then, when she started receiving chemo, she asked that it be cut and shaved really short like some of her boy friends in her class. Our local coach came over and shaved it for her. It was only about a quarter of an inch long at that point. Then when it fell out a week later, it was no big deal for her, because she had already taken it off. That was her way of controlling the situation.

Now we celebrate her baldness by painting henna designs on her head and using face paints to paint fancy designs whenever we go somewhere special, or visit the hospital. On July 4th, we painted stars and rockets in red, white, and blue. On our last visit to the hospital, we painted a floral vine with flowers and lightning bolts above her ears to show she's hot stuff. She even had her sisters add two eyes at the back of her head—to watch the doctors and nurses when her back is turned. Everyone loves to check out her head when she comes in the hospital, and she receives tons of attention as a result of it. Also, now she's beginning to play with the rub-on tattoos and is placing them where the doctors like to inspect, just to surprise them when they pull up her shirt.

She also loves to dress up her head with funny wigs and masks. Last week she was dancing in the front yard with a black/blue fright wig, monster ears, a Grateful Deadhead shirt and black platform heels. She literally stopped traffic! It was a riot. She absolutely refuses to talk to most of her doctors and nurses, and is extremely shy, but this is her silly way of poking fun at them and the whole situation with her cancer.

Nausea and vomiting

The effects of anticancer drugs vary from person to person and dose to dose. A drug that makes one child violently ill often has no effect on other children. Some drugs produce no nausea until several doses have been given, while others cause nausea after a single dose. Because the effects of chemotherapy are so variable, each child's treatment must be tailored to her individual needs. There is no relationship between the amount of nausea and the effectiveness of the medicine.

Following is a list of suggestions for helping children and teenagers cope with nausea and vomiting:

• Give your child antiemetic (antinausea) medications as prescribed. Do not skip any doses.

• Ask your doctor whether a drug that blocks gastric secretions, such as Pepcid® or Zantac®, would be helpful.

- Your child should wear loose clothing, because it is both more comfortable and easier to remove if soiled.

- Parents should try to have at least one change of clothes for their child in the car.

- Large zip-lock plastic bags provide an easily used container if your child gets sick in the car. They can be sealed and disposed of quickly and neatly, ridding the car of unpleasant odors that could make your child's nausea worse.

- Carry a bucket, towels, and baby wipes in the car in case of vomiting.

- Try to keep your child in a quiet, well-ventilated room after chemotherapy.

- Smells can trigger nausea. Try not to cook in the house when your child feels ill. If possible, open windows to provide plenty of fresh air.

- If your child is nauseated by smells, use a covered cup with a straw for liquids.

- Do not serve hot foods if the odor aggravates your child's nausea.

- Serve dry foods such as toast, pretzels, or crackers in the morning or whenever your child is feeling nauseated.

- Serve several small meals rather than three large ones.

- Have your child keep his head elevated after eating. Lying flat can induce nausea.

- Provide plenty of clear liquids such as water, juice, Gatorade®, and ginger ale.

- Avoid serving sweet, fried, or very spicy food. Instead, stick with bland foods such as potatoes, cottage cheese, soup, or toast when your child feels nauseous.

- Watch for any signs of dehydration, including dry skin and mouth, sunken eyes, dizziness, and decreased urination. Call the physician if your child appears dehydrated.

- Use distractions such as TV, videos, music, games, or reading aloud to divert attention from nausea.

- After your child vomits, rinse her mouth with water or a mixture of water and lemon juice to help remove the taste.

- If your child develops a metallic taste in his mouth, chewing gum or sucking on popsicles may help.

> Meagan has always had problems in every phase of treatment with stomachaches, especially in the morning. She will often vomit once and then be over it. She is frequently soothed with just rubbing her tummy or laying a hot towel on it.

If the various antinausea medications do not work well for your child, investigate the Food and Drug Administration (FDA)-approved Relief Band®. This wrist band gives an electrical stimulation (too faint to feel) to a nerve in the wrist that affects the portion of the brain that controls nausea. Information about the band is available online at *www.reliefband.com.*

Low blood counts

Bone marrow—the spongy material that fills the inside of the bones—produces red cells, white cells, and platelets. Chemotherapy drugs damage or destroy the cells inside the bone marrow and dramatically lower the number of cells circulating in the blood. Frequent blood tests are crucial in determining whether your child needs transfusions. Most children treated for leukemia require many transfusions of red cells and sometimes platelets. When the number of infection-fighting white cells is low, your child is in danger of developing serious infections.

Absolute neutrophil count (ANC)

The activities of families of children with leukemia revolve around the sick child's white blood cell (WBC) count, specifically the absolute neutrophil count (ANC). The ANC provides an indication of the child's ability to fight infection.

When a child has blood drawn for a complete blood count (CBC), one section of the lab report will state the total WBC count and a "differential." This means each type of WBC will be listed as a percentage of the total. For example, if the total WBC count is 1500 mm^3, the differential might appear as follows:

White Blood Cell Type	Percentage of Total WBC
Segmented neutrophils (also called polys or segs)	49%
Band neutrophils (also called bands)	1%
Basophils (also called basos)	1%
Eosinophils (also called eos)	1%
Lymphocytes (also called lymphs)	38%
Monocytes (also called monos)	10%

To calculate the ANC, add the percentages of segmented and band neutrophils, then multiply by the total WBC. Using the example above, the ANC is 49% + 1% = 50%; 50% of 1,500 (.50 x 1500) = 750; so the ANC is 750.

> *Erica ran a fever whenever her counts were low, but nothing ever grew in her cultures. They would hospitalize her for 48 hours as a precaution. She was never on a full dose of medicine because of her chronically low counts. She's 2 years off treatment now and doing great.*

How to protect the child with a low ANC

Generally, an ANC of 500 to 1,000 provides children enough protective neutrophils to fight off exposure to infection due to bacteria and viruses. With an ANC this high, you can usually allow your child to attend all normal functions such as school, athletics, and parties. However, it is wise to keep close track of the pattern of the rise and fall of your child's ANC. If you know the ANC is 1,000, but is on the way down, it will affect what activities are appropriate for your child. Each hospital has different guidelines concerning activities for children with low ANCs.

Following are parent suggestions to prevent and detect infections:

- Insist on frequent, thorough hand washing for every member of the family. Use plenty of soap and warm water, lather well, and rub all portions of the hands. Children and parents need to wash before preparing meals, before eating, after playing outdoors, and after using the bathroom.

    We always had antibacterial baby wipes in our car. We washed Justin's hands, and our own, after going to any public places such as parks, museums, or restaurants. They can also be used to wipe off tables or high chairs at restaurants.

- Make sure all medical personnel at the hospital or doctor's office thoroughly wash their hands before touching your child.

    Nurses and doctors frequently come into the room and don't wash their hands. I make them wash their hands, change their gloves, or squirt Purell® on them. I always had a bottle of Purell® with me. They would say that they washed their hands before they came into the room. Well, you just touched the doorknob and you have to wash them again. I had a situation like this with our oncologist. He washed his hands, and then right before starting Zoe's spinal, his cell phone rang and he answered it. He started to proceed, and I stopped him and told him to wash his hands again because he touched the cell phone. He was taken aback for a second, and then agreed. Fortunately, he is a great guy and has fun ribbing me about my overprotective nature and attention to detail (I doubt these are the exact words he uses to describe me).

- Keep your young child's diaper area and skin creases clean and dry.

- When your child's ANC is low, make arrangements with your pediatrician to use a back entrance to the office to avoid exposure to sick kids in the waiting room. It sometimes helps to make all appointments for early morning so your child can be seen in a room that hasn't already had several sick children in it.

- Whenever your child needs a needle stick, make sure the technician cleans your child's skin thoroughly with both betadine and alcohol.

- If your child gets a small cut, wash it with soap and water, rinse it with hydrogen peroxide, and cover it with a small bandage.

- When your child is ill, take his temperature every 2 to 3 hours. Call the doctor if your child's temperature is 101° F (38.5° C) or above.

- Do not permit anyone to take your child's temperature rectally (in the anus) or use rectal suppositories, as these may cause anal tears and increase the risk of infection and bleeding.

> Believe it or not, we once stopped the nursing assistant from doing a rectal temp during an inpatient admission. When we had a room on the pediatric oncology side, this never happened. But for that admission those rooms were full, and we were on the other side of the floor.

- Do not use a humidifier, as the stagnant water can become a reservoir for contamination.

- Apply sunscreen whenever your child plays outdoors. Children taking certain chemotherapy drugs, such as methotrexate, or who have recently received cranial radiation therapy are sun sensitive, and a bad sunburn can easily become infected.

- Your child should not receive routine immunizations while on chemotherapy. Your physician or nurse can prepare medical exemption cards for your child's school.

- Siblings should not be vaccinated with the live polio virus (OPV); they should get the killed polio virus (IPV). Verify that your pediatrician is using the appropriate vaccine for the siblings.

> Katy was diagnosed just a week after her younger sister, Alison, had been given the live polio vaccine. Because there was a small risk that Alison could infect any immunosuppressed child with polio, she was not allowed to visit the cancer floor of the hospital.

- If your child's ANC is low, an infected site may not become red or painful.

> My daughter kept getting ear infections while on chemotherapy. They would find them during routine exams. I felt guilty because she never told me her ears were hurting. I told her doctor that I was worried because she didn't complain of pain, and he reassured me by telling me that she probably felt no pain because she didn't have enough white cells to cause swelling inside her ear.

• • • • •

> Shawn had continual ear infections while on treatment. He had two sets of tubes surgically implanted while on chemotherapy.

- Never give aspirin for fever. Aspirin or drugs containing aspirin interfere with blood clotting. Ibuprofen may be given if approved by your child's oncologist. If your child has a fever, call the doctor before giving any medication.

- Ask your child's oncologist about using a stool softener if your child has problems with constipation. Stool softeners can help prevent anal tears.

- Call the doctor if any of the following symptoms appear: fever above 101° F (38.5° C), chills, cough, shortness of breath, sore throat, severe diarrhea, bloody urine or stool, and pain or burning while urinating.

> *Some people choose to keep their kids away from everything and everyone during treatment, while others restrict their activities when they're neutropenic or receiving a particularly heavy dose of chemo. You will learn how to trust your instincts and your doctor's advice, and also learn how to take your cues from your child. For us, we try to walk a fine line between keeping Hunter's life as normal and stimulating as possible, while not taking any foolish risks with his health. When he's neutropenic (ANC below 500), when he's in a particularly heavy round of chemo, or when there's chicken pox going around we keep him at home. When he's doing well then we take him out a bit more, but sensibly: no shopping malls on Saturdays, no contact with anyone who's sick, and limited contact with other kids. During the week, I will take him with me to the grocery store, or to see his grandparents or cousins, provided everyone is healthy. When he's feeling well we also go to the park, ride our bikes, and do normal kid stuff. I carry around antibacterial hand wipes with me so I can keep him clean after playgrounds.*

Serious illnesses

Two illnesses that are especially dangerous for children during treatment are pneumonia and chicken pox.

Pneumonia

Pneumonia is inflammation of the lungs caused primarily by bacteria, viruses, or other organisms. The symptoms of pneumonia are rapid breathing, chills, fever, chest pain, cough, and bloody sputum. Children with low blood counts can rapidly develop a fatal infection and must be treated quickly and aggressively. Most cancer centers recommend an annual influenza (flu) shot to help prevent pneumonia.

> *My son received his high-dose methotrexate and vincristine injection just days before he was scheduled to go to the American Cancer Society's camp. His ANC was 1,200 and he looked so sick, but he begged to go and I let him. It was early in his treatment, and I didn't realize the pattern of his blood counts. They called me from camp on Friday to say he had a temperature of 103° and needed to go to the hospital. He*

was very weak and feverish; his WBC was 140, and his ANC was 0. Both lungs were full of pneumonia. I was furious at the doctor for giving him permission to go to camp and at myself for not paying closer attention to how quickly his counts dropped. I'm sure he had the pneumonia before he even went to camp. They started him on five different antibiotics, and his fever went up to 106° that night. We didn't know if he would live or die. He started to improve the next morning and was completely recovered in a week.

• • • • •

At the beginning of interim maintenance, Justin developed a fever. His oncologist said to give him Tylenol® and to call if it didn't go down. The next day he was breathing faster and his little hands and feet were turning purple. We rushed him to the hospital, and the chest x-rays showed pneumonia in both lungs. He rapidly deteriorated over the next 48 hours, so they tried an experimental constant flow ventilator that had only been used on premature infants. It was the last-ditch effort to save his life. He gradually improved. He spent a total of 5 months in the hospital, 4 more months on a portable ventilator at home with full-time nursing care, and he breathed through his tracheostomy until he completed his treatment 2 years later. It was a miracle.

• • • • •

Erica complained that her back hurt for 2 days. Then she woke up in the night crying, and she couldn't move because it hurt her too badly. She was blazing with fever, and screamed if I touched her. Her x-ray showed that her left lung was half full of fluid. They put her on antibiotics, and within 24 hours she was on the mend.

Children taking steroids (e.g., prednisone, dexamethasone) are at increased risk for contracting serious and potentially life-threatening lung infections from an organism called Pneumocystis jiroveci. In most cases, the infection can be prevented by taking trimethoprim-sulfamethoxazole (brand names Septra®, Bactrim®) 2 or 3 days per week.

Chicken pox

Chicken pox is a common childhood disease (although less so than it used to be because of the vaccine) caused by a virus called varicella zoster. The symptoms are headaches, fever, and tiredness, followed by eruptions of pimple-like red bumps that typically start on the stomach, chest, or back. The bumps rapidly develop into blister-like sores that break open, then scab over in 3 to 5 days. Any contact with the sores can spread the disease. Children are contagious up to 48 hours before breaking out.

Chicken pox can be a fatal disease for immunosuppressed children, so extreme care must be taken to prevent exposure. You will need to educate all teachers and friends so they will vigilantly report any outbreaks. Your child should not go to school or pre-school until the outbreak is over.

Chicken pox can be transmitted through the air or by touch. Exposure is considered to have occurred if a child is in direct contact or in a room for as little as 10 minutes with an infected person. If your child has never had chicken pox, it is better to take him to beaches or parks rather than indoor play areas.

If an immunosuppressed child is exposed to chicken pox, call the doctor immediately. If the doctor gives a shot called VZIG (varicella zoster immune globulin) within 72 hours of exposure, it may prevent the disease from occurring or minimize its effects.

> We knew when Jeremy was exposed, so he was able to get VZIG. He did get chicken pox, but only developed a few spots. He didn't get sick; he got bored. He spent 2 weeks in the hospital in isolation. We asked for a pass, and we were able to go outside for some fresh air between doses of acyclovir.

If a child develops chicken pox while on chemotherapy, the current treatment is hospitalization or, if possible, home therapy for IV administration of acyclovir, a potent antiviral medication that has dramatically lowered the complication rate of chicken pox.

> Kristin broke out with chicken pox on the Fourth of July weekend. Our hospital room was the best seat in the house for watching the city fireworks. She did get covered with pox, though, from the soles of her feet to the very top of her scalp. We'd just give her gauze pads soaked in calamine lotion and let her hermetically seal herself. They kept her in the hospital for 6 days of IV acyclovir; then she was at home on the pump (a small computerized machine that will administer the drug in small amounts for several hours) for 4 more days of acyclovir. She had no complications.

A child who has already had chicken pox may develop herpes zoster (shingles). If your child develops eruptions of vesicles similar to chicken pox that are in lines (along nerves), call the doctor. The treatment for shingles is identical to that for chicken pox.

> Kristin also got a herpes zoster infection, this time on Thanksgiving. It looked like a mild case of chicken pox, limited to her upper right arm, her upper right chest, and her right leg. They kept her overnight on IV acyclovir and then let her go home for 9 more days on the pump.

Untreated chicken pox or shingles can result in life-threatening complications including pneumonia, hepatitis, and encephalitis. Parents must make every effort to prevent exposure and watch for signs of these diseases while their child is on treatment.

Diarrhea

Because chemotherapy destroys all cells that are produced at a rapid rate, such as those that line the mouth, stomach, and intestines, it can cause diarrhea, ranging from mild (frequent, soft stools) to severe (abundant quantities of liquid stool). Diarrhea during chemotherapy can also be caused by some antinausea drugs, antibiotics, and intestinal infections. After chemotherapy ends and immune function returns to normal, the lining of the digestive tract heals and the diarrhea ends.

The following suggestions for coping with diarrhea come from parents:

- Do not give any over-the-counter drug to your child without approval from the oncologist. He may want to test your child's stool for infection prior to treating the diarrhea. Frequently recommended drugs for diarrhea are Kaopectate®, Lomotil®, and Immodium®.

- It is very important that your child drink plenty of liquids. The liquids will not increase the diarrhea, but they will replace the lost fluids.

  My 3 year old had stopped drinking from bottles months before her diagnosis. When she first began her intensive chemotherapy, she had uncontrollable, frequent diarrhea. Liquid would just gush out without warning. It was hard for her to drink from a cup, so one night she said in a small voice, "Mommy, would it be okay if I drank from a bottle again?" I said, "Of course, honey." It was a great comfort to her, and she took in a lot more fluids that way.

- Hot or cold liquids can increase intestinal contractions, so give your child lots of room-temperature clear liquids or mild juices such as water, Gatorade®, ginger ale, peach juice, or apricot nectar.

- Diarrhea depletes the body's supply of potassium, so give your child foods high in potassium, such as bananas, oranges, baked or mashed potatoes without the skin, broccoli, halibut, mushrooms, asparagus, tomato juice, and milk (if tolerated).

- Low potassium can cause irregular heartbeats and leg cramps. If these occur, call the doctor.

- Do not serve greasy, fatty, spicy, or sweet foods.

- Do not serve foods high in fiber such as bran, fruits (dried or fresh), nuts, beans, or raw vegetables.

- Serve bland, low-fiber foods such as bananas, white rice, noodles, applesauce, unbuttered white toast, creamed cereals, cottage cheese, fish, and chicken or turkey without the skin.

  In the middle of maintenance, my son had severe diarrhea for a week. He had large amounts of liquid stools 20 times a day. I felt so sorry for him. The doctor cultured a stool specimen, but they never identified a cause. It cleared up after a week of the BRAT diet (bananas, rice, applesauce, toast). He had a problem with diarrhea almost weekly throughout his treatment.

- Keep a record of the number of bowel movements and their volume to keep the doctor informed. Call the doctor if you notice any blood in the stool, or if your child has any signs of dehydration such as dry skin, dry mouth, sunken eyes, decreased urination, or dizziness.

- Keep the area around the anus clean and dry. Wash with warm water and mild soap after every bowel movement, then gently pat the area dry.

- If your child's anus is sore, check with the doctor before using any non-prescription medicine. She may recommend using Desitin®, A&D ointment®, or Bag Balm® after each bowel movement.

> *While taking ARA-C my daughter had a terribly sore rectum, which was a big problem. It hurt to have bowel movements, she'd cry and have to squeeze our hands to go, then the urine would run back and burn. She was very itchy. We carried around bags with Q-tips® and every known brand of rectal ointment—A&D®, Preparation H®, Desitin®, and Benadryl®. Thank goodness this cleared up quickly on maintenance.*

- Call the doctor if your child has significant pain with bowel movements, especially if your child has low blood counts.

Constipation

Constipation means a decrease in a child's normal number of bowel movements or dry, hard stool that is painful to pass. There are many reasons constipation occurs when children are on chemotherapy. Some drugs, such as vincristine, slow the movement of stool through the intestines, resulting in constipation. Pain medication, decreased activity, decreased eating and drinking, and vomiting can all affect the normal rhythm of the intestine. When movement through the intestine slows, stools become hard and dry, and they can be painful to pass.

Following are parents' suggestions for preventing and helping constipation:

- Encourage your child to be as physically active as possible.

- Encourage your child to drink plenty of liquids every day. Prune juice is especially helpful.

- Serve high-fiber foods such as raw vegetables, beans, bran, graham crackers, whole-wheat breads, whole-grain cereals, dried fruits (especially prunes, dates, and raisins), and nuts.

- Check with the doctor before using any medications for constipation. He may recommend a stool softener such as Colace®. If the doctor suggests liquid Docusate®, be aware that many children don't like the taste. Senokot®, another frequently prescribed stool softener, comes in a tablet or chocolate-flavored liquid and granules that can be mixed into yogurt or ice cream. Metamucil® and Citrucel® increase the volume of the stool, which stimulates the intestine. Milk of Magnesia®, magnesium citrate, and MiraLax® help the stool retain fluid and remain soft.

> *Vincristine constipation resulted in horrible screaming, bottom itching, constant trips to the bathroom with no luck, for days at a time. It is absolutely frustrating! We now have a preventative routine so that never happens again. Beginning the morning of a vincristine injection, I give one Peri-Colace® (stool softener plus laxative) each morning and evening until things improve—which is usually after about a week or so. Then, I taper down to one a day until things seem to be getting on the too soft side, then stop. The Peri-Colace® is manufactured in a brown "soft-gel" thing, and the liquid inside it tastes horrible. If at any time during our Peri-Colace® phase there are 2 consecutive days with no bowel movements, I give bisacodyl in the evening of the second day, and things usually get straightened out the next morning. Unfortunately, if it's a school day, I have to keep him home until mid-morning, as the prednisone diet and laxatives lead to a very busy morning in the bathroom.*

- Do not give enemas or rectal suppositories. These can cause anal tears that can be dangerous for a child with a weakened immune system.

- When your child feels the need to have a bowel movement, sipping a warm drink can help the feces come out.

> *My 4-year-old daughter either had diarrhea or severe constipation for the entire 8 months of intensive treatment. Her bowel habits returned to normal during maintenance. When constipated, she would just sob and try to hold it in. This made her stool even harder and more painful. One time she cried, "Why is my anus round and my poop square?" We ended up just putting her in a warm bathtub, gave her warm drinks, and let her go in the bathtub.*

Fatigue and weakness

Fatigue, a feeling of weariness, is an almost universal side effect of treatment for cancer. General weakness, while different from fatigue, is caused by many of the same things and is treated the same way. Fatigue and weakness may be constant throughout therapy or intermittent. They can be minor annoyances or totally debilitating. Many parents worry that if fatigue is present, so is the cancer. But, fatigue and weakness are usually caused by one, or a combination, of the following things:

- Your child's body working overtime to heal tissues damaged by treatment and to rid itself of dead and dying cancer cells

- Medications to treat nausea or pain

- Mineral imbalances caused by chemotherapy, diarrhea, or vomiting

- Infections

- Emotional factors such as anxiety, fear, sadness, depression, or frustration

- Malnutrition caused by nausea, vomiting, loss of appetite, or taste aversions

- Anemia (low red cell count)

- Cranial radiation

- Disruption of normal sleep patterns (common when hospitalized or when taking some drugs, such as steroids).

> My son is almost 19 and is just beginning his third year of maintenance for ALL (acute lymphoblastic leukemia). He is a quiet and studious young man, has never dated, and does not go about partying and the like. The last 3 months, he appears to be all right, but he is, in his own words, always "exhausted." In college and living in the dorm, he can get up in the morning at 6 a.m., but if he has two classes in a row, he is quite likely to fall asleep during the second class. He's too tired to concentrate on homework for more than an hour at a time. Before diagnosis, a 50-mile bike ride was nothing to him. Even 6 months ago he could ride 30 miles, although he did feel some fatigue. Now, his beloved bike rests gathering dust. It breaks my heart that my son cannot feel the exuberance of young adulthood that I experienced at his age, but I am so very thankful that the treatment for leukemia has saved his life. I hope that when he is off treatment he will finally feel good again.

Following are suggestions from parents:

- Make sure your child gets plenty of rest. Naps or quiet times spaced throughout the day help.

> Erica took a 2½ hour nap every afternoon throughout therapy. She's 4 now and off treatment, but her endurance is low and she still tires easily.

- Limit visitors if your child is weak or fatigued.

> While in the hospital, my daughter was very weak. She had too many visitors, yet didn't want to hurt anyone's feelings. We worked out a signal that solved the problem. When she was too tired to continue a visit, she would place a damp washcloth on her forehead. I would then politely end the visit.

- Serve your child well-balanced meals and snacks, but don't get upset if he doesn't eat them (see next point about stress).

- Parents and children should try to avoid physical and emotional stress.

- Encourage your child to pursue hobbies or interests, if able. For example, if your child is too weak to play on his athletic team, let him go to cheer the team on.

My eighth-grade daughter was a fabulous athlete prior to her cancer diagnosis. When she went back to school after missing a year, she wasn't very competitive, but she managed the softball team and dressed for basketball. So she was still part of the social scene and was able to do things with the teams.

• Help your child make a prioritized list of activities. If he feels strongly that he wants to attend a certain event and you think he may run out of energy, throw a wheelchair or stroller into the car and go.

• Encourage your child to attend a kid or teen support group, and go to the parent group yourself. Seeing that others have the same problems and talking about how you are feeling can lighten the load.

Many children go through the low- or average-risk protocols for leukemia without fatigue or weakness, while other children are not so lucky. The following are two typical stories.

Before Brent was diagnosed at age 6, he was exceptionally well coordinated and a very fast runner. During treatment, he slowed down to about average. He played soccer and T-ball throughout, and was very competitive.

· · · · ·

Jeremy has had some major, persistent problems with weakness and loss of coordination. When he was 9 years old, a year off therapy, he still could not catch a ball. When he ran, he was like a robot, and the trunk of his body stayed straight. Some kids made fun of him, and he got very frustrated with himself. He had lots of physical therapy, and now, 3 years off chemotherapy, his skills have improved, but he still has to work harder than the other kids. We put him into martial arts in hopes of further increasing his motor skills and his confidence.

Bed wetting

Bed wetting can be a very upsetting side effect of chemotherapy. Some drugs increase thirst, while others disrupt normal sleep patterns, both of which can make bed wetting more likely. Lots of IV fluids at night are a problem for some children. When the bed wetting is caused by drugs or IVs, time will cure the problem. Once the drug or extra fluid is no longer needed, the bed wetting will stop.

There are also psychological reasons for bed wetting during chemotherapy. The trauma of cancer treatment causes many children to regress to earlier behaviors such as thumb sucking, baby talk, temper tantrums, and bed wetting. Punishment for this type of bed wetting only adds to the child's trauma and rarely solves the problem. Following are parents' suggestions:

- Use super-absorbant and disposable undersheets, or double-sheet the bed. Put down one plastic liner with fitted and flat sheets, then put another plastic liner with a fitted and flat sheet on top of it. During the night, simply pull off the wet top sheets and plastic and there are fresh sheets below.

- For younger children, you can use disposable, absorbant underwear.

- Keep a pile of extra-large or beach towels next to the bed. Cover the wet spot with towels and save the bed change for the morning.

- Give the last drink 2 hours before bedtime so the child's bladder can be totally emptied right before bed.

- Change sleeping arrangements.

> *Prednisone caused my child to have nightmares and frequent bed wetting. I felt if she could sleep through the night, the bed wetting might stop. I told her she could sleep with me for the month that she was on prednisone, but that after that she would move back into her own bed. It calmed her to sleep with me. The nightmares and bed wetting decreased, and she moved back into her own bed without complaint when the time came.*

- Adopt an attitude that lets your child know bed wetting is "no big deal." There should be no shaming or punishment.

- If your child is extremely distressed by his bed wetting, ask if he wants you to set the alarm for the middle of the night so he can get up and go to the bathroom.

> *Alex was potty-trained during consolidation. He would get major hydration with the high-dose methotrexate, but he never had an accident. We brought his potty with us to the hospital and kept it right next to his bed. If he had to go during the night he would just get out of bed and go. It worked out really well, and you can empty it in the morning.*

- Give extra love and reassurance.

> *When my daughter started bed wetting, I didn't think it was the drugs. I thought long and hard about any additional worries that she might have, and I realized that because her dad had emotionally withdrawn from her during her illness, she might be worried that I would do the same. So I told her one night, "You know, I just real- ized that every day I tell you how much I love you. But I've never told you that no matter how hard life gets and no matter how mad we get at each other, I will always love you. I love you now as a child, I will love you as a teenager, and I will love you when you are all grown up." She started to sob and hugged and hugged me. She has never wet the bed again.*

My teenaged son wet the bed whenever he was given antinausea medicine prior to high doses of chemotherapy. He was so embarrassed. I stayed with him every night at the hospital. He was so groggy that even if he woke up in time, I had to help him out of bed and support him while he stood, half asleep, to use the urinal.

. . . . .

My son wet the bed before, during, and after the 3 years of his treatment for ALL. We just kept him in diapers at night. He would absolutely flood the bed while on prednisone. After he completed treatment, they put him on a drug called DDAVP to help cure the bed wetting.

Dental problems

Both cranial radiation and chemotherapy can cause changes in the mouth and teeth. Awareness of the potential problems, coupled with good preventive care, can help maintain oral health during treatment.

Some anticancer drugs and radiation can cause changes in children's ability to salivate. Plaque may build up rapidly on your child's teeth, increasing the chance for both cavities and gum infections. Take your child to the dentist for a cleaning and check-up every 3 to 4 months, as long as his counts are good (an ANC of more than 1,000 and platelets of more than 100,000). If your child has a central venous catheter, he should be given antibiotics before and after each visit to the dentist. Ask your dentist to refer to the current issue of the *Pediatric Dentistry Reference Manual* to formulate a dental plan.

Ask your child's oncologist and dentist for advice about tooth care when counts are very low. Often parents are advised to use a sponge or damp gauze to gently wipe off their child's teeth after meals instead of brushing.

> *My daughter had problems with thick yellow saliva during the entire time she was treated. It coated her teeth and formed a lot of plaque. I brought her to an excellent pediatric dentist every 3 months to have the plaque removed. She took antibiotics half an hour before treatment and then again 6 hours afterward. He also put sealants on all of her molars and, even though there were many weeks when her teeth could not be brushed, she never got a cavity.*

Some parents report delays in the arrival of their child's permanent teeth. Children who receive chemotherapy or cranial radiation therapy may also have poorly developed or absent permanent teeth and blunted tooth roots, increasing the possibility of premature tooth loss.

Mouth and throat sores

The mouth, throat, and intestines are lined with cells that divide rapidly and can be severely damaged by chemotherapy drugs. This is more common for children on very intensive protocols and for those having stem cell transplants. The sores are extremely painful and can prevent eating and drinking. Check your child's mouth periodically for sores, and if any are present ask the oncologist for advice. Following are some suggestions from parents:

- To prevent infection, the mouth needs to be kept as clean and free of bacteria as possible. After eating, have your child gently brush teeth, gums, and tongue with a soft, clean toothbrush.

- If your child is old enough, the doctor may recommend a rinse to decrease the amount of bacteria in your child's mouth, which may help prevent mouth sores.

> When David was told to use Peridex®, I asked the doctor if we could substitute 0.63 percent stannous fluoride rinse. He said yes. As a dentist, I knew Peridex® kills bacteria and lasts up to 8 hours, but it tastes terrible and stains teeth. Children do not like using it. The 0.63 percent stannous fluoride has the same bacteria-killing properties and also lasts up to 8 hours, but has a better taste and does not stain as badly. The fluoride also helps prevent cavities and makes the teeth less sensitive. It comes in a variety of flavors like mint, tropical, and cinnamon. It is a prescription drug that a lot of dentists dispense.
>
> Mix ⅛ ounce of concentrate with warm water, making 1 ounce. A measuring cup comes with the bottle. I have David swish with half the mixture for 1 minute. (Time it, because it's longer than you think!) This can only be used by kids who are old enough not to accidentally swallow it. Six-year-old David has no problem taking this once a day before he goes to bed. If and when he starts developing mouth sores, he will take it morning and evening. It's important not to eat or drink for 30 minutes after rinsing. That is why David rinses before bedtime, after he has taken his meds and brushed his teeth.

- Keep a record of what your child eats and drinks. Your child may need prescription pain medication to allow him to swallow and take adequate fluids.

- Serve bland food, baby food, or meals put through the blender.

- Use a straw with drinks or blender-processed foods.

> Preston got bad mouth sores every time he was on high-dose methotrexate. He could not swallow, but we were supposed to be forcing fluids to flush the drugs out. The only thing that felt good on his throat was guava nectar. It was very expensive and hard to find, and he would drink several quarts a day. Unfortunately, my daughter and husband both developed a liking for it, too. At one point we cornered the market on guava nectar at three grocery stores in our neighborhood.

- There are several prescription products available to treat mouth sores. One common product is called "magic mouthwash," which contains an antibiotic, an antihistamine, an antifungal, and an antacid. Some formulations add dexamethasone. More information about this product is available at *www.mayoclinic.com/health/magic-mouthwash/AN02024*. If your child has painful mouth sores, ask the oncologist for a prescription. Because large amounts of lidocaine can numb the back of the throat and cause difficulty swallowing, this medication should be used at a dose recommended by the oncologist.

Glutamine, a nutritional supplement available at most drug and health food stores, may help prevent or minimize mouth sores in some children. If your child is receiving chemotherapy with a high probability of causing mouth sores, you may want to try glutamine as a prophylactic measure. The powder can be mixed in juice and should be started 1 or 2 days before your child receives a cycle of chemotherapy. Be sure to get your oncologist's approval before starting this treatment.

Changes in taste and smell

Chemotherapy can cause changes in the taste buds, altering the brain's perception of how food tastes. Meats often taste bitter, and sweets can taste unpleasant. Even foods that children crave can taste bad. The sense of smell is also impacted by chemotherapy, heightening smells that other family members do not notice and sometimes causing nausea in a child on chemotherapy.

Both the senses of smell and taste can take months to return to normal after chemotherapy ends.

> *Once Katy begged me to make her my special double chocolate sour cream cake. Surprisingly, it smelled really good to her as it baked. She took a big bite, spit it out all over the table, and ran back to her room sobbing. She cried for a long time. She told me later that it had tasted "bitter and horrible."*

Skin and nail problems

Minor skin problems are frequent while on chemotherapy. The most common problems are rashes, redness, itching, peeling, dry skin, and acne. Following are suggestions for preventing and treating skin problems:

- Avoid hot showers or baths, as these can dry the skin.
- Use moisturizing soap.
- Apply a water-based moisturizer after bathing.

- Avoid scratchy materials such as wool. Your child may feel more comfortable in loose, cotton clothing.

- Have your child use sunscreen with a sun protection factor of at least SPF 30. This is especially important for areas that have been irradiated.

- Insist on head coverings or sunscreen every time your child goes outdoors if she child is bald, especially if she has had cranial radiation.

- Buy your child lip gloss with sunscreen.

   Matthew's lips would get very dry and eventually start to peel. It irritated him, and he developed a habit of biting on his lips. To minimize the problem I learned that wiping a cool, wet cloth over his mouth many times a day worked well. I would then apply a light coating of Vaseline® to his lips to keep them moist.

- Rub cornstarch on itchy skin to help sooth it.

If your child has chemotherapy drugs injected into the veins (rather than a central catheter), you may notice a darkening along the veins; this will fade after treatment ends. However, skin and underlying tissues can be damaged or destroyed by drugs that leak out of a vein. If your child feels a stinging or burning sensation, or if you notice swelling at the IV site, call a nurse immediately.

Call the doctor anytime your child gets a severe rash or is very itchy. Scratching rashes can cause infections, so you need to get medications to control the itching.

Chemotherapy affects the growing portion of nails located under the cuticle. After chemotherapy, you may notice a white band or ridge across the nail as it grows out. These brittle bands are sometimes elevated and feel bumpy. As the white ridge grows out toward the end of the finger, the nail may break. Keeping your child's fingernails trimmed can help prevent breakage.

Steroid problems

Most children with leukemia require therapy with steroid medications at intervals throughout treatment. Prednisone, dexamethasone, hydrocortisone, and others in this category can cause many unpleasant side effects, including fluid retention, high blood pressure, elevated blood sugar, sleep disturbances, muscle weakness, cataracts, and loss of bone mass. Most children and teens experience profound mood swings and are very emotional. For more information about steroids, see Chapter 9, "Chemotherapy."

Learning disabilities

Some children who have been treated for leukemia are at risk for developing learning disabilities as a consequence of their treatment. Those at highest risk are children under 5 years old who receive both cranial radiation and intrathecal methotrexate, children who received high-dose methotrexate, and young children who are given significant amounts of intrathecal methotrexate. There is considerable research about the types of learning difficulties exhibited by these children. This topic is covered in Chapter 15, "School."

Uncommon but serious side effects

Intracranial hypertension (IH)

This condition, also known as pseudotumor cerebri, is rare but serious. IH is an excess of cerebral spinal fluid, resulting in increased intracranial pressure in the absence of a tumor. IH has not been well researched in children. While no specific causes have been identified, steroids are known to temporarily raise intracranial pressure. Symptoms can include, but are not limited to: debilitating pain in the head; changes in vision; a whooshing noise in one or both ears; profound fatigue; changes in personality and behavior (e.g., irritability, obsessiveness, rage, excessive crying) that get worse as the intracranial pressure rises; problems with short-term memory; and difficulties maintaining balance. The condition is initially treated by decreasing or eliminating doses of methotrexate and steroids, and giving one of two drugs that decrease the amount of cerebrospinal fluid—Diamox® and Neptazane®. If this condition is suspected, the child or teen should immediately be seen by a neuro-ophthalmologist with expertise in IH, because permanent damage may occur if the condition is not diagnosed and treated quickly. General information is available from the Intracranial Hypertension Research Foundation at *www.ihrfoundation.org*.

> *My daughter, Avalon, was diagnosed with ALL at 17 months old. During the delayed intensification phase of treatment, Avalon developed a line infection, which was unsuccessfully treated with antibiotics. During one of the resulting hospitalizations, Avalon became very sound-sensitive and began grabbing at her ears. Being only 22 months old, Avalon was incapable of verbally communicating her issues, and we were left scrambling, trying to understand them.*
>
> *For the next year, Avalon displayed what can be considered common chemo side effects: lethargy, sound/light sensitivities, poor balance, irritability. One interesting side note though, Avalon's poor balance was blamed on vincristine, yet she exhibited no tightening of her tendons. Finally, nearly a year after the original symptoms, Avalon began to fall asleep at inappropriate times. When this happened in clinic in front of the attending, it was deemed that Avalon may have a problem.*

During a scheduled lumbar puncture, Avalon's intracranial pressure was measured at 32, roughly 3 times normal parameters. Following examination of Avalon's optic nerves by a neuro-ophthalmologist, she was officially diagnosed with intracranial hypertension. By that time, she had lost nearly 70% of her peripheral vision. The pressure affects various other nerves, resulting in poor balance and irregular heart rates. Avalon experiences tinnitus that increases in severity as her intracranial pressure increases. Through the years we have learned to gauge Avalon's intracranial pressures by how loud she is, or how often she complains of an inability to hear the television; both are signs of increased tinnitus. We also look for increased agitation and frustration. Avalon also seems to slow down cognitively when pressure is high. She becomes tired easily, and has difficulty focusing on detailed tasks.

In children, IH will often resolve after the stressor on the body is removed (i.e., when chemo ends). Avalon's pressure did not respond as such. She has had three surgeries, including temporal decompressions—holes in the side of her skull to increase the size of her cranial vault. So far, Avalon's vision has been maintained, but energy, cognition, and hearing have all been affected. She continues to fight the increasing pressures.

Osteonecrosis

Osteonecrosis, also called avascular necrosis (AVN), is a condition caused by the death of small blood vessels that nourish the bones and joints. In children and teens treated for leukemia, it is caused by the use of steroids; it is more commonly caused by dexamethasone than prednisone (except when prednisone is given in high doses for long periods of times, such as for children who relapse or who are treated with stem cell transplants). AVN is much more common in children older than 10; however, on protocols that use dexamethasone exclusively, it is being seen in younger children more often. The course of the disease is variable. Some children and teens have the condition for years with only minor problems with pain and movement, but others require one or more surgeries soon after the condition is diagnosed. The website for an international support group is *http://avnsupport.org*.

At the beginning of long-term maintenance (COG trial AALL0331 augmented therapy), my 6-year-old daughter, Emilie, said that her arms hurt at night, so we did some research and learned quite a bit about AVN from the ALL-KIDS list on www.acor.org. Our nurse practitioner is very good, but we had to push to get an x-ray done. When substantial AVN was confirmed in Emilie's left shoulder, she had an MRI of both shoulders and finally a nuclear bone scan of her entire body to see if it was in any of the other joints. The bone scan did not show any damage to other joints, but Emilie's knees hurt after an active day, so it may be starting there as well. Our oncologist took her off the steroids, and I had to get my head wrapped around that, which was hard for me. But, he believed her body had probably had enough and he was not concerned regarding her prognosis. We met with an orthopedic surgeon and he recommended that a procedure called small-diameter percutaneous decompression be done on both shoulders. She had the surgery 2 months ago. Within 2 weeks her symptoms disappeared in both shoulders and the x-rays 6 weeks later showed stabilization, so it was very effective. I am so glad that we did it.

Can pets transmit diseases?

It is very unlikely that your child will be harmed from living with a household pet, but several common-sense precautions are needed to protect a child with a low ANC from disease, worms, or infection:

- Make sure your pet is vaccinated against all possible diseases.

- Have pets checked for worms as soon as possible after your child is diagnosed, and then every year thereafter (more often for puppies). Give preventative treatments to your pets as directed by your veterinarian.

- Do not let pets eat off plates or lick your child's face.

- Keep children away from the cat litter box and any animal feces outdoors.

- Have all of your children wash their hands after playing with the pet.

- Make sure your pet has no ticks or fleas.

- If you have a pet that bites or scratches, consider finding another home for it. But if you have a gentle, well-loved pet, do not give it up.

> *I think parents should know that you should not automatically get rid of your dog because your child has a low ANC. We went through a small crisis trying to decide whether to give away our large but beloved mongrel. The doctors wouldn't really give us a straight answer, but a parent in the support group said, "DO NOT get rid of your dog. Your son will need that dog's love and company in the years ahead." She was right. The dog was a tremendous comfort to our son.*

If your child wants to buy a pet while undergoing cancer treatment, follow these guidelines:

- Do not get a puppy. All puppies bite while teething, increasing the chance that your child may contract an infection.

- Do not get a parrot or parakeet, as these species can transmit an infection called psittacosis to humans.

- Do not get a turtle or other reptile (e.g., snake, iguana) as they sometimes carry salmonella.

- Avoid buying any animal that is likely to bite or scratch.

We bought Sarah an older puppy. We were very selective about the breeder and the breed. The dog has given my little girl back to me. After she got the dog, she started to want to walk again. She started to laugh. She had reason to think beyond herself and how terrible this illness is. She had someone who needed her. Someone who was delighted to see her and made her feel special in a way no human can. It literally transformed my child.

The dog's name is Libbe, and after having Libbe for about a week, Sarah started asking when Libbe was going to die. She knew Libbe was just a puppy, but she really was asking about herself. We were able to tell her that Libbe will be around when she is a teenager and she can take Libbe with her on those big-girl sleepovers. Heck, she could take Libbe in the car for a ride, if she wanted. She beamed. It put the death and dying issue to rest.

If you have any concerns or questions about pets you already own or are thinking about purchasing, ask your oncologist and veterinarian for advice.

There were times during my son's protocol that I felt he suffered more from the side effects of treatment than from the disease. It was emotionally painful for me to watch him go through so much. I think one of the hardest moments for me was the day he lost all his hair. Up until that point I had been living in a semi-state of denial. His bald head was more proof of our reality—he really did have cancer.

I had to learn how to accept our situation, because I needed to be strong for my child. To get through, I reminded myself every day that the treatments were necessary, and that without them he would die. It was a struggle, but the unpleasant side effects soon passed, and he was able to resume his normal activities. I was constantly amazed at his resilience.

Chapter 11

Radiation Therapy

Nothing is so strong as gentleness,
and nothing is so gentle as true strength.

— St. Francis De Sales

RADIATION THERAPY has improved survival rates of children with high-risk leukemia. However, radiation therapy to the brain, spine, or testes can cause mild, short-term side effects; it can also lead to permanent damage that may not be evident until months or years after treatment. The benefits and risks of radiation treatment must be carefully weighed by both doctors and parents.

This chapter describes radiation therapy, explains when and how it is used, and outlines its potential side effects. It also contains stories to help prepare parents and children for treatment.

Radiation

Radiation treatment, also called irradiation or radiotherapy, is the use of high-energy x-rays to kill cancer cells. A large machine called a linear accelerator directs x-rays to the precise portion of the body needing treatment. The radiation is given in doses measured in units called centigrays (cGy).

Radiation is usually given every day for a specific number of days, excluding weekends; this schedule is called standard or conventional fractionation. Radiation given more than once a day is called accelerated fractionation, or hyperfractionation; this schedule uses smaller amounts of radiation during each treatment.

Children who need radiation therapy

Because of the possibility of long-term side effects from radiation, only a small percentage of children with leukemia receive radiation treatment. Some of the children for whom radiation is prescribed are:

- Children who have leukemia blasts in their central nervous system (CNS) at diagnosis.

- Children who are determined to be at extremely high risk for relapse in the CNS.

- Children who have relapsed in their CNS or testes.

- Children who require certain types of stem cell transplants.

Treatment for childhood leukemia is constantly evolving. Several ongoing clinical trials are evaluating alternative methods for preventing the spread of disease to the CNS. Perhaps in the near future, no child with leukemia will need radiation. But for now, although side effects occur, radiation to the brain provides children with certain types of very high-risk leukemia or CNS leukemia the best chance to be cured.

Questions to ask about radiation treatment

If radiation treatment has been recommended for your child, some questions you can ask the oncologist include:

- Why does my child need radiation?

- What type of radiation does she need?

- What part of his body will be treated with radiation?

- What is the total dose of radiation she will receive?

- How many treatments of radiation will he get?

- How much experience does this institution have with administering this type of radiation to children?

- How will she be positioned on the table?

- Will any restraints be used?

- Will anesthesia or sedation be needed?

- How long will each treatment take?

- What are the possible short-term and long-term side effects?

- Could this type and dosage of radiation cause cancer later?

- What are the alternatives to radiation?

- Are there any precautionary procedures that should be done prior to radiation therapy (such as moving the ovaries out of the radiation area or sperm banking) to prevent infertility?

Radiation therapy facilities

For optimal treatment, children should receive radiation therapy only at major medical centers with experience treating children with cancer. Do not go to a local radiation center or the radiation department in your community hospital. All treatments should be supervised by physicians who are board-certified or equally experienced in pediatric radiation oncology. State-of-the-art equipment, expert personnel, and vast experience with pediatric cancers are what you should look for when choosing a center.

Radiation oncologist

A radiation oncologist is a medical doctor with years of specialized training in using radiation to treat disease. Other names for this type of specialist are radiotherapist or therapeutic radiologist. In partnership with the pediatric oncologist, the radiation oncologist develops a treatment plan tailored specifically for each child.

The radiation oncologist will explain to you and your child what radiation is, how it will be administered, and any possible side effects. She will also answer all your questions regarding the proposed treatment. You will be given a consent form to review prior to the first treatment. Take the consent form home if you need extra time to read it. Parents should not sign the consent form until they thoroughly understand all benefits, risks, and possible side effects of the radiation. The radiation oncologist will meet at least weekly with the child and parents to discuss how the treatment is going and to address concerns or answer questions.

Radiation therapist

The radiation therapist is a specially trained technologist who operates the machine that delivers the radiation dose prescribed by the radiation oncologist. This member of the medical team will give your child a tour of the radiation room, explain about the equipment, and position your child for treatment. The technologist will operate the x-ray machine and monitor your child via a closed-circuit TV and a two-way intercom.

> When 3-year-old Katy was being given the tour of the radiation room by her technologist, Brian, he was just wonderful with her. He gave her a white stuffed bear, which he used to demonstrate the machine. He immobilized the bear on the table using Katy's mask (device to hold the head still during treatment), then moved the machine all around it so that she could hear the sounds made by the equipment. He then took a Polaroid® picture of the bear on the table, in the mask, for Katy to take home with her.

Masks

Because children need to hold perfectly still during cranial radiation treatment, a mask of the child's face is made and used to immobilize the head during treatments. Great care should be taken to ensure the mask-making procedure isn't traumatizing for your child. This can often be accomplished by using play therapy to demonstrate the procedure beforehand.

Masks are made from a lightweight, porous, mesh material. First, the technologist should explain and demonstrate the entire mask-making process to the child. The technologist can make a mask of your child's hand to demonstrate how it looks and feels. The child lies down on a table, and the technologist puts a sheet of the mask material in warm water to soften it. This warm mesh sheet is then placed over the child's face and quickly molded to her features. The child can breathe through the mesh material the entire time but must hold still for several minutes as the mask hardens. The mask is lifted off the child's face, and the technologist cuts holes in the mask for the eyes, nostrils, and mouth.

Very young children, or those who have difficulty holding still, are sedated while the mask is being made.

> *The cancer center staff had scheduled 2 hours for mask-making for my 3-year-old daughter. I asked them to explain very quietly every step in the process. I told her I would be holding her hand, and I promised that it would not hurt, but it would feel warm. I asked her to choose a story for me to recite as they molded the warm material to her face, to make the time go faster. She picked* Curious George Goes to the Hospital. *She held perfectly still; I recited the story; the staff were gentle and quick; and the entire procedure took less than 20 minutes.*

> • • • • •

> *Shawn (2 years old) needed to be sedated for his 10 doses of radiation. They also made his mask while he was anesthetized.*

During the cranial radiation treatment, your child will lie on his back, the mask will be placed over his face, and the mask will be clamped to the table to keep your child's head perfectly still.

Other immobilization devices

Different institutions use a variety of devices to immobilize children to ensure the radiation beam is directed with precision; these devices are also used on adults who receive radiation. Some of the products used are custom-made plaster of Paris casts, thermal plastic devices, vacuum-molded thermoplastics, and polyurethane foam forms. Custom fitting the forms on a child who has already undergone numerous painful procedures requires skill and patience. Immobilization devices can be fitted without difficulty on well-prepared, calm, or sedated children. The following are suggestions from parents about how to prepare a child for the fitting of a immobilization device:

• Give the child a tour of the room where the fitting will take place.

• Explain each step of the process in clear language.

• Be honest in describing any discomfort the child may experience.

- For small children, fit the device onto a mannequin or stuffed animal to demonstrate the process.

- For older children or teenagers, show a video or read a booklet describing the procedure.

> *Seventeen-month-old Rachel was fitted with two immobilization devices. They made a mask to hold her head in position, as well as a body mold from her neck to her thighs.*

More time spent on preparation will mean less time spent on fitting the device. Also, if the fitting goes well, it establishes trust and good feelings that will help make the actual radiation treatments proceed smoothly.

> *After relapsing while on treatment, Stephan (7 years old) needed cranial and spinal radiation. I took him on a tour and explained in detail what would happen. All of his questions were answered. He would go in, have the black marks put on, and lie face down on a bed. There was a thing for his forehead to rest on, but he didn't require any other supports. He would just hold perfectly still. We kept a bucket next to the bed, because he was on high-dose ARA-C, and after his radiation session, he would often need to lean over and vomit.*

> *He was so wonderful about it. He would go up to all of the older patients who were awaiting treatment and chat. He really reached out to them, and their eyes would just sparkle.*

Sedation

All infants, most preschoolers, and some school-age children require sedation or anesthesia to ensure they remain perfectly still during radiation treatment. Most radiation facilities use a combination of anesthetics that are effective and that allow the child to recover quickly.

The radiation facility should give you written instructions concerning pediatric anesthesia, including guidelines about when your child needs to stop eating and drinking before sedation or anesthesia. After treatment, children can eat and drink as soon as they are alert enough to swallow.

Anesthesia is given through a mask or through the child's catheter or intravenous line (IV). Sometimes the parent can hold or comfort the child while anesthesia is administered, but the parent must leave the room when the radiation treatment takes place. Once your child is easily aroused and can swallow, you can take her home. The entire procedure generally takes from 30 to 90 minutes. Nausea and vomiting are occasional side effects of anesthesia, but they are usually well controlled by anti-nausea drugs such as ondansetron (Zofran®).

Shawn was almost 3 years old when he needed his cranial radiation. He is an extremely active child, and we agreed with the medical team that he would have to be sedated. His appointment was always at 1 p.m., and we were told that he could have apple juice or Jell-O® at 6 a.m. but nothing to eat or drink after that. Every single morning he would drink the juice and then throw up. At the radiation room, I would hold him while he was anesthetized, then wait in the waiting room. They would bring him out to me in 30 to 45 minutes.

During a course of radiation therapy, the dose, drugs, and methods used to sedate or anesthetize the child may need to change, because some children develop a tolerance to certain drugs. Good communication between parents and members of the treatment team should prevent unnecessary anxiety about increased dosages or the use of a different drug. In some cases, less anesthesia is needed if the child is gently coached about ways to hold still.

Each time my young son came in for radiation, part of the routine was to place the hard plastic mesh mask over his face while he was awake, just for an instant, to get him used to the idea of trying to wear it for treatments without sedation. No pressure was ever put on him about it; it was just mentioned as a possibility of something he could try, something that would let him keep eating and drinking all through the day instead of having to fast for a few hours before each sedation, which was very hard for such a small boy who was getting sedation twice a day.

They left the mask on him for a tiny bit longer each time, until he was tolerating it for several seconds, and then close to a minute. His fifth birthday was at the exact middle of treatment, and he decided that since he was such a big boy now, he would try to do it without sedation. I know he was trying to please and impress all these kind people. He worked it out quietly with a favorite technician, asked the "sleepy medicine doctor" to wait outside the treatment room, let them screw the mask down to the table, and did the whole thing awake.

I've never been more proud in my life. Everyone cheered and hugged him. He finished the rest of the treatments without sedation, sometimes eating and drinking on his way in the door just to show off that he could!

Types of radiation treatments

Radiation treatments can be very stressful for both children and parents. Knowledge and preparation, however, can make the entire process much easier. This section describes radiation simulation and the various types of radiation therapy.

Radiation simulation

Prior to receiving any radiation therapy, many measurements and technical x-rays are taken to map the precise area to be treated. This preparation for therapy is called the "simulation." The simulation generally takes longer than any other appointment—from 30 minutes up to 2 hours. Because simulation does not involve high-dose radiation, parents are often allowed to remain in the treatment room to help and comfort their child. Some children will need to be sedated for the simulation.

During simulation, the radiation oncologist and technologist use a specialized x-ray machine to outline the treatment area. They will adjust the table your child lies on, the angle of the machine, and the width of the x-ray beam needed to give the exact dosage in the proper place. In addition, the oncologist or technologist will put small ink marks on the skin to pinpoint the area that will be treated. These marks should not be scrubbed in the bath or shower. They do fade with time, so the technologist may need to add more ink at some point in the child's treatment.

Children who wear masks during treatment will have these ink marks put on the mask instead of their skin. At some institutions, children who require spinal radiation may have tiny black dots permanently tattooed on their skin. These tattoos are made by putting a drop of India ink on the skin, then pricking the skin with a pin. The dots look like tiny black freckles.

After the simulation, the child can go home while the radiation oncologist carefully evaluates the developed x-ray film and measurements to design the treatment field.

Cranial radiation

To receive cranial radiation, children are given 8 to 10 weekday appointments for the same time each day. The children usually have the weekend off. At some institutions, children go twice a day. When the parent and child arrive, they must check in at the front desk. Then, the technologist comes out to take the child into the treatment room. Often, the parent accompanies the young child into the room. If the child requires anesthesia, it is usually given in the treatment room.

The technologist will secure children or teens in place with an immobilization device. Measurements are taken to verify that the child's body is perfectly positioned. Frequently, the technologist will shine a light on the area to be irradiated to ensure the machine is properly aligned. The technologist and parents leave the room, closing the door behind them.

At some institutions, parents are allowed to stay and watch the TV monitor and talk to their child via the speaker system. If this is the case, you should be careful not to distract the technologist as he administers the radiation. At other institutions, parents are asked to stay in the waiting room. It's important that you understand the department's policies; ask the therapist if anything is unclear.

I desperately wanted my 3 year old to be able to receive the radiation without anesthesia. I asked the center staff what I could do to make her comfortable. They said, "Anything, as long as you leave the room during the treatment." So I explained to my daughter that we had to find ways for her to hold very still for a short time. I said, "It's such a short time, that if I played your Snow White tape, the treatment would be over before Snow White met the dwarves." Katy agreed that was a short time, and asked that I bring the tape for her to listen to. She also wanted a sticker (a different one every day) stuck on the machine for her to look at. I brought her pink blanket to wrap her in because the table was hard and the room cold. Each day, she chose a different comfort animal or doll to hold during treatment. So we'd arrive every day with tapes, blanket, stickers, and animals. She felt safe, and all treatments went extremely well.

· · · · ·

There was something about the radiation or the anesthesia that frightened Shawn terribly. He would scream in the car all the way to the hospital. It was a scream as if he was in pain. He had nightmares while he was undergoing radiation and every night after it was over. We decided a month after radiation ended to bring a box of candy to the staff who had been so nice. Shawn asked, "Do I have to go in that room?" When I explained that it was over and he didn't need to go in the room anymore, he asked if he could go in to look at it once more. He stood for a long time and just looked and looked at the equipment. Somehow he made his peace with it, because he never had any more nightmares.

The function of the thyroid gland is sometimes impaired by cranial radiation, so blood tests are periodically needed for the rest of the child's life.

Spinal radiation

If your child receives spinal radiation, the back of the heart may be affected. A baseline electrocardiography (EKG) and echocardiogram should be performed prior to treatment and on a regular basis thereafter. Spinal radiation may also damage the thyroid gland, which is located in the neck. The oncologist should periodically evaluate the functioning of this gland if spinal radiation has been given.

Testicular radiation

For male children or teens with leukemic cells in their testes, radiation may be included in the treatment plan; however, current clinical trials are evaluating the effectiveness of using intensive chemotherapy rather than testicular radiation. Radiation treatment is usually only given Monday through Friday, with weekends off. Treatment plans and the amount of radiation used vary among protocols and institutions.

Prior to your son's radiation to the testes, the technologist or child life specialist will give him a tour of the facility, describe the machines, and explain exactly how the radiation sessions will be done. Usually, only older boys require radiation to the testes, so anesthesia is rarely needed. The male child or teen will lie on the table, the technologist will support the testicles on a small piece of lead, and the penis will be taped up to keep it out of the radiation field. Each treatment will last less than 5 minutes, during which time the boy must hold perfectly still. As with cranial radiation, the technologist will watch your son through a window and will be in verbal contact through a two-way intercom system.

> We told our 5-year-old son that he needed to have some special photos done, like x-rays, and he needed to lie very still to have them taken. A special mold was made of his bottom to hold him in the correct position. This was like a beanbag, and when he was in it at the radiation planning appointment, the air was sucked out of the cushion, leaving a firm cast of his bottom and legs, which he sat in for the radiation sessions. We had a dry run to be sure he didn't need sedation (which was a possibility and a team was on call for the first session). He had to lie on the cushion, and his penis was taped up and out of the way to enable the machine to be focused on the testes. Each session was very short, about 15 minutes from set up to finish.

> There were already stickers on the machine for him to look at, and he liked those. He took his favorite "pilly" into the room with him and that was nestled around his neck for the session. He also was covered up with a blanket until the very last second, as I think little people's dignity is just as important as adults. We took a book along with us so I could read to him through the microphone while the radiation was happening. He had a reward after each session, which we supplied and the nurses gave him a chart to stick them to. We displayed this proudly in his room and I still have it!

Radiation therapy to the testes causes sterility. For all sexually mature males, sperm banking should be done prior to treatment. Sperm can be kept viable for 10 to 15 years, and this may allow some teens the opportunity to become fathers later in life.

Total body radiation

Total body radiation (also known as total body irradiation, or TBI) is sometimes given prior to stem cell transplantation. There are numerous protocols, each with a different treatment schedule. Two examples are: 200 cGy given twice a day for 3 days, or 120 cGy given three times a day for 4 days. The treatments are usually 5 to 6 hours apart. Prior to treatment, the child will be measured by the radiation therapist using tape measures. The therapist will give the family a tour and will show them the two machines that will be on either side of the stretcher in the middle of the room.

On the first day of treatment, the child will be brought to the room (at some institutions, small children ride a tricycle or are pulled in a wagon) and may choose to watch

TV or a movie, or listen to an iPod® or the radio. He will lie on the stretcher between the two machines, and the therapist will position him on his side or on his back. These positions will alternate with each treatment—once on the back, then once on the side. It doesn't matter which side the child lies on, so if a child has a sore left side, he can always lie on his right. The child can move a bit to scratch his nose or cross his ankles, but he cannot get off the stretcher.

The therapist will remove all metal from the child's body and clothing—watches, rings, zippers, clamps. Anything with tight elastic—diapers or tight socks—will also be loosened or removed. Treatment time lasts from 18 to 35 minutes, depending on the size of the child.

Antinausea drugs are given to prevent vomiting, and these often make the child drowsy enough to doze through the treatment. Some young or extremely active children will need to be sedated.

> *The radiation was easy. When I wasn't sleeping, I watched TV or listened to the radio. I threw up once, but they gave me Benadryl® and I never was sick again from the radiation. The room was neat; it was painted lots of bright colors and had two big blue machines, one on each side of me.*

Possible short-term side effects

Generally, radiation treatments given to children with leukemia are completed in less than 2 weeks. Many children have no short-term side effects. If side effects do occur, it is often hard to differentiate those caused by radiation and those caused by the high-dose chemotherapy that is usually given at the same time. Possible short-term side effects are:

- Loss of appetite

- Nausea and vomiting

- Fatigue

- Slightly reddened or itchy skin

- Hair loss

- Low blood counts

- Changes in taste and smell (sometimes during the treatment)

- Sleepiness (somnolence syndrome)—from cranial radiation

- Swollen parotid (salivary) glands—from TBI.

Methods of coping with most of the above side effects are contained in Chapter 10, "Common Side Effects of Chemotherapy."

Somnolence syndrome is uniquely associated with cranial radiation and is characterized by drowsiness, prolonged periods of sleep (up to 20 hours a day), fever, headaches, nausea, vomiting, irritability, loss of appetite, difficulty swallowing, and difficulty speaking. It tends to occur 5 to 7 weeks after radiation treatment ends and can last from a few days to several weeks.

> *Nine weeks after ending her cranial radiation, my daughter started complaining of severe headaches. She would hold her head and just sob with pain. She also vomited several times. Then she became very sleepy, and dozed on the couch most of the day. She developed a low fever and choked when she tried to swallow liquids or solid food. This lasted for about a week, and I was worried sick. I called her oncologist, her radiation oncologist, and her pediatrician, and they all said they didn't think it was related to the radiation or chemotherapy. I went to the medical library and discovered somnolence syndrome.*

· · · · ·

> *Stephan (8 years old) had no side effects from the cranial and spinal radiation other than sleepiness, but he was very affected by it. First, he just started taking naps and generally slowing down. Then the naps got longer, and he was awake less. Finally, he only woke up to eat. Luckily, that part coincided with Christmas vacation, so he didn't miss much school. Altogether, it lasted about 6 weeks.*

· · · · ·

> *Ryan (14 years old) had his radiation during consolidation when he was very ill from the chemotherapy. He would develop severe headaches and vomiting an hour after each radiation treatment.*

· · · · ·

> *Three weeks after her radiation ended, Rachel (18 months old) slept for 3 days. We tried to wake her to eat, but she literally would fall asleep with her face in her food. After 3 days, she gradually became more alert, with the whole episode lasting only a week and a half. Oddly enough, the oncology people warned me about the possibility of sleepiness, but the radiation staff insisted that it wasn't related to the radiation.*

Possible long-term side effects

Most children and teens with high-risk or relapsed leukemia receive 1,800 cGy or less to the whole brain and sometimes radiation to the spinal cord. Male children or teens with a testicular relapse may be given radiation to the testicles, and some children get total body radiation prior to stem cell transplant. Specific radiation-related disabilities that may later appear in life depend on the age and sex of the child, the dose of radiation, and the location of the radiation.

Although short-term effects appear and subside, long-term side effects may not become apparent until months or years after treatment ends. The effects of radiation on cognitive functioning, bone growth, soft tissue growth, teeth, sinuses, endocrine glands, puberty, and fertility range from no late effects to severe, life-long impacts. Second tumors in the radiation field are also a possible long-term side effect. Detailed information about possible late effects is provided in *Childhood Cancer Survivors: A Practical Guide to Your Future*, 2nd edition by Nancy Keene, Wendy Hobbie, and Kathy Ruccione.

Cognitive problems

Intrathecal and IV methotrexate and/or radiation to the brain can sometimes cause damage to the CNS, resulting in learning disabilities, which can start immediately or several years after treatment. Typically, poor performance is noted in mathematics, understanding visual/spatial relationships, organizational ability, problem solving, attention span, and concentration skills.

My daughter is a year off treatment and 3 years past radiation and seems to have no cognitive problems at all. She is doing well in kindergarten. She reads and writes and has taught herself to add and subtract all of the combinations up to 20. I was worried while she was on chemotherapy that her comprehension was slow. She continually asked me to reread portions of books and didn't seem to understand without constant repetition. But that faded away after the chemotherapy ended, and now she's quick to understand stories read aloud. She does, however, have significant social problems that may be related to the radiation.

· · · · ·

My son turned 3 years old while receiving his cranial radiation. He is now 5 years old and has major cognitive problems. He can't count, and so far he hasn't been able to learn the alphabet. He is in a preschool for the developmentally disabled, and the teacher feels that he has just hit a brick wall. I gave her the Candlelighters book, Educating the Child with Cancer, *and several articles. She is trying different techniques with him. He is a super kid, though, with a great attitude, and we hope for the best.*

· · · · ·

Rachel received 1,800 cGy of cranial radiation when she was 17 months old. She's 6 now, in kindergarten. She has multiple cognitive problems, including problems with letter and number recognition and short-term memory. She is a child who will need extra help in school, including phonics and drilling while learning to read. It is challenging for her to sit quietly in class and listen to the teacher. After much observation, I truly think that these kids have a quirky organizational system for their brain. They seem to have a different way of inputting and outputting information. She will frequently say something completely out of the blue during a conversation that is totally unrelated to what is being discussed. My husband and I both realize that school may be a struggle for her, but we intend to get her all of the help available to persons who are traumatically brain injured. Her self-esteem is high, she is a very bright, verbal child, and we will work with each of her teachers to ensure that she gets the best education possible.

Children at greatest risk for cognitive problems are those treated when younger than 5 years of age, with those under 2 at the highest risk. Chapter 15, "School," discusses in detail the types of educational challenges some children face and methods to deal with the problems.

Problems with growth

The brain contains the hypothalamus and the pituitary gland, which control many body processes, including growth and reproduction. At the dosages of radiation given to children with leukemia, growth is usually not affected, except in younger girls. Effects on growth are usually only seen in children who received 2,400 cGy or more. If the child requires additional cranial radiation or radiation to the spine, growth can be slowed or stopped.

The growth of children who receive cranial radiation or craniospinal radiation should be followed closely. Children should be measured (sitting and standing) at every follow-up visit and have their growth plotted on a chart to measure speed of growth.

If your child is one of the rare individuals who experiences premature puberty (before the age of 8 for girls and 10 for boys), growth may be affected. These children may be given daily growth hormone injections to support their growth until they reach their final height, and then be given a lower dose every day for the rest of their lives.

Children who receive TBI prior to stem cell transplantation also may exhibit delayed growth, especially if they have already had cranial and/or spinal radiation. These children should be under the care of a pediatric endocrinologist who is experienced in follow-up care for pediatric transplant patients.

Mandy (age 16) is a tad short-waisted, but grew 7 inches on growth hormone treatment! The doctors closely monitor wingspan (that is, outstretched arms fingertip to fingertip) to make sure it correlates to height. Otherwise they may have longer arms and be out of balance. The growth hormone adds energy and good spirits as well.

Adrenal and thyroid functions also need periodic, life-long monitoring after spinal radiation.

Early or delayed puberty

Some young children who receive radiation to the brain do not experience puberty at the appropriate age. A very small percentage of children enter precocious puberty, which means that puberty begins several years earlier than normal. This is most common in children who also have impaired growth. Consultation with a pediatric endocrinologist is necessary to delay the puberty to allow children to continue to grow. Conversely, puberty in some children is significantly delayed. Teenage girls who do not show signs of puberty—pubic and underarm hair, breast development—should be evaluated by a pediatric endocrinologist. Similarly, teenage boys who show no signs of puberty—growth of body hair, deepening voice—should also see an endocrinologist with experience treating children who had cancer.

Teeth

Cranial radiation at a young age may result in disrupted tooth development and the blunting of the roots of your child's permanent teeth. This can result in permanent teeth never developing or in early tooth loss because of shortened roots. During radiation treatment and for several years after, it is important to consult with a pediatric dentist. Any child who has received cranial or spinal radiation is at additional risk for dental decay because of diminished function of the salivary glands. Appropriate dental evaluations and treatment with fluoride preparations are necessary.

Secondary cancers

Children who receive radiation have an increased risk of malignancy (cancer) years after treatment. Thyroid, salivary, and brain tumors have been reported in children who survived leukemia. Those at highest risk received 2,400 cGy or more of cranial radiation, spinal radiation, or TBI when younger than 5 years old. Therefore, any child who was treated with radiation should have life-long follow-up from an expert in the late effects of treatment for childhood cancer, which is described in Chapter 19, "End of Treatment and Beyond."

My 18-year-old daughter had AML M5 when she was 8 and does have some late effects. She was a very early bone marrow transplant recipient (1987), so she had total body irradiation. As a result of that, she has ongoing endocrine problems, menstrual difficulties, and cataracts. She also has a reduced ejection fraction of the heart from the anthracyclines and had to deal with a second cancer in her thyroid gland. That said, you'd never pick her out of a crowd. She graduated from high school with a perfect 4.0 GPA and wants to specialize in biology with the intent to go into medicine (pediatric oncology) or molecular genetics with a focus on cancer genetics. There is hope.

Chapter 12

Family and Friends

Shared joy is double joy,
shared sorrow is half sorrow.

— Swedish proverb

THE INTERACTIONS BETWEEN the parents of a child with cancer and their extended family and friends are complex. Potential exists for loving support and generous help, as well as for bitter disappointment and disputes. The diagnosis of leukemia creates a ripple effect, first touching the immediate family, then extended family, friends, coworkers, schoolmates, church members, and sometimes the entire community.

Chapter 3 discussed ways to notify family and friends. This chapter provides scores of ideas for helpful things extended family and friends can do to support your family during this difficult time. To prevent possible misunderstandings, parents also share in this chapter their thoughts about what things are not helpful.

The extended family

Extended family—aunts, uncles, cousins, grandparents—can cushion the shock of a leukemia diagnosis through loving words and actions. Extended family members sometimes drop their own lives to rush to the side of the child with leukemia, and often remain steadfast throughout the years of treatment. Regrettably, some family members may not be helpful, either out of ignorance about what your family needs or simply because they are too overwhelmed by events in their own lives.

Some extended families, and even entire communities, rally around the family, while for other families support never materializes. Several factors affect the strength of support: well-established community ties, good communication within the extended family, physical proximity to the extended family, and clear exchange of information about the needs of the affected family. If any of these elements are missing, support may dissipate or never appear.

> *We had just moved 3,000 miles away from family and friends for my husband to accept a new job. We had no family close by, no friends. Each family member and*

some close friends used their vacations to fly out and take 2-week shifts at our new house to help out. Thankfully, they got us through the first months, but the 2 stressful years of maintenance were lonely.

Families with stronger community ties often receive support throughout treatment:

Shortly after Jesse relapsed, I was praying with my Bible study group. With four children ages 1 to 9, I just didn't know how we would manage with one parent 100 miles away at the hospital and one parent working. The group decided to collect enough money to allow my sister to quit her job and move in to take care of our other three children while I was at the hospital with Jesse. She stayed for 8 months. It was such a wonderful thing. They didn't even ask us; they just said they would support her financially so she could care for my children and keep the household running.

Grandparents

Grandparents grieve deeply when a grandchild has leukemia. They are concerned not only for their grandchild, but for their own child (the parent) as well. Cancer wreaks havoc with grandparents' expectations, reversing the natural order of life and death. Grandparents frequently say, "Why not me? I'm the one who is old." Cancer in a grandchild is a major shock to bear.

Many parents reported that the grandparents responded to the crisis with tremendous emotional, physical, and financial support.

My mother was a rock. She lived far away, but she put her busy life on hold to come help. She took care of the baby and kept the household running through both induction and reinduction when I was living at the hospital with my very ill child. She was strong, and it gave me strength.

Some parents express tremendous gratitude for the role played by the grandparents in providing much-needed stability to the family rocked by cancer. When the grandparents care for the siblings and run the household, the parents can care for the sick child and return to work.

Because Judd had no neutrophils at diagnosis, he was put in isolation at Children's for a month. I stayed with him full time, and my husband took a month off work to be there. Luckily, my mother had moved to our town just the year before and was able to immediately move to our house to take care of Erin, my 10-year-old daughter. Grandma was great because she cooked special meals for Erin and helped with cleaning and transportation.

Other families are not as fortunate. Many grandparents are too old, too ill, estranged from the family, or simply unable to cope with a crisis of this magnitude. Some simply fall apart.

> My mother became hysterical when my daughter was diagnosed with leukemia. She called every day, sobbing. Luckily, she lived far away, and this minimized the disruption. We had to ask her not to come, because we just couldn't handle the catastrophe at home and her neediness too. It hurt her feelings, but we just couldn't cope with it.

Other grandparents allow pre-existing problems with their adult child to color their perceptions of what the family needs or what role they should take on during the crisis. For example, sometimes cancer allows grandparents to renew criticism of the way grandchildren are being raised.

> While we stayed at the hospital, the grandparents moved into our house to care for our 8-year-old daughter. They decided that this was their chance to "whip her into shape, teach her some manners, and get her room cleaned up." Our daughter was in tears, and we ended up saying, "We appreciate your help, but we will take over."

Sometimes grandparents try to blame the parents for the cancer or make other hurtful comments:

> The first day in the hospital my mother told me I had caused the leukemia by coloring my hair blond during the pregnancy. My mother-in-law wasn't helpful either. Throughout the ordeal of treatment, all she did was to tell us to "put it in God's hand."

It is hard to predict how anyone will react to the diagnosis of childhood leukemia. Grandparents are no exception. Some respond with the wisdom gleaned from decades of living, others become needy or overbearing, and some withdraw. It is natural in a time of grave crisis to look to your parents for support and help, but it is important to remember that grandparents' ability to respond also depends on events in their own lives. If problems between family members develop, help can be obtained from hospital social workers or through individual counseling.

Helpful things for family members to do

Families differ in what is truly helpful for them. The suggestions in this chapter are snapshots of what some families appreciated. True listening and working on maintaining your relationship with the family is paramount. Connections can be made in many different, unique, and personally meaningful ways. Try to support the family in ways that respect their wishes while also honoring their privacy.

- Be sensitive to the emotional state of both the sick child and the parents. Sometimes parents want to talk about the leukemia; sometimes they just need a hand to hold.

- Encourage all members of the extended family to keep in touch through visits, calls, mail, e-mail, text messages, videos, audios, or pictures. When visits are welcome, make them brief and cheerful. Not only do long visits sometimes distress sick children, but they can also overtax a tired parent.

  Our relatives who lived close to the hospital had teenagers. One was a candy striper at Children's on Saturdays. Judd's aunts, uncles, and cousins came to visit several times a week any time he was in the hospital during his 3 years of treatment. They were all very supportive, very positive, and fun to be around.

- Be understanding if the parents do not want phone calls in the hospital. Remember that the child can often hear phone conversations when parents talk on the phone in the room.

  The first 3 days in the hospital I spent much of my time crying on the phone when talking to friends and relatives. Then I realized how frightening this must be to my 2-year-old. So I just took the phone off the hook and left it there. Now, each time Jennifer is hospitalized, I call one friend and have her spread the news. Then I take the phone off the hook again and concentrate on my daughter.

- A cheerful hospital room really boosts a child's spirits. Encourage sending balloon bouquets, funny cards, posters, toys, or humorous books. Be aware that some hospitals do not allow rubber balloons, only mylar. Flowers are usually not allowed in children's rooms.

  We plastered the walls with pictures of family and friends, and so many people sent balloons that the ceiling was covered. It was a lovely sight.

- Laughter helps heal the mind and body, so send funny videos or arrive with a good joke if you think it is appropriate.

  My brother Bill and his wonderful girlfriend, Cathy, created an exciting "trip" for my 4-year-old daughter. She was bald, big-bellied from prednisone, and her counts were too low to leave the house, but her interest in fashion was as sharp as ever. Bill and Cathy bought 10 outfits, rigged up a dressing room, and with Cathy as saleswoman, turned Katy's bedroom into a fashion salon. She tried on outfits, discussed all of their merits and shortcomings, and had a fabulous time. It was a real high point for her.

- Puzzles, games, picture books, coloring books, age-appropriate computer games, and crafts are welcome. Remember that attention spans may be shortened by treatment, so keep it simple.

A friend who was a nurse came to my son's room shortly before Christmas and brought an entire gingerbread house kit, including confectioner's sugar for the icing. We had a very good time putting it together.

- Offer to give the parent(s) a break from the hospital room. A walk outside, shopping trip, haircut, dinner out together, or just a long shower can be very refreshing.

- Donate frequent flyer miles to distant family members who have the time but not the money to help.

   A close friend (who lived 3,000 miles away) had just lost her job and wished she could be there for us. My parents gave her their frequent flyer miles. She flew in for 3 weeks during a hard part of treatment and helped enormously.

- If you don't hear from a family member, call. Often silence means that he doesn't know what to do or say.

- Donate blood. Your blood may not be used specifically for the ill child, but it will replenish the general supply, which is depleted by children with cancer.

   Our family friend John is terrified of needles. John always avoided giving blood. John doesn't like going to the doctor. But John showed up to donate platelets once, early on, and we found that he was a great platelet match for Deli. So he kept returning to that awful two-needle machine that you stay hooked onto for 3 hours at a time, probably a couple dozen times, because we needed him. Then we had Beth, who was one of my professional acquaintances. Beth was always pretty nice to us, but she found out that she too was a good "sticky" platelet donor. Probably at least a dozen times she took hours out of her work day and donated platelets whenever Deli needed some. We concentrated on the few "star" friends and relatives, the one or two people whose attitude, abilities, and circumstances allowed them to be the most helpful.

Helpful things for friends to do

Like family, friends can cushion the shock of diagnosis and ease the difficulties of treatment with their words and actions. You may want to share the suggestions that follow with your extended family and friends so they will have a better idea of how to help you.

Mother Theresa once said, "We can do no great things—only small things with great love." It is a given that the family of a child being treated for leukemia is overwhelmed. The list of helpful things to do is endless, but here are some suggestions from parents who have traveled this hard road.

Household

- Provide meals. It is helpful to call in advance to see if anyone in the family has food allergies or if there is something special the child with cancer would like to eat.

  One of the nicest things that friends did was to bring us a huge picnic basket full of food to the hospital. We spread a blanket on the floor, Erica crawled out of bed, and the entire family sat down together and ate. Most people don't realize how expensive it is to have to eat every meal at the hospital cafeteria, so the picnic was not only fun, but helped us to save a few dollars.

- Take care of pets or livestock.

- Mow grass, shovel snow, rake leaves, water plants, and weed gardens.

  We came home from the hospital one evening right before Christmas, and found a freshly cut, fragrant Christmas tree leaning next to our door. I'll never forget that kindness.

- Clean the house.

  My husband's cousin sent her cleaning lady over to our house. It was so neat and such a luxury to come home to find the stove and windows sparkling clean.

- Grocery shop (especially when the family is due home from the hospital).

- Do laundry. Drop off and pick up dry cleaning.

- Provide a place to stay near the hospital.

  One of the ladies from the school where I worked came up to the ICU (intensive care unit) waiting room where we were sleeping and pressed her house key into my hand. She lived 5 minutes from the hospital. She said, "My basement is made up, there's a futon, there's a TV; you are coming and staying at my house." I hardly knew her, but we accepted. Every day when we came in from the hospital there was some cute little treat waiting for us like a bowl of cookies, or two packages of hot chocolate and a thermos of hot milk.

Siblings

It takes an entire chapter to deal with the complex feelings that siblings confront when their brother or sister has cancer. Chapter 14, "Siblings," provides an in-depth examination of the issues from the perspective of both siblings and parents. Below is a list of suggestions about how family and friends can help with siblings.

- Baby-sit whenever parents go to the clinic or emergency room, or need to be with their child for a prolonged hospital stay.

> *The mother of a secretary from my office called me, introduced herself, and offered to care for my newborn daughter while I spent time at the hospital. I had never met this woman, but she turned out to be a real lifesaver and a jewel. She would come every day, bathe, dress, and feed my daughter, clean up the house, and stay from morning until evening. She did this for several months. I will never forget her for being so kind. I would not have been able to get through those first few difficult months without this type of support—and to find it in a complete stranger certainly renewed my faith in mankind!*

- When parents are home with a sick child, take sibling(s) somewhere fun to get their minds off of the stresses at home. Find out what they would enjoy, such as going to the park, a sports event, miniature golfing, bowling, the zoo, or a movie.
- Invite sibling(s) over for meals.
- If you bring a gift for the sick child, bring something for the sibling(s), too.

> *Friends from home sent boxes of art supplies to us when the whole family spent those first 10 weeks at a Ronald McDonald house far from our home. They sent scissors, paints, paper, and colored pens. It was a great help for Carrie Beth and her two sisters. One friend even sent an Easter package with straw hats for each girl, and flowers, ribbons, and glue to decorate them with.*

- Offer to help sibling(s) with homework.
- Drive sibling(s) to lessons, games, or school.
- Listen to how they are feeling and coping. Siblings' lives have been disrupted; they have limited time with their parents, and they need support and care.

Psychological support

There is much that can be done to help the family keep on an even emotional keel.

- Call frequently, and be open to listening if the parents want to talk about their feelings. Also talk about non-cancer-related topics, such as sharing neighborhood and school news.
- Visit the hospital and bring fun stuff like bubbles, silly string, water pistols, joke books, funny videos, rub-on tattoos, and board games.
- If one parent has to leave work to stay in the hospital with the sick child, coworkers can send messages by mail, tape, text, or fax.

One very neat thing that was an emotional boost was that my friends and former coworkers from Kansas faxed us messages and pictures and sent things to Meagan while we were in the hospital. It was very nice to get such fresh messages—it really shortened the miles.

- If you think the family might be interested, call Candlelighters or the social worker at the local hospital to find out if there are support groups for parents and/or kids in your area.

- Offer to take the children to the support groups or go with the parents. For most families, the parent support group becomes a second family with ties of shared experience as deep and strong as blood relations.

- Drive the parent and child to clinic visits.

- Buy books (uplifting ones) for the family if they enjoy reading.

- Send e-mail, cards, or letters.

    Word got around my parents' hometown, and I received cards from many high school acquaintances who still cared enough to call or write and say we're praying for you, please let us know how things are going. It was so neat to get so many cards out of the blue that said, "I'm thinking about you."

- Baby-sit the sick child so the parents can go out to eat, exercise, take a walk, or just get out of the hospital or house.

- If the child has a type of leukemia that may require a stem cell transplant, organize a drive to get people typed and entered into the marrow registry. For more information contact the National Marrow Donor Program online at *www.marrow.org*, or by calling (800) 627-7692.

- Ask what needs to be done, then do it.

    A close friend asked what I needed the week after Michelle was diagnosed. I asked if she could drive our second car the 100 miles to the hospital so my husband could return in it to work. She came with her family to the Ronald McDonald House with two big bags containing snack foods, a large box of stationery, envelopes, stamps, books to read, a book handmade by her 3-year-old daughter containing dozens of cut-out pictures of children's clothing pasted on construction paper (which my daughter adored looking at), and a beautiful, new, handmade, lace-trimmed dress for my daughter. It was full-length and baggy enough to cover all bandages and tubing. She wore it almost every day for a year. It was a wonderful thing for my friend to do.

- Give lots of hugs.

Grandpa Fred is a 71-year-old retiree who has been visiting pediatric oncology patients at Children's for almost 12 years. He begins his day at 9:30 every morning on the teens' ward, then he moves on to visit the younger patients, the playroom, and the clinic. Grandpa Fred always takes pictures of his young friends, very good ones, and has filled 23 photo albums with them. Fred has two prints made of each picture he takes and gives one to the families. He also helps Santa on Christmas and visits on Halloween. He has been the camp manager at Camp Goodtimes every summer for 8 years. Fred feels that a hug is more important than anything he can say to someone. "Listening and giving a hug," he says, "That's the best I can do."

Financial support

Helping families avoid financial disaster can be the next greatest gift after the life of the child and the strength of the family. It is estimated that even fully insured families spend 25 percent or more of their income on co-payments, travel, motels, meals, and other uncovered items. Uninsured or underinsured families may lose their savings or even their homes. Even families with full health insurance, such as those in Canada, have additional expenses that are not covered. Most families need financial assistance, so here are some suggestions for helping:

• Start a support fund.

> *A friend of mine called and asked very tentatively if we would mind if she started a support fund. We felt awkward, but we needed help, so we said okay. She did everything herself, and the money she raised was very, very helpful. We did ask her to stop the fund when people started calling us to ask if they could use giving to the fund as an advertisement for their business.*

• Help the family apply for financial aid from the Leukemia and Lymphoma Society at *www.leukemia-lymphoma.org/all_page.adp?item_id=4599* (or go to the main page and type "financial support" in the search box).

• Share leave with a coworker. Governments and some companies have leave banks that permit people who are ill or taking care of someone who is ill to use other coworkers' leave so they won't have their pay docked.

> *My husband's coworkers didn't collect money, they did something even more valuable. They donated sick leave hours so he was able to be at the hospital frequently during those first few months without losing a paycheck.*

• Job share. Some families work out job-share arrangements in which a coworker donates time to perform part of the parent's job; this way the parent can spend extra time at the hospital. Job sharing allows the job to get done, keeps peace at the job site, and prevents financial losses for the family. Another possibility is for one or more friends with similar skills (e.g., word processing, filing, sales) to rotate through the job on a volunteer basis to cover for the parent of the ill child.

After my son's diagnosis, the Board of Directors requested that the balance of my school year contract be paid—even though I was unable to fulfill my obligations. It was handled by using my sick days (I had only been on the job a little over 6 months) and then maternity/ disability. I was expecting a baby 8 weeks after Matt's diagnosis, so I went right into the maternity/disability benefit. How they figured it on paper to carry the rest of my contract, I don't know. I did not return to my job until the second school year into Matt's illness. I then began to work on a job-share basis, which I still do. To this day, I have not used any family medical leave time. My agency has been absolutely the exception, and it has been one of our blessings to be working for such a compassionate agency.

- Collect money at church or work to give the family informally.

The day my daughter was diagnosed, my husband's coworkers passed the hat and gave us over $250. I was embarrassed, but it paid for gas, meals, and the motel until there was an opening in the Ronald McDonald House.

• • • • •

Finances were a main concern for us because I wanted to cut back on work to be at home with Meagan. Sometimes my coworkers would pool money and present it with a card saying, "Here's a couple of days work that you won't have to worry about."

- Collect money by organizing a bake sale, dance, or raffle.

Coworkers of my husband held a Halloween party and charged admission, which they donated to us. We were very uncomfortable with the idea at first, but they were looking for an excuse to have a party, and it helped us out.

- Keeping track of medical bills is time-consuming, frustrating, and exhausting. If you are a close relative or friend, you could offer to review, organize, and file (or enter into a computer) the voluminous paperwork. Making the calls and writing the letters over contested claims or errors in billing are very helpful.

Help from schoolmates

The friendships and social lives of children often revolve around school. Trying to maintain ties with school, teachers, and friends will help your child make a smooth transition back as soon as he is able.

- Encourage visits (if appropriate), cards, e-mails, text messages, and phone calls from classmates.

- Ask the teacher to send the school newspaper and other news along with assignments.

- Classmates can sign a brightly colored banner to send to the hospital.

> *Brent's kindergarten class sent a packet containing a picture drawn for him by each child in the class. They also made him a book. Another time they sent him a letter written on huge poster board. He couldn't wait to get back to school.*

- School friends and civic groups can show their support by doing volunteer work at their local hospital or by participating in, or organizing, cancer-awareness events.

> *Ethan's school read* Sadako and the Thousand Paper Cranes, *which is a story about a Japanese girl from Hiroshima who contracted leukemia after World War II. The crane is the sign of health, good fortune, and long life in Japan. There is a legend that if you fold a thousand origami cranes, you will be granted one wish. Sadako's wish was that she live a long and healthy life, but she died of cancer 386 cranes short of her goal. Her classmates finished her cranes for her, and paper cranes subsequently became a symbol of peace.*
>
> *So, the kids at Ethan's school began to fold cranes for him. Each crane has a wish written on the wing (things like "Cancer Be Gone" and "Ethan I love your spirit"). Kids used favorite music, the school newsletter, or copied favorite poems, in addition to using fancy paper or decorating the finished crane. Some are the size of a robin, and some are smaller than a dime.*
>
> *They reached their goal of a thousand last week and they are now hanging (on strands, from one to 10 cranes per strand) on the ceiling over Ethan's bed. They are absolutely magical to look at, all rotating and casting shadows; and you can actually read each one's wish on the lower hanging ones. I thought it was a beautiful thing to do.*

Religious support

Following are a few suggestions for families who have religious affiliations:

- If the family goes to church, synagogue, mosque, or other house of worship, contact a member of the clergy and alert him or her to the family's situation.

- Arrange for church members and clergy to visit the hospital, if that is what the family wants.

- Arrange prayer services for the sick child.

> *The day our son was diagnosed, we raced next door to ask our wonderful neighbors to take care of our dog. The news of our son's diagnosis quickly spread, and we found out later that five neighborhood families gathered that very night to pray for Brent.*

- Have the child's religious education class send pictures, posters, letters, balloons, or audio or video tapes to the sick child.

Accepting help (for parents)

As a parent of a child with cancer, one of the kindest things you can do for your friends is to let them help you. Let them channel their time and worry into things that will make your life easier. Think of the many times you have visited a sick friend, made a meal for a new mom, baby-sat someone else's child in an emergency, or just pitched in to do what needed to be done. These actions probably made you feel great and provided a good example for your children. When your child is diagnosed with cancer, both you and your friends will benefit immensely if you let them help you and if you give them guidance about what you need.

One father's thoughts about accepting help:

> *Fathers have a deep-seated need to protect their family. Yet here I was with a child with leukemia, and there wasn't a single thing that I could do about it. The loss of control really bothered me. The very hardest thing I had to learn was to let go enough to let people help us.*

One mother's thoughts about accepting help:

> *The most important advice I received as the parent of a child newly diagnosed with cancer came from a hospital nurse whom I turned to when I was overwhelmed with all the advice being offered by family and friends. This wise nurse said, "Don't discount anything. You're going to need all the help you can get." I think it is very important for families to remain open and accept the help that is offered. It often comes when least expected and from unlikely sources. I was totally unprepared at diagnosis for how much help I would need, and I'm glad that I remained open to offers of kindness. This is not the time to show the world how strong you are.*

What to say (for friends)

Following are some suggestions about what to say and how to offer help. Of course, much depends on the type of relationship that already exists between you and the family you want to help; but a specific offer can always be accepted or graciously declined.

- "Our family would like do your yard work. It will make us feel as if we are helping in a small way."

- "We want to clean your house for you once a week. What day would be convenient?"

- "Would it help if we took care of your dog (or cat, or bird)? We would love to do it."

- "I walk my dog three times a day. May I walk yours, too? "

- "The church is setting up a system to deliver meals to your house. When is the best time to drop them off? "

- "I will take care of Jimmy whenever you need to take John to the hospital. Call us anytime, day or night, and we will come pick him up. "

Things that do not help

Sometimes people say things to parents of children with cancer that aren't helpful. If you are a family member or friend of a parent in this situation, please do not say any of the following:

- "God only gives people what they can handle." (Some people cannot handle the stress of childhood leukemia.)

- "I know just how you feel." (Unless you have a child with cancer, you simply don't know.)

- "You are so brave," or "so strong," etc. (Parents are not heroes; they are normal people struggling with extraordinary stress.)

- "They are doing such wonderful things to save children with leukemia these days." (Yes, the prognosis is usually good, but what parents and children are going through is not wonderful.)

- "Well, we're all going to die one day." (True, but parents do not need to be reminded of this fact.)

- "It's God's will." (This is just not a helpful thing to hear.)

- "At least you have other kids," or "Thank goodness you are still young enough to have other children." (A child cannot be replaced.)

> A woman whom I worked with, but did not know well, came up to me one day and out of the blue said, "When Erica gets to heaven to be with Jesus, He will love her." All I could think to say was, "Well, I'm sorry, but Jesus can't have her right now."

Parents also suggest the following things:

- Rather than say, "Let us know if there is anything we can do," make a specific suggestion.

> Many well-wishing friends always said, "Let me know what I can do." I wish they had just "done," instead of asking for direction. It took too much energy to decide, call them, make arrangements, etc. I wish someone would have said, "When is your

clinic day? I'll bring dinner," or "I'll baby-sit Sunday afternoon so you two can go out to lunch."

- Do not make personal comments about sick children in front of them. For instance, "When will his hair grow back in?" "He's lost so much weight." Or, "She's so pale."

- Do not do things that require the parents to support you (for example, repeatedly calling them up and crying about their child's illness).

- Do not ask "what if" questions: "What if he can't go to school?" "What if your insurance won't cover it?" Or, "What if she dies?" The present is really all the parents can deal with.

Losing friends

It is an unfortunate reality that most parents of children with leukemia lose some of their friends. For a variety of reasons, some friends just can't cope and either suddenly disappear or gradually fade away. Many times this can be prevented by calling them to keep them involved; but sometimes, they just can't handle the stress.

> *I had a friend who really thought herself to be empathetic, except that she just couldn't "deal with" hospitals. She said they made her uncomfortable, so she wouldn't visit. I also got tired of her talking about the silver lining of the dark cloud that has been hanging over my head. So we stopped communicating.*

> • • • • •

> *We had friends and family we thought would be the greatest sources of support in the world. Yet, they pulled away from us and provided nothing in the way of help, emotional or otherwise. We also had friends that we never expected to understand step up in surprising ways. My wife's friend, Leslie, a busy single woman who we would never expect to do such a thing, actually negotiated time off with a new employer so she could fly from her home in Tampa and help out after Garrett's bone marrow transplant (BMT). She stayed with us for over a week, then came back a few months later to do it again.*

> *A couple of my "dive buddies" who we liked, but didn't know well, have since become our best friends. They would visit us in the hospital, bringing both our kids gifts, and giving us a much-needed break. They were the only folks who regularly came by when Garrett was home after the BMT and who always followed our strict rules without complaint.*

> *Of course, the best support we had was from other parents of kids with serious illnesses or problems.*

Restructuring family life

Childhood cancer doesn't just strike families of brave children and heroic parents. In the United States, the popular press has responded to people's terror of cancer by churning out story after story about people who faced the diagnosis with almost superhuman hope and strength. Families rally round, the community cheers, and human will triumphs over the evil of cancer. This simply is not always the case. Cancer strikes all types of families: single-parent families, families with two parents in the home, financially secure families, families with no insurance, families with strong community ties, and families who have just moved to a new community. Families of every size, type, and ethnicity are affected. Most parents do find unexpected reserves of strength to deal with the crisis. They survive the years of stress and pain, emerging different and sometimes stronger. Still, expectations of heroism are unrealistic and inappropriate.

Keeping the household functioning

Every family of a child with leukemia needs massive assistance. It helps if parents recognize this early and learn not only to accept aid gracefully but also to ask for help when needed. As discussed earlier in the chapter, most family members, friends, and neighbors want to help, but they need direction from the family about what is helpful but not intrusive.

In families where both parents are employed, decisions must be made about the jobs. It is better, if possible, to use all available sick leave and vacation days prior to deciding whether one parent needs to terminate employment. Parents need to be able to evaluate their financial situation and insurance availability; this requires time and clarity of thought—both of which are in short supply in the weeks following diagnosis.

> *I was 8 months pregnant when my 2-year-old son was diagnosed. I went on maternity leave, but we needed to make arrangements quickly with my husband's employer to allow him time off to care for Carl in the hospital after I had the baby. Even worse, I knew that I would need to deliver by caesarian section. Carl's protocol required him to be in the hospital for 1 week, then home for 1 week from September through January. My husband worked out a schedule where he worked 70 hours the week that Carl was home, then was off work the week Carl was hospitalized. He then only needed to use 10 hours of leave and was able to stay at the hospital with Carl.*

· · · · ·

> *When Garrett got sick, I used up all of my vacation. At that time, our head of Human Resources called me in and informed me that I now had to take unpaid leave if I wanted to stay out of the office any longer. He then added that in order to continue my benefits, I had to pay "my share" of all benefits costs during this leave.*

This included insurance, retirement, and other contributions. The weekly outlay was not insignificant. I was dismayed to say the least.

Fortunately, our senior management and common sense prevailed. We came to an informal arrangement where I "made up" lost time by working weekends and extended days when Garrett was home and doing okay. When he was inpatient (most of the first year and the first 3 months of the second), I would stay with him in the hospital on the weekends (Friday night through Sunday evening) and on Tuesday night and all day Wednesday. This would give my wife a break from the hospital and let me spend time with my son.

It worked very well. Pam later calculated that I worked more hours in make-up than I missed for Garrett. The company came out ahead. Every situation is different and every solution will be different in these circumstances. There is only one constant: You will never ever regret the precious time you spent with your child.

Family and Medical Leave Act

In August 1993, the Family and Medical Leave Act (FMLA) became federal law in the United States. FMLA protects job security of workers in large companies who must take a leave of absence to care for a seriously ill child, to take medical leave because the employee is unable to work because of his or her own medical condition, or for the birth or placement of a child for adoption or foster care. The FMLA:

- Applies to employers with 50 or more employees within a 75-mile radius.

- Provides 12 weeks of unpaid leave during any 12-month period to care for a seriously ill spouse, child, or parent, or to care for oneself. In certain instances, the employee may take intermittent leave, such as reducing his or her normal work schedule's hours.

- Requires employers to continue providing benefits, including health insurance, during the leave period.

- Requires employers to return employees to the same or equivalent positions upon return from the leave. Some benefits, such as seniority, need not accrue during periods of unpaid FMLA leave.

- Requires employees to give 30-day notice of the need to take FMLA leave when the need is foreseeable.

- Is enforced by complaints to the Wage and Hour Division, U.S. Department of Labor, or by private lawsuit. The nearest office of the Wage and Hour Division may be located by calling (866)-4-USWAGE (487-9243) or visiting its website at *www.dol.gov/ESA/WHD*.

I have never used FMLA. Yes, our bills got bigger than they would have if I had continued to work, but the hospital billing rep has always made sure none of those bills went to collection. The doctor's group, on the other hand, has sent our bills to collection, and it takes a long time to straighten things out.

The regular bills, utility, mortgage, car, etc., get first priority. I do some of our grocery shopping at the cheap cash-n-carry store, which really eases the budget. We go out very seldom, and we still use support from family and friends for incidental baby-sitting. I hire a person to come to my home when I work. My son's care/baby-sitting is paid for by the state Home Services program and I supplement her for my daughter's care.

In Canada, a parent may be entitled to benefits under the Employment Insurance Act. Consideration is provided in the act for a parent having to leave work to care for an ill child. Entitlement to benefits is made on a case-by-case basis. Should a parent qualify, benefits are determined by the number of hours the parent has worked prior to making the claim. For further information, parents should contact the nearest Human Resources and Skills Development Canada office, listed in the Government of Canada pages of the telephone directory, or visit its website at *www.hrsdc.gc.ca.*

Marriage

Cancer treatment places enormous pressure on a marriage. Couples may be separated for long periods of time, emotions run high, and coping styles and skills may differ. Initially, family life may be shattered; couples then must work together to rearrange the pieces into a new pattern. Here are parents' suggestions and stories about how they managed:

• Share medical decisions.

> *My husband and I shared decision-making by keeping a joint medical journal. The days that my husband stayed at the hospital, he would write down all medicines given, side effects, fever, vital signs, food consumed, sleep patterns, and any questions that needed to be asked at the next rounds. This way, I knew exactly what had been happening. Decisions were made as we traded shifts at our son's bedside.*

· · · · ·

> *I made most of the medical decisions. My husband did not know what a protocol was, nor did he ever learn the names of the medicines. He came with me to medical conferences, however, and his presence gave me strength.*

· · · · ·

> *Curt and I discuss every detail of the medical issues. It is so helpful to hash things over together to get a clearer idea of what our main concerns are.*

- Take turns staying in the hospital with the ill child.

   We took turns going in with our son for painful procedures. The doctors loved to see my husband come in because he's a friendly, easygoing person who never asked them any medical questions. We shared hospital duty, also. I would be there during any crisis because I was the person better able to be a strong advocate, but he went when our son was feeling better and needed entertaining company. It worked out well.

   • • • • •

   My husband fell apart emotionally when our daughter was diagnosed, and he never really recovered. He stayed with her once in the hospital and cried almost the whole time. She never wanted him there again, so I did all of the hospital duty.

   • • • • •

   Whenever Brent was in the hospital, we both wanted to be there. We were able to be there most of the time because our children have a wonderful aunt and uncle who stayed with them when needed. During Brent's second extended stay in the hospital, we both let go a little, and we each took turns sleeping at the Ronald McDonald House. That way we each got a decent night's sleep (or some sleep) every other night.

   • • • • •

   My wife took care of most of the medical information gathering because she had a scientific background. But my work schedule was more flexible, so I took my son for almost all of his treatments and hospitalizations. I cherish my memories of those long hours in the car and waiting room, because we were always so very close.

- Share responsibility for home care.

   My husband worked long hours, and therefore I had to do almost all of the home care. It was very hard on me, especially in the beginning when my daughter was so ill and needed so many medications. I felt like I was doing all the horrible things to her; I wish that he could have done some of it.

   • • • • •

   We had a traditional relationship in which I took care of the kids and he worked. I didn't expect him to cook or clean when I was staying at the hospital—it was all he could do to ferry our daughter to her various activities and go to work.

   • • • • •

   We both worked full time, so we staggered our shifts. He worked 7 to 3 during the day; I worked 3 to 11 at night. He did every single dressing change for the Hickman® catheter—584 changes, we counted them up. Wherever I left off during the day, he took over. He was great, and it really worked out well for us. We shared it all.

My husband really didn't help at all. I couldn't even go out because he wouldn't give the pills. He kept saying that he was afraid he would make a mistake.

- Accept differences in coping styles.

   We both coped differently, but we learned to work around it. I didn't want to deal with "what if" questions, but he was a pessimist and constantly asked the fellow questions about things that might happen. I felt that it was a waste of energy to worry about things that might never happen. I didn't want to hear it and felt that it just added to my burden. It was all I could do to survive every day. We worked it out by going to conferences together, but I would ask my questions and then leave. He stayed behind to ask all of his questions.

   • • • • •

   My husband didn't have the desire to read as much as I did. However, whenever I read something that I felt he should read, he always took the time to do so and then we discussed it.

- Seek counseling.

   I went for counseling because I couldn't sleep. At night, I got stuck thinking the same things over and over and worrying. I ended up spending 2 years on antidepressants, which I think really saved my life. They helped me sleep and kept me on an even keel. I'm off them now, my son is off treatment, and everything is looking up.

   • • • • •

   My husband and I went to counseling to try to work out a way to split up the child rearing and household duties because I was overwhelmed and resenting it. I guess it helped a little bit, but the best thing that came out of it was that I kept seeing the counselor by myself. My son wanted to go to the "feelings doctor," too. I received a lot of very helpful, practical advice on the many behavior problems my son developed. And my son had an objective, safe person to talk things over with.

Most marriages survive, but some don't. It is usually marriages with serious pre-existing problems that are further strained by cancer treatment.

My husband had a lot of problems that really brought my daughter and me down. The cancer really opened my eyes to what was important in life. We stayed together through treatment, but we divorced after the bone marrow transplant. I just realized that life is too short to spend it in a bad relationship.

My husband went to work rather than go with us to Children's when our son was diagnosed. It went downhill from there. He started using drugs and mistreating us, so we divorced.

Blended families

Many children diagnosed with leukemia live in blended families. Parents may be separated or divorced, remarried, or living as single parents. There may be foster parents, biological parents, stepparents, or legal guardians. Communication between involved adults may be open and amiable or stressed and uncooperative. It is best for the child when all parents/guardians involved put their differences aside and work together to provide an environment focused on curing and supporting the ill child. Counseling helps, too.

> *I have a blended family (although my husband and I have been married for 20 years now) and have two teenagers in the house. My recommendation is counseling. Both of my teenagers and I see a therapist individually. My husband and I also had to go to marriage counseling at various times during our marriage. Serious illness will put a strain on any marriage. If you have issues before cancer strikes, they will become exacerbated. We have good insurance and it pays for most of our sessions. I paid about 20 percent out of pocket. It is so worth it. Raising a family is hard work. Add cancer on top of it and, quite frankly, it can become overwhelming. Family counseling helps each member of the family have an outlet to express their concerns and worries.*

If the child with cancer has two homes due to a blended family, it often helps to have a journal that goes with the child to each set of parents. It keeps everyone involved up to date. It can contain medications given, dose changes, doctor's appointments, blood test results, and current symptoms.

Unfortunately, the diagnosis of cancer in a child can make strained family relations even worse. It is important that all parents/guardians with a legal right to information about all aspects of the illness receive that information and are able to participate in the decision-making process. In some situations a social worker, nurse practitioner, primary physician, or psychologist will work with all parties to set up family meetings (together as a group or separately, depending on family dynamics) with healthcare providers to make this possible.

Telling your friends about cancer is difficult, but it's not as hard as keeping it a secret would be. Fighting this cancer has been a family effort and, frequently, an effort involving our larger circle of friends. The more people we've been able to call on for support, the better. We've had to keep in mind that we've had an opportunity to adjust. But, the news is brand new to our friends, and it can be a shock. People often don't know what to do or say when they've been told that someone they care about has cancer.

After we've given them some time, and when they ask what they can do, we tell them something constructive: mow the lawn, take back the recyclables, go to the store, bring over a pizza on Friday night, whatever would help.

Before my son was diagnosed, I had no idea what this experience was like, and I try to remember that my friends don't really know either, unless I tell them. They can't know the sleepless nights, the anxiety over tests, the fear when your child says he doesn't feel well, or the terror that we might lose our precious child. Some of us have found great support and others none. I hope your family and friends come to your side.

I want to say that I hope that cancer does not become your life. For us, it used to be an "elephant in the living room," and now it's maybe a "zebra in the kitchen." There are times when it demands everything you can give, no doubt, but there will be moments when there is time for the rest of your life.

Chapter 13

Communication
and Behavior

When I approach a child, he inspires in me two sentiments:
tenderness for what he is, and respect for what he may become.

— Louis Pasteur

UNDER THE BEST OF CIRCUMSTANCES, child rearing is a daunting task. When parenting is complicated by an overwhelming crisis such as leukemia, communication within the family may suffer, and both children and parents may have difficulty adjusting to the new stressors in their lives. Prior to the diagnosis, children usually know the family rules and the consequences for breaking them. After diagnosis, normal family life is disrupted, and all sorts of confusing and distressing feelings and behaviors may appear. When people are under great stress, they often behave in ways they would not under normal circumstances. In response, parenting styles may need to change to the frequently shifting needs and behaviors of the ill child and affected siblings.

This chapter covers feelings that many children have about their disease and some emotional and behavioral changes that may arise in both children and parents. Suggestions for maintaining effective communication and appropriate behavior within the family are also offered. The stories included describe what many parents experienced and how they coped with their and their ill child's powerful, and sometimes overwhelming, emotions. For stories about the emotions of siblings, please see Chapter 14, "Siblings."

Communication

Chapter 1, "Diagnosis," lists many of the feelings parents may experience after their child's leukemia diagnosis. It is helpful to remember that children, both siblings and the ill child, are also overwhelmed by strong feelings, and they generally have fewer coping skills than adults. At different times and to varying degrees, children and teens may feel fearful, angry, resentful, powerless, violated, lonely, weird, inferior, incompetent, or betrayed. Children have to learn strategies to deal with these strong feelings to prevent "acting out" behaviors (aggression, risk taking) or "acting in" behaviors (depression, withdrawal).

Good communication is the first step toward helping your family identify how child behavior and family functioning are being impacted and how family members can work with each other and with professionals to restore order and a nurturing climate. Clear and loving communication with your child or teen is the foundation for trust. Children need to know from the very beginning that you will answer questions truthfully and take the time to talk about feelings.

Honesty

Above all else, children need to be able to trust their parents. They can face almost anything, as long as they know their parents will be at their side. Trust requires honesty. For your ill child and her brothers and sisters to feel secure, they must always know that they can depend on you to tell them the truth, be it good news or bad. This trust you build with your children reduces feelings of isolation and disconnection within the family.

> We were always very honest. We felt that if she couldn't trust us to tell her the truth, how scary that would be. I've seen a few incidents in the clinic of people with totally different styles who don't tell their kids the truth. I ran into the bathroom at the clinic crying after overhearing a mother who had deceived her child into coming to the clinic. Then he found out he needed a back poke and completely lost it. It makes me cringe. Children just have to be prepared. If they can't trust their parents, who can they trust?

Listening

Just trying to get through each day consumes most of a parent's time, attention, and energy. Consequently, one of the greatest gifts parents can give their children is time—a special time when they really focus on what children are saying; a time when they listen to not only the words, but the feelings that generate them.

> After my relapse at age 13, the chemotherapy was much more difficult to tolerate. My appearance changed dramatically due to hair loss and rapid weight gain from prednisone. The L-asparaginase made my legs stiff and sore, so that it was difficult to walk. After a 2-month absence, when I returned to school, the treatment I received from the other students was unbearable. I finally refused to go to school. I felt so strongly about not going to school that once, on the way there, I jumped out of the car at an intersection. This helped mom and dad make the decision to send me to a private school. The kids and staff at the new school knew my situation and were very compassionate. The decision to change schools was one of the best things my parents ever did for me.

· · · · ·

*When my daughter was 7 years old (3 years after her treatment ended), I realized
how important it was to keep listening. She was complaining about a hangnail and
I told her that I would cut it for her. She started to yell that I would hurt her. I asked
her, "When have I ever hurt you?" and she said, "In the hospital." I sat down with
her in my arms, rocked her, and explained what had happened in the hospital during
her treatment, why we had to bring her, and how we felt about it. I told her how I
felt when she was hurt by procedures. I asked her to tell me about her memories and
feelings about being in the hospital. We cleared the air that day, and I expect we will
need to talk about it many more times in the future. Then she held out her hand so I
could cut off her hangnail.*

Talking

If you are not in the habit of sharing your feelings with your children, it is hard to start
doing so in a crisis. But now, more than ever, it's important to try. Parents can provide an
opening for discussion by simply stating how they are feeling, for example, "I have lots
of different feelings at the same time. Sometimes I really get mad at the cancer because
it is making you life so tough but I am also happy that the medicine is working." Telling
your healthy children how you feel can strengthen your connection and reassure them
of your love: "I really miss you when I have to take your sister to the hospital. I'll call
you every night just so I can hear your voice," or "I wish the family didn't have to be
separated so much, and I feel sad that you have to go through this."

It is also helpful to tell your child with leukemia how the illness is affecting her siblings,
for example, "It is very hard for Jim to stay at home with a babysitter when I bring you
to the hospital. Let's try to think of something nice to do for him." Such statements reassure children of your continued love for them and distress about being separated from
them; they also create an opportunity for children to share with you how they feel about
what is happening to the family.

*My daughter, diagnosed at 1 year old and now entering fifth grade, has three older
siblings, so we have been through many developmental stages as far as communication goes. I try to answer their questions honestly, but I only tell them what I think
they can understand without overwhelming them with information. I remember one
of my boys, soon after my daughter's diagnosis, asked me if she was going to die, and
I said "no" emphatically. I regretted it immediately, and realized that I would have
to deal with my fears about the possibility of her dying, then go back and tell him
the truth. So, later, I told him that I hadn't given an accurate answer because I was
scared and that we didn't know if she was going to die. We hoped not, but we would
have to wait and see.*

I have found that as their understanding deepens, they come back with more questions, needing more detailed answers. So, my motto is, be honest, but don't scare them. If you say everything is okay, but you are crying, they know something is wrong, and that they can't trust you for the truth.

Common behavioral changes in children

Discipline can be challenging, even when family life is going well. But when a child has leukemia, parents are stressed, siblings are angry, and the ill child is scared and upset. Parents may find themselves reaching their emotional breaking points, and children may begin behaving in negative ways, making the situation unmanageable. The first step to reestablishing order is to decide whether the ill child is going to be treated as if she only has a few months to live, or as if she will survive and needs to learn strategies for how to self-regulate difficult emotions. Step two is to examine your own behavior to see if you are modeling the conduct that you expect from your children. Step three is to develop a consistent, healthy response to the angry or destructive child to help her develop social and emotional competence.

Barbara Sourkes, a respected child psychologist, wrote in her book *Armfuls of Time: The Psychological Experience of the Child with a Life-Threatening Illness:*

> *While loss of control extends over emotional issues, and ultimately over life itself, its emergence is most vivid in the child's day-to-day experience of the illness, in the barrage of intrusive, uncomfortable, or painful procedures that he or she must endure. The child strives desperately to regain a measure of control, often expressed through resistant, noncompliant behavior or aggressive outbursts. Too often, the source of the anger—the loss of control—goes unrecognized by parents and caregivers. However, once its meaning is acknowledged, an explicit distinction may be drawn for the child between what he or she can or cannot dictate. In order to maximize the child's sense of control, the environment can be structured to allow for as much choice as is feasible. Even options that appear small or inconsequential serve as an antidote to loss, and their impact is often reflected in dramatic improvements in behavior.*

In the following sections, parents share how they handled their children's range of emotions and behaviors.

Anger

Parents respond to the diagnosis of leukemia with anger, and so do children. Not only is the child angry at the disease, but also at the parents for bringing her in to be hurt, at having to take medicine that makes her feel terrible, at losing her hair, at losing her friends, and on and on. Children with cancer and their siblings have good reasons to be angry.

I think that much anger can be avoided by giving choices and letting kids have some control. Parents need to clearly explain that there are some things that simply have to be done (spinal taps) but that the child or teen is in control of positions, people present, music, even timing. For example, if your teen gets bad headaches after spinals, help him negotiate the date and time when the spinal will be done so that sports or social life will not be impacted.

• • • • •

We have a case of the halo or the horns. Our son is either very defiant or an absolute angel. He argues about every single thing. I really think that it is because he has had so little control in his life. I have very clear rules, am very firm, and put my foot down. But I also try to choose my battles wisely so we can have good times, too. My husband reminds me when I get aggravated that if he weren't this type of tough kid, he wouldn't have made it through so many setbacks. Then I am just glad to still have him with us.

Tantrums

Healthy children have tantrums when they are overwhelmed by strong feelings, and so do children with leukemia. In some cases, tantrums can be predicted by parents paying close attention to what triggers the outburst (for example, a missed nap or anxiety about an upcoming procedure). This knowledge can help parents prevent tantrums by avoiding situations that create emotional overload for their child; but sometimes there is no warning of the impending tantrum. Knowledge can also help parents understand that many tantrums and behavioral changes are due to medication side effects (for example, steroids) and are out of the child's control.

We never knew what would set off 3-year-old Rachel, and to tell the truth, she didn't know what the problem was herself. She was very verbal and aware in many ways, but she had no idea what was bothering her and causing the anger. I would just hold her with her blanket, hug her, and rock until she calmed down. Later she would say, "I was out of control," but she still didn't know why.

Of course, if the child is destructive, he needs help learning safer ways to vent his anger. For a child who is frequently destructive, professional counseling is necessary. *The Misunderstood Child* by Larry Silver has a chapter that explains in detail how parents can initiate a behavior modification program at home:

My son had frequent, violent rages that sometimes caused damage (toys thrown at the walls, books ripped up). He was small, but strong. I talked to him when he was calm about how the tantrums would be handled. Tantrums with no damage would be ignored; afterwards we would cuddle and talk about what prompted the anger and other ways for him to handle the anger. If he began to break things or hurt people, I would wrap him in a blanket and rock him until he relaxed. I would tell him, "I need to hold you because you are out of control. This is so hard. I know. I love you." All of the tantrums ended after he went off treatment, but dealing with his destructive anger was one of the hardest things I have ever experienced.

• • • • •

When my son needed to get out a good old temper tantrum just to unload, I'd let him. Then he'd fall into my reassuring arms and soak up some good ole momma lovin' and just whimper till he slept...my hand stroking his hair, and I'm whispering things like, "I know, honey, I know. It's just so wrong. I'm here, baby. I love you. I know. I know. Just sleep for now. I'll be here when you wake. I'm not moving. I'm not going anywhere. I love you. There now."

Withdrawal

Some children deal with their feelings by withdrawing rather than blowing up in anger. Like denial, withdrawal can be temporarily helpful as a way to come to grips with strong feelings. However, too much withdrawal is not good for children, and it can be a sign of depression. Parents or counselors need to find gentle ways to allow withdrawn children to express how they are feeling.

My daughter became very depressed and withdrawn as treatment continued. She started to talk only about a fantasy world that she created in her imagination. She seemed to be less and less in the real world. She didn't ever talk to her therapist about her feelings, but they did lots of art work together. At the beginning, she only drew pictures of herself with her body filling the whole page. After EMLA® (local anesthetic) became available, and she was less terrified of being hurt, she began to draw her body more normal sized. As she got better, she began to draw the family again. When she drew a beautiful sun shining on the family, I cried. She just couldn't talk about it, but she worked so much out through her art.

The emotional impact of cancer is very pronounced during the teenage years, a time when appearance is particularly important. When adolescents look different from their peers, they may feel sad, angry, embarrassed, bewildered, helpless, and scared. Thus, depression is common during and after treatment. Children and teens may go through a period of withdrawal and/or grieving; it is crucial that children and teens receive support and counseling during these times.

I had cancer when I was 15. I tried so hard as a freshman in college to put it all behind me and get on with my life. It just didn't work. Next to treatment, that was the worst year of my life. It showed me that if I didn't deal with it consciously, I was going to deal with it subconsciously. I had nightmares every night. I'd wake up feeling that I had needles in my arms. I decided to start taking better care of myself in a different kind of way. I do something fun every day. I try to see the positive side of situations. I read more and write a lot. I unplug from the cancer community whenever I feel overwhelmed. I try to explore my feelings with my counselor rather than shove them in the back corner. It's like garbage; if you don't take it out, it starts to stink. Once I started dealing with these feelings, things really improved.

Comfort objects

Many parents worry when, after diagnosis, children regress to using a special comfort object. Many young children ask to return to using a bottle, or cling to a favorite toy or blanket. It is reasonable to allow your child to use whatever he can to find comfort against the terrible realities of treatment. The behaviors usually stop either when the child starts feeling better or when treatment ends.

My daughter was a hair twirler. Whenever she was nervous, she would twirl a bit of her hair around her finger. As her hair fell out, she kept grabbing at her head to find a wisp to curl. I told her that she could twirl mine until hers grew back. She spent a lot of time next to me or in my lap with her hand in my hair. It was annoying for me sometimes, but it had a great calming effect on her. When hers grew back, I would gently remind her that she had her own hair to twirl. She also went back to a bottle, although we did limit the bottle use to home or hospital. Both behaviors, hair twirling and drinking from a bottle, disappeared within 6 months of the end of treatment, when she was 6 years old.

• • • • •

My son was a blanket baby. I remember getting so much advice about how to take the blanket away from him, when actually I was not at all concerned. He eventually cuddled it less and less, and it finally was packed into my memory box—until he was diagnosed with leukemia. He was 15, and he actually asked me to bring it to the hospital. In tears, I dragged that pitiful-looking, raggedy blanket to the hospital.

Talking about death

Part of effective parenting is allowing children to talk about topics that may cause feelings of discomfort in parents and children. No parent wants to talk, or even think, about the possibility of a child's death. In some cultures, the subject of death is taboo. But a diagnosis of cancer forces both parents and children to acknowledge that death is a very real possibility. Even children as young as 3 years old may think about death and what it means. They need to be able to talk about their feelings, fears, or questions without the parents shutting down the conversation.

Eighteen months into treatment, 5-year-old Katy said, "Mommy, sometimes I think about my spirit leaving my body. I think my spirit is here (gesturing to the back of her head) and my body is here (pointing to her belly button). I just wanted you to know that I think about it sometimes."

• • • • •

After my first relapse at age 13, my parents always kept the focus on the future. On the way to every procedure, we would plan the wonderful things that we were going to do afterwards. They never discussed death. But when I asked if leukemia could kill people, my father was honest and he told me, "Yes, some kids die." I appreciated him being straight with me, and I went right back to being optimistic.

After my third relapse, my nurse said something to me about death and dying. I clearly remember my reaction. I told her, "I know kids die from this, but I'm not going to!"

Trusting your child

Sometimes children will tell you what they need to do to persevere through this trial. Their coping choices may not be what the parents would choose—the decisions may even make the parents nervous. But, it is the child or teen's way to make peace with the day-to-day reality of diagnosis and treatment.

Early one summer morning, 12-year-old Preston and I left the hospital after a week-long stay for his high-dose methotrexate infusion. He had been heavily sedated and was groggy and shaky on his feet. My husband and daughter were getting ready to go on a boat trip, and I felt Preston was too sick to go. We sadly saw them off, then returned to the car. Preston said, "Mom, I really need to go fishing. I know you don't understand, but I really need to do this."

It made me very uncomfortable, but we went home to get his equipment. We then drove up to the mountains to a very deserted spot on the river, and Preston said that he needed to be out of my sight. So I watched him put on his waders, walk into the swift river, and disappear around a bend upstream. I went out into the river and sat on a rock. I waited for 2 hours before Preston came back. He said, "That's what I needed; I feel much better now."

There is a fine line between providing adequate protection for our children or teens and becoming overly controlling because of worry about the disease. You might ask yourself, "If she didn't have cancer, would I let her do this?"

Coping well

Many children develop emotional competence from facing and coping with the difficulties of cancer. Others, because of both temperament and the environments in which they have lived, are blessed with good coping abilities. They understand what is required, and they do it. Many parents express great admiration for their child's strength and grace in the face of adversity.

Stephan has not had any behavior problems while being treated for his initial diagnosis (age 5) or his relapse (age 7). He has never complained about going to the hospital and views the medical staff as his friends. He has never argued or fought about painful treatments. Unlike many of the parents in the support group, we've never had to deal with any emotional issues. We are fortunate that he has that confident personality. He just says, "We've got to do it, so let's just get it done."

Common behavioral changes in parents

It's impossible to talk about children's behavior without discussing parental behavior. Your child's development does not occur in a vacuum; it occurs within the context of your family, and you set the tone for your home's atmosphere. At different times during their child's treatment, parents may be under enormous physical, emotional, financial, and existential stress. The crisis can cause parents to behave in ways of which they are not always proud—ways in which they would not behave under normal circumstances. Some of the common problem behaviors mentioned by parents follow.

Dishonesty

As stated earlier, children feel safe when their parents are honest with them. If the parents start to keep secrets from the child to protect her from distressing news, the child feels isolated and fearful. She might think, "If mom and dad won't tell me, it must be really bad," or, "Mom won't talk about it. I guess there's nobody I can tell about how scared I am."

Denial is a type of unconscious dishonesty. This occurs when parents say things to children such as, "Everything will be just fine," or, "It won't hurt a bit." This type of pretending just increases the distance between child and parent, leaving the child with no support. However horrible the truth, it seldom is as terrifying to a child as a half-truth upon which his imagination builds.

> *I try so hard to be honest with my 5-year-old son, but blood draws, which he thinks of as "shots," are just so hard for him. Every doctor's visit, that's his first question, "I'm going to get a shot?" and I just want to say no. My husband's the one who started saying, "It'll be fine," but the anxiety that came up later at the appointment was so much worse that I put an end to that pretty quickly. Now I say, "Yes, but just once," because if I say, "I don't know," it just makes him worry.*

Depression

Parents of children with cancer often feel sad or depressed. If you or your child are consistently experiencing any of the following symptoms, it would probably be helpful to get professional help: changes in sleeping patterns (sleeping too much, waking up frequently during the night, early morning awakening), appetite disturbances (eating too little or too much), loss of sex drive, fatigue, panic attacks, inability to experience pleasure, feelings of sadness and despair, poor concentration, social withdrawal, feelings of worthlessness, suicidal thoughts, or drug or alcohol abuse. Depression is extremely common and very treatable, and it should be dealt with early.

> *Find a counselor you click with. Stick with that person until you truly feel some peace about your experiences and strength for dealing with the ongoing stress of treatment or whatever else might come up. I regret that I toughed it out and didn't recognize the depression I was experiencing for such a long time. I think finding sources of support in a variety of ways at the earliest moment possible can greatly mitigate long-term difficulties in coping.*

Losing your temper excessively

All parents lose their temper sometimes. They lose their tempers with spouses, healthy children, pets, and even strangers. But it is especially painful for parents, the sick child, and siblings when the target of the anger is a very sick child or a brother or sister.

Abuse of children and spouses increases at times when either or both spouses feel incompetent and powerless. If you find yourself unable to manage your temper, seek professional counseling.

> *I had my share of temper tantrums. The worst was when he was having his radiation. I tried to make him eat because it would be so many hours before he could have any more food. He always threw up all over himself and me, several times, every morning. It seemed like we changed clothing at least three times before we even got out of the house each day. I remember one day just screaming at him, "Can't you even learn how to throw up? Can't you just bend over to barf?" I really flunked mother of the year that day. I can't believe that I was screaming at this sick little kid, who I love so much.*

• • • • •

> *I had always taught my children that feeling anger was okay, but we had to make good choices about what to do with it. Hitting other people or breaking things was a bad choice; hitting pillows, running around outside, or punching pillows were good choices. But, as with everything else, they learned the most from watching how I handled my anger, and during the hard months of treatment my temper was short. When I found myself thinking of hitting them, I'd say, in a very loud voice, "I'm afraid I'm going to hurt somebody so I'm going in my room for a time-out." If my husband was home, I'd take a warm shower to calm down; if he wasn't, I'd just sit on the bed and take as many deep breaths as it took to calm down.*

Unequal application of household rules

You will guarantee family problems if the ill child enjoys favored status while the siblings must do extra chores. Granted, it is hard to know the right time to insist that your ill child resume making his bed or setting the table, but it must be done. Siblings need to know from the beginning that any child in the family, if sick, will be excused from chores, but that this child will have do them again as soon as he is physically able.

> *I spoiled my sick daughter and tried to enforce the rules for my son. That didn't work, so I gave up on him and spoiled them both. He was really acting out at school. What he needed was structure and more attention, but what he got was more and more things. They both ended up thinking the whole world revolved around them, and it was my fault.*

Overindulgence of the ill child

Overindulgence is a very common behavior of parents of children with cancer.

> *I bought my daughter everything I saw that was pretty and lovely. I kept thinking that if she died she would die happy because she'd be surrounded by all these beautiful things. Even when I couldn't really afford it, I kept buying. I realize now that I was doing it to make me feel better, not her. She needed cuddling and loving, not clothes and dolls.*

· · · · ·

> *Four days into Selah's diagnosis, we were doing anything to keep her happy. Our sweet little 4-year-old had turned into a demon child in that short time. Luckily, my very dear friend took me outside into the hallway, pushed me against the wall, and demanded to know exactly what I was doing. I just looked at her and said, "I have no idea." I just didn't want my daughter to die and that was my only focus. She then told me I was giving my daughter no boundaries, no behavior expectations, and she had no respect for anyone who walked into the room. She was so right, and I couldn't see it for fear that Selah would die. Through my tears and our hugs, she assured me that the way we were going, if she didn't die from leukemia, we were going to want to kill her because of the monster we were creating. I am still so grateful that she wasn't afraid to tell me what I needed to hear.*

One aspect of overindulgence that is quite common is parents' reluctance to teach life skills to sick children. After years of dealing with a physically weak and sometimes emotionally demanding child, parents may forget to expect age-appropriate skills.

> *I realized that I had formed a habit of treating my child as if she were still young and sick. I was still treating her like a 3 year old, and she was 7. One day, when I was pouring her juice, I thought, "Why am I doing this? She's 7. She needs to learn to make her own sandwiches and pour her own drinks. She needs to be encouraged to*

grow up." Boy, it has been hard. But I've stuck to my guns, and made other extended family members do it, too. I want her to grow up to be an independent adult, not a demanding, overgrown kid.

Overprotection of sick child

For a child to feel normal, he needs to be treated as if he is normal. Ask the doctor what changes in physical activity are necessary for safety, and do not impose any additional restrictions on your child. Let the child be involved in sports or neighborhood play. And even though it is hard, stop yourself from constantly reminding your child to be careful.

> *My 6-year-old son finished his radiation and is still on chemo for his cancer. I feel like I have to lighten up in order for life to go on. So I just let the nanny take all four kids on a 4-hour drive to spend 8 hours at Six Flags®. It just about drove us nuts with worry, but they all came home safe and sound. They felt like they had a normal sibling outing.*

Not spending enough time with the sibling(s)

While acknowledging that there are only so many hours in a day, parents interviewed for this book felt the most guilt about the effect leukemia had on the siblings. They wished they had asked family and friends to stay with the sick child more often, allowing them to spend more of their precious time with the siblings. Many expressed pain that they didn't know how severely affected the siblings had been.

> *I try to find some time in each holiday, weekend, or whenever it is just for Christopher and me. No matter how ill Michael is, someone else can cope with it for an hour or two, and nothing is allowed to interfere with that. We still go out, even if it is only Christopher and me at McDonald's®.*

> *Bottom line is that all mothers have to accept that along with the baby is delivered a large package of guilt, and whatever we do for one we will wish we had done for the other.*

> *But I don't think you can put one child on hold for the duration of the other's illness, because the year that Christopher has lost while Michael has been ill won't ever come again. He'll only be 11 once, just as surely as Michael will only be 14 once (or possibly forever), and we owe it to our healthy kids to allow them to be just that.*

Using substance abuse to cope

Some parents find themselves turning to alcohol or drugs to help them cope. Not only illegal drugs are abused; overuse of over-the-counter sleeping pills or prescription medications also occurs. If you find yourself drinking so much that your behavior is affected, or using drugs to get through the day or night, seek professional help.

Coping

Many parents find unexpected reserves of strength and are able to ask for help from friends and family when they need it. They realize that different needs arise when there is a great stress to the family, and they alter their expectations and parenting accordingly. These families usually had strong and effective communication prior to the illness and pull together as a unit to deal with it.

The majority of families, however, have periods of calm alternating with times when nerves are frayed and tempers are short. And in the end, most families survive intact and are often strengthened by the years of dealing with cancer.

Improving communication and discipline

Parents suggest the following ways to keep the family more even keeled.

- Make sure the family rules are clearly understood by all of the children. Stressed children feel safe in homes with regular, predictable routines.

    After yet another rage by my daughter with leukemia, we held a family meeting to clarify the rules and consequences for breaking them. We asked the kids (both preschoolers) to dictate a list of what they thought the rules were. The following was the result, and we posted copies of the list all over the house (which created much merriment among our friends):

    1. No peeing on rug.

    2. No jumping on bed.

    3. No hitting or pinching.

    4. No name calling.

    5. No breaking things.

    6. No writing on walls.

    If they broke a rule, we would gently lead them to the list and remind them of the house rules. It really helped.

- Have all caretakers consistently enforce the family rules.

    We kept the same household rules. I was determined that we needed to start with the expectation that Rachel was going to survive. I never wanted her to be treated like a "poor little sick kid," because I was afraid she would become one. We had to be careful about babysitters, because we didn't want anyone to feel sorry for her or treat her differently. I do feel that we avoided many long-term behavior problems by adopting this attitude early.

- Give all the kids some power by offering choices and letting them completely control some aspects of their lives, as appropriate.

> For a few months we ignored Shawn's two brothers as we struggled to get a handle on the situation. We just shuttled them around with no consideration for their feelings. When we realized how unfair we were being, we made a list of places to stay, and let them choose each time we had to go off to the hospital. We worked it out together, and things went much smoother.

· · · · ·

> My bald, angry, 4-year-old daughter asked me for some scissors one day. I asked what she was going to do, and she said "Cut off all the Barbies'® hair." I told her those were her dolls and she could cut off their hair if she chose. I asked her to consider leaving one or two with hair, because when she had long hair again, she might want dolls that looked like her then, too. But I said it was up to her. She cut off the hair (down to the plastic skull!) of all but one of the dolls. It really seemed to make her feel better. A few months later, she dismembered them. Fifteen years later, we occasionally find Barbie® legs and arms lying around the house, and we all laugh.

- Take control of the incoming gifts. Too many gifts make the ill child worry excessively ("If I'm getting all of these great presents, things must be really bad") and make the siblings jealous. Be specific if you want people not to bring gifts, or if you want gifts for each child, not just the sick one.

- Recognize that some problems are caused solely by the drugs. (See the prednisone section of Chapter 9, "Chemotherapy.") It helps to remember that children with cancer are not naturally defiant or destructive. They are feeling sick, powerless, and altered by massive doses of toxic drugs, and parents need to try to help by sympathizing, yet setting limits. Remember, when they get off the drugs, their real personalities will return.

> In the beginning, my 2-year-old daughter was incredibly angry. She would have massive temper tantrums, and I would just hold her and tell her that I wouldn't let her hurt anybody. I would continue to hold her until she changed from angry to sad. When she was on the dexamethasone, she would either be hugging me or pinching, biting, or sucking my neck. It drove me crazy. Now, on maintenance, she's not having as many fits, but she still pushes her sisters off swings or the trampoline. She has a general lack of control. Sometimes, when I can't stand it anymore, I swat her on the bottom, and then I feel really bad.

- Even though some oncologists tell parents that during the maintenance phase of treatment life will return to normal, it usually does not. It is often better than the intensive parts of treatment, but emotional and behavioral difficulties often arise during maintenance when the child regains his strength. Be glad if your child's difficulties subside during maintenance, but don't expect them to.

Our kids go along okay for a while, dealing with stuff. Then suddenly (because they're tired, have reached a new point developmentally, or are not feeling well in a way they can't describe), they lose it. It seems that every kid needs something different at these times, but what works best for Cami is for us to help her find words for her frustration. We talk about how unfair cancer is, how terrible treatment is, how no one else really knows what she's going through. Sometimes she just bursts out crying with relief that someone understands!

Recently, when Cami was going through another "This-is-the-last-time-I'm-going-to-the-doctor" outburst, we spent the waiting time writing a list of all the horrible things we want to do to cancer (step on it; put needles in its eye; not let it have cake). I also draw cells—good and bad. We give lollipops to the good cells and scribble out the bad ones. It sounds simplistic, but it really helps.

• If your child likes to draw, paint, knit, collage, or do other artwork or crafts, encourage it. Art is both soothing and therapeutic, and it gives the child a positive outlet for feelings and creativity.

When Jody was in the laminar airflow (isolation) room for weeks after his bone marrow transplant, he passed the time by doing many collages. I kept him well supplied with all sorts of materials, and he created beautiful things.

• Allow your child to be totally in charge of his art. Do not make suggestions or criticisms (e.g., "stay inside the lines" or "skies need to be blue not orange"). Rather, encourage them and praise their efforts. Display the artwork in your home. Listen carefully if your child offers an explanation about the art, but do not pry if she says it is private. Above all, do not interpret it yourself or disagree with your child about what the art represents. Being supportive will allow your child to explore ways to soothe himself and clarify strong feelings.

Jody was continually making projects. We kept him supplied with a fishing box full of materials, and he glued and taped and constructed all sorts of sculptures. He did beautiful drawings full of color, and every person he drew always had hands shaped like hearts. If we asked him what he was making, he always answered, "I'll show you when I'm done."

• If your child does artwork or likes to write, recognize that powerful emotions may surface for both child and parents.

At my daughter's preschool, once a week each child would tell the teacher a story, which the teacher wrote down for the child to take home. Most of my daughter's stories were like this: "There was a rhinoceros. He lived in the jungle. Then he went in the pool. Then he decided to take a walk. And then he ate some strawberries. Then he visited his friend." But the week before or after a painful procedure, she would dictate frightening stories (and this from a kid who wasn't allowed to watch TV and had never seen any violence). Two examples are: "Once there were some bees and they stung someone and this someone was allergic to them and then they got hurt by some monkeybars and the monkeybars had needles on them and the lightning came and hit the bees," and, "Once upon a time there were six stars and they twinkled at night and then the sun started to come up. And then they had a serious problem. They shot their heads and they had blood dripping down."

- Come up with acceptable ways for your child to physically release her anger. Some options are: ride a bike, run around the house, swing, play basketball or soccer, pound nails into wood, mold clay, punch pillows, yell, take a shower or bath, or draw angry pictures. In addition, teach your child to use words to express his anger, for example, "It makes me so angry when you do that," or "I am so mad I feel like hitting you." Releasing anger physically and expressing anger verbally in appropriate ways are both valuable life skills to master.

    Shawn was very, very angry many times. We had clear rules that it was okay to be angry, but he couldn't hit people. We bought a punching bag, which he really pounded sometimes. Play-Doh® helped, too. We had a machine to make Play-Doh® shapes, which took a lot of effort. He would hit it, pound it, push it, roll it. Then he would press it through the machine and keep turning that handle. It seemed to really help him with his aggression.

- Treat the ill child as normally as possible.

    When Justin was in the hospital, I could never stand to see him in those little hospital gowns. I asked if we could dress him in his own outfits, and they said yes. So even when he was in the ICU (intensive care unit) with all the tubes coming out of his body, we dressed him every day in something cute. It just felt better to see him in his clothes. Several months later my mother said she really admired us for doing that, because we were sending the message to Justin that everything was going to be okay. That even though he couldn't breathe on his own, he was still going to get up every day and get dressed. Now I think it probably did communicate to him that things were going to be normal again.

- Get professional help whenever you are concerned or run out of ideas about how to handle emotional problems. Mental health care professionals (see Chapter 16, "Sources of Support") have spent years learning how to help resolve these kinds of problems, so let them help you.

    My daughter and I both went to a wonderful therapist throughout most of her treatment for ALL (acute lymphoblastic leukemia). My daughter was a very sensitive, easily overwhelmed child, who withdrew more and more into a world of fantasy as cancer treatment progressed. The therapist was skilled at drawing out her feelings through artwork and play. She also helped me with very specific suggestions on parenting. For instance, when I told the therapist that my daughter thought that treatment would never end (a reasonable assumption for a preschooler), she suggested that I put two jars on my daughter's desk. One was labeled "ALL DONE," and the other was labeled "TO DO." We put a rock for every procedure and treatment already completed in the ALL DONE jar, and one rock for every one yet to do in the TO DO jar. (Only recommended if the child is more than halfway through treatment.) Then, each time we came home, my daughter would move a rock into the ALL DONE jar. It gave her a concrete way to visualize the approach of the end of treatment. She could see the dwindling number of pebbles left. On the last day of treatment, when she moved the last pebble over and the TO DO jar was empty, I cried, but she danced.

- Most emotional problems resulting from cancer treatment can be resolved through professional counseling. However, some children and parents also need medications to get them through particularly rough times.

   My daughter was doing really well throughout treatment until a combination of events occurred that was more than she could handle. Her grandmother died from cancer during the summer, one of her friends with cancer died on December 27, then another friend relapsed for the second time. She was fine during the day, but at night she constantly woke up stressed and upset. She had dreams about trapdoors, witches brewing potions to give to little children, and saw people coming into her room to take her away. She would wake up smelling smoke. She was awake 3 or 4 hours in the middle of the night, every night. Her doctor put her on sleeping pills and anti-anxiety medications, and the social worker came out to the house twice a month.

- Teach children relaxation or visualization skills to help them cope better with strong feelings. (See Appendix C, "Books, Websites, and Videotapes" for books about developing such skills.)

- Have reasonable expectations. If you are expecting a sick 4 year old to act like a healthy 6 year old, or a teenager to act like an adult, you are setting your child up to fail.

   It seemed like we spent most of the years of treatment waiting to see a doctor who was running hours behind schedule. Since my child had trouble sitting still and was always hungry, I came well prepared. I always carried a large bag containing an assortment of things to eat and drink, toys to play with, coloring books and markers, books to read aloud, and Play-Doh®. He stayed occupied and we avoided many problems. I saw too many parents in the waiting room expecting their bored children to sit still and be quiet for long periods of time.

- As often as possible, try to end the day on a positive note. If your child is being disruptive, or if you are having negative feelings about your child, here is an exercise you can use to end the day in a pleasant way. At bedtime, parent and child each tell one another something they did that day that made them proud of themselves, something they like about themselves, something they like about each other, and something they are looking forward to the next day. Then a hug and a sincere "I love you" bring the day to a calm and loving close.

Checklist for parenting stressed children

A group of parents compiled the following checklist to help you parent your stressed child(ren).

- Model the type of behavior you desire. If you talk respectfully and take time-outs when angry, you are teaching your children to do so. If you scream or hit, that is how your children will handle their anger.

- Seek professional help for any behaviors that trouble you.

- Teach your children to talk about their feelings.

- Listen to your children with understanding and empathy.

- Be honest and admit your mistakes.

- Help your children examine why they are behaving the way they are.

- Distinguish between feelings (always okay) and acting on strong feelings in destructive or hurtful ways (not okay).

- Have clear rules and consequences for violations.

- Teach children to recognize when they are losing control.

- Discuss acceptable outlets for anger.

- Give frequent reassurances of your love.

- Provide plenty of hugs and physical affection.

- Notice and compliment your child's good behaviors.

- Recognize that the disturbing behaviors result from stress, pain, and drugs.

- Remember that with lots of structure, love, time, and sometimes professional help, the problems will become more manageable.

> Every possible grouping of our family has been in therapy at one point or another. We have all done individual therapy, family therapy, and my husband and I did couples therapy. I feel that each of these sessions was a gift to our family. It helped us vent, cry, plan, and forge stronger bonds. We are all happy together many years after our daughter's cure, and every single penny we spent was worth it.

Our children look to us to learn how to handle adversity. They learn how to cope from us. Although it is extremely difficult to live through your child's diagnosis and treatment for cancer, it must be done. So we each need to reach deep into our hearts and minds to help our children endure and grow.

Children Learn What They Live

If a child lives with criticism, he learns to condemn.
If a child lives with hostility, he learns to fight.
If a child lives with ridicule, he learns to be shy.
If a child lives with shame, he learns to feel guilty.
If a child lives with tolerance, he learns to be patient.
If a child lives with encouragement, he learns confidence.
If a child lives with praise, he learns to appreciate.
If a child lives with fairness, he learns justice.
If a child lives with security, he learns to have faith.
If a child lives with approval, he learns to like himself.
If a child lives with acceptance and friendship,
He learns to find love in the world.

— Dorothy Law Nolte

Chapter 14

Siblings

*Why was his hair falling out? Why was he going to the
hospital all the time? Why was he getting bone marrows all
the time? It never occurred to me that he might die. What was
happening? I didn't get to go to the hospital to see him. What
was leukemia? Why was he getting so many presents???*

— Chet Stevens
Straight from the Siblings:
Another Look at the Rainbow

CHILDHOOD CANCER TOUCHES all members of the family, with especially long-lasting
effects on siblings. The diagnosis creates an array of conflicting emotions in siblings;
not only are the siblings concerned about their ill brother or sister, but they usually
resent the turmoil that the family has been thrown into. They feel jealous of the gifts
and attention showered on the sick child, yet feel guilty for having these emotions. The
days, months, and years after diagnosis can be extremely difficult for the sibling of a
child with leukemia.

Ways to explain the leukemia diagnosis to siblings are discussed in Chapter 3, "Telling
Your Child and Others." This chapter discusses common emotions and behaviors of the
siblings and provides insights about how to cope from parents and siblings who have
been through this.

Emotional responses of the siblings

Brothers and sisters are shaken to the very core by leukemia in the family. Their parents,
the leaders of the family clan, sometimes have no time, and little energy, to focus on the
siblings. During this major crisis, siblings sometimes feel they have no one to turn to for
help. They may feel concerned, worried, fearful, guilty, angry, sad, abandoned, or many
other powerful emotions. If you recognize these ever-changing emotions as normal, you
will be better able to help your children talk about and cope with their strong feelings.

Although the years of treatment are emotionally potent for every member of the family,
research has shown that siblings have good psychological outcomes, particularly if they

have been made to feel that they remain valuable contributing members of the family whose thoughts and feelings matter. In many cases, siblings report the experience as life-changing in many positive ways. Following are descriptions and stories about the emotions felt by siblings.

Concern for sick brother or sister

Children really worry about their sick brother or sister. It is difficult for them to watch someone they love be hurt by needles and sickened by medicines. It is scary to see a brother or sister lose weight and go bald. It is hard to feel so healthy and energetic when the brother or sister has to stay indoors because of weakness or low blood counts. The siblings may be old enough to know that death is a possibility. There are plenty of reasons for concern.

> Christine's younger sister has really developed the nurturing side of her personality as a result of the leukemia. She frequently puts her arm around her sister, comforts her with soothing words or touches, and seems to feel her pain.

• • • • •

> I'm the mother of three children. Logan was 19 months old when diagnosed. It was very hard on all of us. Kathryn (5½ at the time of diagnosis) felt that she had to take so much on herself. She was there with us the entire time Logan was in the hospital. She had a cot right next to Logan's bed, and only she and I were the ones who could take care of "our Logan."

> She used to love to visit the other kids on the hospital floor and entertain them. She hated to go home. She would get so involved with the other kids and didn't want to leave them. She actually got very close to two little girls that lost the battle, so here she was at 6, dealing with the loss of two friends.

Fear and worry

It is extremely common for young siblings of children with cancer to think that the disease is contagious, that they can "catch it." Many also worry that one or both parents may get cancer. The diagnosis of cancer changes children's view that the world is a safe place. They feel vulnerable, and they are afraid. Depending on their age, siblings worry that their brother or sister may get sicker or may die.

Fears of things other than cancer may emerge: fear of being hit by a car, fear of dogs, fear of strangers. Many fears can be quieted by accurate and age-appropriate explanations from the parents or medical staff.

> My 3-year-old daughter vacillated between fear of catching cancer ("I don't ever want those pokes") to wishing she was ill so that she would get the gifts and attention ("I want to get sick and go to the hospital with Mommy"). She developed many

fears and had frequent nightmares. We did lots of medical play, which seemed to help her. I let her direct the action, using puppets or dolls, and I discovered that she thought there was lots of violence during her sister's treatments. She continues to ask questions, and we are still explaining things to her, 4 years later.

Jealousy

Despite feeling concern for the ill brother or sister, almost all siblings also feel jealous. Presents and cards flood in for the sick child, Mom and Dad stay at the hospital with the sick child, and most conversations revolve around the sick child. When the siblings go out to play, the neighbors ask about the sick child. At school, teachers are concerned about the sick child. Is it any wonder brothers and sisters feel jealous?

The siblings' lives are in turmoil and they sometimes feel a need to blame someone. It's natural for them to think that if their brother didn't get sick, life would be back to normal. Some siblings develop symptoms of illness in an attempt to regain attention from the parents.

> *Our 9-year-old son seemed to be dealing with things so well until one evening as I was tucking him in, he confided that he had tried to break his leg at school by jumping out of the swing. He began to cry and told me he doesn't want his brother to be sick anymore; that he needs some attention, too. As parents, we were always so concerned with our sick child that we didn't realize how much our healthy child was suffering, too.*

Guilt

Young children are egocentric; they are not yet able to see the world from any viewpoint but their own. It is logical to them to believe that because their sister has cancer, they caused it. They may have said in anger, "I hope you get sick and die," and then their sister got sick. This notion should be dispelled right after diagnosis. Children need to be told, many times, that cancer just happens, and no one in the family caused it. They need to understand that no one can make something happen just by thinking or talking about it.

Virtually every sibling feels guilt for their normal responses to cancer, such as anger and jealousy. They think, "How can I feel this way about my brother when he's so sick?" Assure them that the many conflicting feelings they are experiencing are normal and expected. As a parent, share some of your conflicting feelings (such as anger at the behavior of a child on prednisone, guilt about being angry).

It is also common for some children (and parents) to feel guilt for being healthy. It is important for parents to provide many opportunities to remind their healthy children that there is no connection between their health and their sibling's illness and that no one, including the sick brother or sister, wants them to feel bad about feeling good.

Abandonment

If parental attention revolves around the sick child, siblings may feel isolated and resentful. Even when parents make a conscious effort not to be so preoccupied with the ill child, siblings sometimes still perceive that they are not getting their fair share of attention and may feel rejected or abandoned.

Sometimes it is necessary to have the siblings stay with relatives, friends, or babysitters. Parents may have to miss activities, such as soccer games or school events, they would otherwise have attended. Vacation plans may be scrapped. The reasons may seem obvious to parents, but the siblings may interpret these changes as evidence that they are not as well-loved as the sick child. Parents should explain in detail the reasons for any alterations in routines, solicit feelings about the changes from the siblings, and try to find solutions that work for everyone in the family.

> *One day when my 4-year-old son was in day care, we unexpectedly had to bring Erica in for emergency surgery on a septic hip. (It turned out to be a life-threatening surgery, and she ended up staying in for weeks.) I called the day care and said that I couldn't pick up Daniel by closing time, and the teacher said, "No problem, I live right across the street and I'll take him home for dinner." We went to get Daniel that evening, and he was very withdrawn. Later, he exclaimed, "All the mommies came. Then teacher turned out the lights, and you didn't come to get me." Then he burst into tears. In hindsight, one of us should have gone to bring him to the hospital to just sit with us. It was tense there, but at least he would have been with us, included as part of the family.*

Sadness

Siblings have many very good reasons to be sad. They miss their parents and the time they used to spend with them. They miss the life they used to have, the one they were comfortable with. They worry that their brother or sister may die. Some children show their sadness by crying often; others withdraw and become depressed. Often children confide in relatives or friends that they think their parents don't love them anymore.

> *When Jeremy was very sick and hospitalized, we sent his older brother Jason to his grandparents for long periods of time. We thought that he understood the reasons, but a year after Jeremy finished treatment, Jason (9 years old) said, "Of course, I know that you love Jeremy more than me anyway. You were always sending me away so that you could spend time with him." It just broke my heart that every time he made that long drive over the mountains with his grandparents, he was thinking that he was being sent away.*

Months after his 4-year-old sister's treatment ended, my 6-year-old son confided to his grandmother that his parents loved her more than him. He still has never told his father or me, but he does sometimes ask if his sister is going to die. When I say no, he looks sort of disappointed.

Anger

Children's lives are disrupted by the diagnosis of a sister or brother with cancer, and siblings often feel very angry. Questions such as "Why did this happen to us?" or "Why can't things be the way they used to be?" are common. Children's anger may be directed at their sick brother, their parents, relatives, friends, or doctors. Children's anger may have a variety of causes. They may resent being left with babysitters so often or having additional responsibilities at home, or they may notice that the sick child isn't always held to the same standards of behavior as the other children. Because each member of the family may have frayed nerves, explosions of temper can occur.

As we were driving home from school one day, Annie was talking, and I was only half listening. All of a sudden I realized that she was yelling at me. She screamed, "See, this is what I mean. You never listen, your mind is always on Preston." I pulled the car over, stopped, and said, "You're right. I was thinking about Preston." I told her that from now on I would try to give her my full attention. I realized that I would really have to make an effort to focus on what she was saying and not be so distracted. This conversation helped to clear the air for a while. I tried to take her out frequently for coffee or ice cream to just sit, listen, and concentrate on what she was saying.

Worry about what happens at the hospital

Children have vivid imaginations, and when they are fueled by disrupted households and whispered conversations between teary parents, children can imagine truly horrible things. Seeing how their ill sister looks upon returning from a hospital stay can reinforce their fears that awful things happen at the clinic or hospital. Or, the sibling may think they are missing some grand parties when they see their sister and parent come home from the hospital with presents and balloons.

My son is only in kindergarten. He has separation anxiety worse than a 6 month old. He doesn't want to go to bed alone. The last time Karissa had the flu, I thought he was going to die from worrying so much. He cried himself to sleep every night and woke up crying. He was so worried. He hasn't gotten much better since she has started feeling better, either. He doesn't even want to go near the hospital with his sister.

Age-appropriate, verbal explanations can help children be more realistic in what they think happens at the hospital, but nothing is as powerful as a visit. Of course the effectiveness of a visit depends on your child's age and temperament, but many parents say that bringing the siblings along helps everyone. The sibling gains an accurate understanding of hospital procedures, the sick child is comforted by the presence of the sibling, and the parent gets to spend more time with all the children.

Another way to help a worried sibling is to read age-appropriate books together. Many children's hospitals have coloring books for preschoolers that explain hospital procedures with pictures and clear language. School-age children benefit from reading books with a parent (see Appendix C, "Books, Websites, and Videotapes"). Adolescents might be helped by seeing videos about the subject or joining a sibling support group.

Veteran parents suggest that another way to reduce siblings' worries is to allow even the youngest children to help the family in some way. As long as children have clear explanations of the situation and concrete jobs to do that will benefit the family, they tend to rise to the occasion. Make them feel they are a necessary and integral part of the family's effort to face leukemia together.

Concern about parents

Exhausted parents are sometimes not aware of the strong feelings of their healthy children. They sometimes assume children understand they are loved, and that they would be getting the same attention if they were the one who had cancer. Siblings frequently do not share their powerful feelings of anger, jealousy, or worry because they love their parents and do not want to place additional burdens on them. It is all too common to hear siblings say, "I have to be the strong one. I don't want to cause my parents any more pain." But burdens are lighter if shared. Parents can help themselves and the siblings by acknowledging their own conflicting feelings and overtly encouraging the children to share their feelings, especially the difficult ones. Try to listen non-defensively and use those moments as an opportunity to grow together and strengthen each other.

Sibling experiences

Simply understanding the pain and fears of your healthy children eases their journey. Being available to listen, to say, "I hear how painful this is for you," or "You sound scared. I am, too," makes siblings feel they are still valued members of the family and that even though their brother or sister is absorbing the lion's share of parents' time and care, they are still cherished. Siblings need to hear that what they feel matters, especially if parents do not have large amounts of time to spend with them. If parents understand that these overwhelming emotions are normal, expected, and healthy, they can provide solace.

Brothers and sisters of children with cancer shared the following stories about some of the difficulties they face.

Silent hurting heart

Dayna E. is 13 years old. One of Dayna's brothers died of a brain tumor, and her other brother is in remission from ALL. This poem was published in *Bereavement* magazine and is reprinted with permission.

"Oh, nothing's wrong," she smiled,
grinning from ear to ear.
The frown that just was on her face
just seemed to disappear.

But deep down where secrets are kept,
the pain began to swell.
All the hurt inside of her
just seemed to stay and dwell.

All the pain in her heart
was too much for her to take.
Pretending everything's OK
is much too hard to fake.

She'd duck into the bathrooms
and hide inside the stalls.
Because no one could see her tears,
behind those dirty walls.

She was sick and tired of losing
and things never turning out right.
She had no hope left in her.
She was ready to give up the fight.

But she wiped away the teardrops,
put a smile back on her face,
pulled herself together, and
walked out of that place.

Life went on and things got better.
She thought that was a start.
But still, no one could see inside
her silent hurting heart.

Alana's story

Alana F. (11 years old) remembers how family life changed when her sister, Laura, had cancer.

My sister was in fifth grade and had been sick for the last week or so. Laura always seemed to be my hero. Although we got into arguments, all siblings get into fights, so I didn't worry. I didn't know what was about to happen, but neither did anyone else.

I don't quite remember how my parents told me she had cancer, but I do remember a lot of tears.

As time progressed, my life changed. I lived with my best friend and her parents, Catherine and Bill, but that changed too. Kelsie (my friend) and I got into a lot of arguments, but we still do. I don't know if that is why my grandmother and grandfather moved up to live in our house so that they could take care of me. Living with them was different. My grandmother had different expectations of me than my mother did.

My parents would each take turns staying at the hospital. Some nights I would live with my mom, grammy, and grandpy; and the next it would be with my dad and them.

Of course going through this dilemma I felt left out. Here I was living with my grandparents, and my sister got to live with our parents. She got lots of flowers, cards, and gifts, and all I got was the feeling of love from my relatives. I know that love is better than material things, but when you are 6 years old, you don't think so.

Things stayed the same for a long time. Then my sister went into remission and started living at home. I had to get used to my parents again and missed my grandparents.

My sister was spoiled at home, too. They bought her a waterbed, so she wouldn't get cold. What did I get? A heating blanket; a used heating blanket.

Having a sister with leukemia

Alison L. (6 years old) describes the experience of having a sister with leukemia:

I think having a sister with leukemia is not fun. My mom paid more attention to Kathryn, my sister. I had to stay with Daddy! Mommy picked Kathryn up and not me! I wanted my sister's PJs. Guess what? I did not get them! Although my mommy wanted to stay with me, she did not want to leave my sister alone. Sometimes I felt like I was going to throw up. But now it has been 2 years since she has stopped having medicine, and she is completely better. To celebrate we are going to Disneyland.

My brother's a legend

To Erin H. (18 years old), her brother has become a "legend" by surviving childhood cancer.

I'm really proud of my brother Judson for handling everything so well. During those years, there were times when I was jealous of him, not only for the attention he received, but for his courage as well. This little boy was going through so much, and I still cowered at getting my finger pricked. As I look back, I wonder if I would have been able to make it through, not only physically, but emotionally as well.

According to some people, a person needs to be dead in order to be a legend, or to have been famous, or well liked. A legend to me, though, is someone who has accomplished something incredible, enduring many hardships and pains, and still comes out of it smiling.

Judd is a legend to me because he didn't give up in a time that he might have. He is a legend because he survived an illness that many do not. Now I look at him after being in remission for almost 5 years, and I hope that someday if I am ever faced with a challenge like his, I will have the same strength and courage he had.

My brother has leukemia

Eight-year-old Amanda M. experienced many ups and downs when her brother had cancer.

Sometimes having a brother with leukemia is fun, like when my family goes on the Fantasy Flight to the North Pole, and going to the special summer camp, and getting special privileges at Disney World.

But other times, it can be really hard, especially when William gets put in the hospital. Right now, he can't leave his room in the hospital, and the doctors wear masks when they come in. I HATE seeing that. And he stays in for very long periods of time. The first time, he was there for almost 3 weeks! It comes so suddenly. He has stayed out for 5 months, then BAM! He's back in. And the worst of it is, people are always pitying us. "Poor little boy." "Poor William." I guess they like pitying us.

So, leukemia has ups and downs like everything else, but to me it's mostly downs.

For brothers and sisters

Ellen Z. discusses the impact that her cancer had on her siblings. (Reprinted with permission from *Candlelighters Youth Newsletter.*)

I am the first of four children and the only girl. When I was diagnosed with ALL at the age of 14, it affected all our lives. My brother Wes was 13, Matthew was 4, and Erik was 2. They and my parents were my support system.

When I was first diagnosed and in the hospital, Dr. Plunkett asked if I wanted anyone besides my parents present when he gave us the diagnosis. I told him I wanted Wes with me. Wes is only 14 months younger than I am, and we have always been very close. He took it all in, and we all decided that we would face this thing, and beat it, as a family. Then he and I sent our parents off so we could have some private time together.

Wes was my support at school and at home. He stuck up for me and kept an eye on me. I lost some of my "friends" after I was diagnosed because of my illness and their fear of it. Wes was always there for me. That's not to say we didn't have our fights. Poor Wes—I could hit him, but he couldn't hurt me physically because of my low blood counts. Sometimes I took advantage of that.

Matt and Erik were also a great source of comfort and support. They would accompany my mom and me to treatments and hold my hand when I got stuck. If one of them wasn't with me when I went in, the nurses would ask me where they were. These little boys made it easier for me to be brave.

I hope my brothers know how much I appreciate, too, the extra time they gave me with our parents during my illness. My parents were very good about splitting time between me and my brothers. If one was with me at treatment or the hospital, then the other was spending time with the boys. Family and friends were also a big help.

I've been out of treatment for 10 years now. I teach second grade and spend a week of my summer as a counselor at a camp for kids with cancer. I am the proud sister of three Eagle Scouts. Wes is married now and lives in another state. I realize how much he meant to me during that trying time and how much he means to me now.

If you are a sibling to someone with cancer and wonder if you make a difference to your sick brother or sister, I would like to tell you that you make a very big difference.

When my brother got cancer

Annie W. (15 years old) relates some ways she benefited from her brother's battle with childhood cancer.

One experience in my life that was in no way comfortable for my family or myself and caused me a lot of confusion and grief was when my brother had leukemia. Along with the disruption of this event, it also caused me to grow tremendously as a person. The Thanksgiving of my third-grade year, Preston, my brother, became very ill and was diagnosed a few weeks later with having cancer.

This event helped me to grow to become a better person in many ways. When my brother had very little hair or was puffed out from certain drugs, I learned to respect people's differences and to stick up for them when they're made fun of. Also, when Preston was in the hospital, I was taught to deal with a great amount of jealousy that I had. He received many gifts, cards, flowers, candy, games, and so many other material things that I envied. Most of all though, he received all the attention and care of my mother, father, relatives, and friends. This is what I was jealous of the most. As I look back now, I can't believe that I was that insensitive and self-centered to be mad at my brother at a time like that.

The thing that made this a "graced" experience was the fact that it enabled me to be very close to my brother as we grew up. My brother and I are now good friends and are able to talk and share our experiences with each other. I don't think that we would have this same relationship if he never had leukemia, and I think that has been a very positive outcome. Another thing that has been a positive outcome of this event is the people I've been able to meet. Through all the support groups, camps, and events for children with cancer and their siblings, I have met some people with more courage and more heart than anyone could imagine. In no way am I saying that I'm glad my brother had cancer, but I will say I'm very glad with some of the outcomes from it.

My sister had cancer

Eleven-year-old Jeff P. explains what happened when "My Sister Had Cancer." (Reprinted with permission from CCCF Canada CONTACT newsletter.)

My sister Jamie got cancer when she was 23 months old. I was 8, and my two other sisters were 6 and 4.

My sisters and I were scared that Jamie was going to die. We weren't able to go to public places and also weren't allowed to have friends in our house. We missed a lot of school when there was chicken pox in our school. I got teased in school sometimes because my sister had no hair. Once an older kid called my sister a freak. My mom was sad most of the time. It was very hard.

We are all pleased that Jamie is doing well, and our lives are getting back to normal. It was an experience I'll never forget, and I hope it has made me a stronger person.

From a sibling

Fifteen-year-old Sara M. won first prize in the 1995 Candlelighters Creative Arts Contest with her essay, "From a Sibling."

Childhood cancer—a topic most teens don't think much about. I know I didn't until it invaded our home.

Childhood cancer totally disrupts lives, not only of the patient, but also of those closest to him/her, including the siblings. First, I was numbed with unbelieving shock. "This can't be happening to me and my family." Along with this came a whole dictionary full of incomprehensible words and a total restructuring of our (up to that time) fairly normal lifestyle.

One day in July 1988, I was waiting for my parents to pick me up from summer camp and anticipating the start of our family vacation to Canada. When they arrived, they informed me that my older brother Danny was very sick, and we wouldn't be taking that trip after all. The following day, the call came that confirmed the diagnosis. Instead of packing for vacation, we packed our bags and headed for Children's Hospital in Denver, 200 miles away, where Danny was scheduled for surgery and chemotherapy.

I developed my own disease (perhaps from fear I would "catch" what Danny had) with symptoms similar to my brother's:

Sympathy pains. I asked, "Why him?" when he came home from the hospital, exhausted from throwing up a life-saving drug for three days.

Fear. "How much sicker is Danny going to get before he gets well? He is going to get well, isn't he?"

Resentment. My parents seemed so worried about him all the time. They didn't seem to have time for me anymore.

Confusion. Why couldn't Danny and I wrestle around like we used to? Why couldn't I slug him when he made me mad?

Jealousy. I felt insignificant when I was holding down the fort at home.

The parts I hated the most were: not understanding what was being done to him, answering endless worried phone calls, and hearing the answers to my own questions when my parents talked to other people.

I was helped to sort out these feelings and identify with other siblings when I attended a program held just for teens who had siblings with cancer. We got together, tried to learn how to cross-country ski, and talked about our siblings and ourselves.

Perhaps you remember this story: "US [speed skating] star Dan Jansen, 22, carrying a winning time into the back straightaway of the 1,000 meter race, inexplicably fell. Two days earlier, after receiving word that his older sister, Jane, had died of leukemia, Dan crashed in the 500 meter" (Life Magazine). Having a sibling with cancer can immobilize even an Olympic athlete. Dan was expected to bring home two gold medals, but cancer in a sibling intervened. He became, instead, the most famous cancer sibling of all time. He shared his grief before a television audience of two billion people. Dan later went on to win the World Cup in Norway and Germany, and capture the gold at the Olympics. He is the first to tell you the real champions can be found in the oncology wards of children's hospitals across our nation, and the siblings who are fighting the battle right along beside them.

Siblings: Having our say

Naomi C. gives advice to parents and siblings of those with childhood cancer.

Twelve young people aged 7 to 29 met at the 25th Anniversary Candlelighters Conference to talk about what it is like having a sibling with cancer in the family. We talked about our families, our anger, jealousy, worries, and fears, and thought about what we wanted to tell others about our experiences. In fact, we made lists of things we wanted other people to know: one for parents, one for other children or young adults in our position, and one for the child who has been diagnosed with cancer.

Some parts of these lists reflect anger and bitterness, but that was not the overriding feeling in the session. I hope it isn't the only message you take away. If nothing else, the issues raised here may provide you with a good starting point for discussions in your own family.

To parents:

- *We know you are burdened and trying to be fair. But try harder.*

- *Give us equal time.*

- *Be tough on disciplining the child with cancer. No free rides.*

- *Put yourself in our shoes once in a while.*

- *If you are away from home a lot, at least call and tell us, "I love you."*

- *Tell us what is going on. Don't just sit us in front of a video (about cancer); talk with us about it.*

- *Keep special time with us like lunch once a week or something. Time for just us. And if you can't be with us, find someone who can.*

- *When you talk to family members, say how everyone is doing—what we are doing is important, too.*

- *Ask how we are feeling. Don't assume you know.*

To siblings of newly diagnosed kids:

- *Keep a diary if you don't want to talk to your parents.*

- *Expect to not get as much attention.*

- *Expect that your parents are going to be extra cautious about what your brother/ sister does, who he/she hangs out with, etc.*

- *Hang in there. You're all you've got for now.*

- *Don't feel like you have to think about the illness all the time.*

- *Be understanding of your parents and stay involved.*
- *Tell someone how you are feeling—don't bottle it up.*
- *Go to the hospital to visit when you can.*
- *Make as many friends as possible at school.*

To our siblings who struggled or are struggling with cancer:

- *The world does not revolve around you.*
- *Stop feeling sorry for yourself.*
- *Not everything is related to cancer. Stop using that as an excuse for everything.*
- *I'm jealous of you sometimes, but I'm not mad. I know it sometimes seems like I'm mad, but I'm not.*
- *Don't take advantage of all the extra attention you get.*
- *Tell mom and dad to pay attention to me sometimes, too.*
- *Now that you are feeling better, where's the gratitude for all those chores that I did?*
- *I really admire your strength and courage. I wouldn't have gotten through your illness without you.*

Helping siblings cope

The following are suggestions from several families about ways to help brothers and sisters cope.

- Make sure you explain leukemia and its treatment to the siblings in terms that they understand. Create a climate of openness so they can ask questions and know they will get answers. If you don't know the answer to a question, write it on your list to ask the doctor at the next appointment, or ask your child if he would like to go to the appointment with you and ask the question himself.

    We drew a lot of pictures of red cells, white cells, and platelets. We showed each doing its job: red cells carrying oxygen around, white cells gobbling up cold germs as well as leukemia blasts, and platelets clumping up to form scabs. Drawing opened the floodgates of questions, and I was always amazed at how each child understood some things so clearly, and was confused and frightened by other things.

- Make sure all the children clearly understand that cancer is not contagious. They cannot catch it, nor can their ill brother give it to anyone else. Impress upon them that nothing the parents or brothers and sisters did caused the cancer.

- Bring home a picture of the brother or sister in the hospital, and carry a tape recorder back and forth to relay songs and messages. Encourage the children to talk on the phone or e-mail messages when your child is in the hospital.

- It is extremely hard for mothers and babies or toddlers to be separated when the mothers need to be at the hospital with the sick child and the baby or toddler sibling must stay at home.

   My daughter was 18 months old when her 3-year-old sister was diagnosed. Each member of the family flew in to stay at the house for 2-week shifts, so she had a lot of caregivers. A friend of mine gave her a big key chain that held eight pictures. We put a picture of each member of the family (including pets) on her key chain, and she carried it around whenever we were away. It seemed to comfort her.

- Try to spend time individually with each sibling.

   We began a tradition during chemotherapy that really helped each member of our family. Every Saturday each parent would take one child for a 2-hour special time. We scheduled it ahead of time to allow excitement and anticipation to grow. Each child picked what to do on their special day—such as going to the park, eating lunch at a restaurant, riding bikes. We tried to put aside our worries, have fun, and really listen.

- If people only comment on the sick child, try to bring the conversation back to include the sibling. For example, if someone exclaims, "Oh look how good Lisa looks," you could say, "Yes, and Martha has a new haircut, too. Don't you think she looks great?"

- Share your feelings about the illness and its impact on the family. Say, "I'm sad that I have to bring your sister to the hospital a lot. I miss you when I'm gone." This allows the sibling an opportunity to tell you how she feels. Try to make the illness a family project by expressing how the family will stick together to beat it.

   I never kept my feelings secret from Shawn's two older brothers (5 and 7 years old). If I was scared, I talked about it. Once when we thought he was relapsing, my stomach was so knotted up that I could barely walk. Kevin said, "Mom, I'm really worried about Shawn." I told him that I was, too, and then we both just hugged and cried together. They really opened up when we didn't hide our feelings.

- Include siblings in decision-making, such as giving them choices about how extra chores will be divided up or devising a schedule for parent time with the healthy children.

   We always gave the boys choices about where they would stay when Shawn had to be in the hospital. I felt like it gave them a sense of control to choose babysitters. They usually stayed at a close neighbor's house where there were younger children.

It allowed them to ride the same bus to school and play with their neighborhood friends. Their lives were not too disrupted. They also really pitched in and helped with the younger kids. I think it helped them to help others.

- Allow siblings to be involved in the medical aspects of their brother's illness, if they want to be. Often the reality of clinic visits and overnight stays is easier than what siblings imagine. Many siblings are a true comfort when they hold their brother's hand during spinal taps or bone marrows.

    Just yesterday, Spencer (who screamed and shrieked at the blood draw for the BMT typing, and didn't match) out of the blue said "Mom, I wish I could have donated my marrow to Travis." And he's 5! He also donated money to plant a tree in Israel today at Sunday school and asked us to write that it was "In honor of God and my brother, Travis." Oh man, we can never forget how this experience is seared in the memory of our children who don't have cancer. I am convinced that for Spencer, too, we will be seeing effects of this entire experience in many ways, long into the future.

- Give lots of hugs and kisses.

    We assumed everything was fine with Erin because she had her grandma, who adored her, staying with her. We made a conscious decision to spend lots of time with her and include her in everything. But we realized later that she felt very left out. My advice is to give triple the affection that you think they need, including lots of physical affection such as hugs and kisses. For years, Erin felt jealous. She thought her brother got more of everything: material things, time with parents, opportunities to do things she was not allowed to do. She finally worked it out while she was in college.

- Be sure to alert teachers of siblings about the tremendous stress at home. Many children respond to the worries about cancer by developing behavior or academic problems at school. Teachers should be vigilant for the warning signals and provide extra support or tutoring for the stressed child or teen. Continue to communicate frequently with the teachers of the siblings to make sure you are aware of any developing problems.

- Expect your other children to have some behavior problems as part of living with cancer in the family. This is a normal response.

    When my 4-year-old healthy child screams and sobs over a minor skinned knee, she gets as much sympathy as my child with leukemia does during a bone marrow aspiration. I put a bandage on the knee, rock her, sing a song, and get her an ice pack. The injuries are not equal, but the needs of each child are. They both need to be loved and cared for; they both need to know that mom will help, regardless of the severity of the problem. I even let Alison use EMLA® for routine shots. My pediatrician laughs at me, but I just tell him, "Sibs need perks, too."

- The child with cancer receives many toys and gifts, resulting in hurt feelings or jealousy in the siblings. Provide gifts and tokens of appreciation to the siblings for helping out during hard times, and encourage your sick child to share.

> My daughter Jacqueline is 7 years old. We have three other children, ages 14, 8½, and 3. We found (through trial and error) that letting them know as much as they were able to handle, and making sure they felt comfortable asking any questions they might have, helped a great deal. We also made sure we called them two or three times a day from the hospital, and talked to them about how THEIR day was. We let them come to the hospital any time they wanted, after checking that it was okay with the docs. The second time around, we made sure that anyone coming to visit, or sending her something through the mail, either brought something small for the other three kids, or didn't bring anything at all. We also kept a small stock of wrapped presents for those who didn't remember our "rule."

- Encourage a close relationship between an adult relative or neighbor and your other children. Having a "someone special" when the parents are frequently absent can help your child feel cared for and loved.

- Take advantage of any workshops, support groups, or camps for siblings. These can be of tremendous value for siblings, providing fun and friendships with others who truly understand their feelings.

Positive outcomes for the siblings

After reading about all the difficult emotions your children might experience, it is important to note that many siblings exhibit great warmth and active caretaking while their brother or sister is being treated for leukemia. Their empathy and compassion seem to grow with the crisis.

Some brothers and sisters of children with cancer feel they have benefited from the stressful experience in many ways, such as: increased knowledge about disease, increased empathy for the sick or disabled, increased sense of responsibility, enhanced self-esteem, greater maturity and coping ability, and increased family closeness. Many of these siblings mature into adults interested in the caring professions, such as medicine, social work, or teaching. Character can grow from confronting a personal crisis, and many parents speak of their healthy children with admiration and pride.

> Brothers and sisters of those with cancer go through much adversity, as we parents do. At times, much is overlooked, unintentionally of course, because of the many changes in our lives that we experience at such a difficult time. Well, today, I want to pay a small tribute to Tommy's 15-year-old brother, Matt. From the time Tommy was

diagnosed, Matt has been by his side. The first night Matt wouldn't go to bed, just so he could stand by Tommy's bedside and be close to him. When we got back home, Matt took over and made sure Tommy would get his "daily laugh." Every evening, even when Tommy felt too sick to sit up, Matt would be there and always made us smile and laugh. As we all know, the siblings sacrifice much of their own lives during this time. Whether it be their social activities or school work, much of their "normal" lifestyle is changed. They even show their courage through the wide range of emotions, including much sorrow, that they experience. It is said, "Angels shine their light on us that we may see more clearly." So as our angel on earth, thank you Matt for shining your light on your brother Tommy, and may you also be blessed with the light of angels.

Chapter 15

School

*Most of us had two feelings at the same time: wanting
to go back to school and being scared of going back.*

— Eleven children with cancer
There Is a Rainbow Behind Every Dark Cloud

CHILDREN WITH CANCER often experience disruptions in their education due to repeated hospitalizations or side effects from the disease or treatment. As their health improves and when their treatment schedule allows, returning to school can be either a relief or a challenge.

For many children, school is a refuge from the world of hospitals and procedures—a place for fun, friendship, and learning. School is the defining structure of children's daily lives and going back to school can signal hope for the future and a return to normalcy. Some children, however, especially teens, may dread returning to school because of temporary or permanent changes to their appearance or concerns that prolonged absences may have changed their social standing with friends. Additionally, school can become a major source of frustration for children who have learning difficulties as a result of treatment.

While educating children with cancer can be a complex process, most issues can be successfully managed through planning and good communication. In this chapter, many parents share their advice and experiences to better help you meet the educational needs of your child. The first part of this chapter deals with educational issues you may encounter while your child is in treatment. The second part of the chapter addresses educational challenges that survivors may face as a result of cancer treatment's toxic effects. The last section describes the role of school in the lives of terminally ill children.

Keeping the school informed

Chapter 3, "Telling Your Child and Others," provides guidance about how and when to inform the school about your child's illness. In the months and years that follow, maintaining an open and amicable relationship with the school will ensure that your child, who may be emotionally or physically fragile, continues to be welcomed and nurtured at school.

After you have informed the school principal in writing of your child's diagnosis, hospitalization, and projected course of treatment, the next step is to designate a person or professional advocate to be the liaison among the hospital, family, and school. Sometimes the person is within the school, such as the child's teacher, guidance counselor, or a special education staff member. Other times, families use an advocate/liaison from the hospital, such as the hospital social worker, a hospital nurse, or a psychologist. The advocate will work to keep information flowing between the hospital and school and will help pave the way for a successful school reentry for your child. The most important qualifications for this role are good communication skills, knowledge of educational programs and procedures, comfort in dealing with school issues, and organizational skills. It must be someone you trust to act fairly on your child's behalf, and someone who is able and willing to advocate for your child's needs.

The liaison should locate a contact person at the school (or hospital) to communicate with about the child's medical condition, treatment, emotional state, and tentative reentry date. The liaison should encourage questions and address staff concerns about having a seriously ill child in school. Privacy laws prohibit these exchanges unless parents sign a release form authorizing the school and hospital to share information. These forms are available at schools.

> We had absolutely no problem keeping the school informed, as we lived directly behind it. The teacher would frequently stop by on her way home to drop off homework assignments and cards or messages from Stephan's classmates. The school nurse, psychologist, and teacher were at my beck and call. Whenever I felt that we needed to talk, I'd call and they would set up a meeting within 24 hours. I gave them the Candlelighters' book, Educating the Child with Cancer, *and they even attended a Candlelighters' meeting. They have been wonderful.*

Keeping the teacher and classmates involved

While your child is hospitalized, it helps to stay connected with his teacher and classmates. The teacher should be getting updates from the liaison, but the parent can help by calling the teacher periodically and bringing notes or taped messages from the sick child to her classmates. Following are suggestions for keeping the teacher and classmates involved with your child's life:

• Give the teacher a copy of *Educating the Child with Cancer* (listed in Appendix C, "Books, Websites, and Videotapes").

• Have the pediatric oncology nurse or social worker give a presentation to the class about what is happening to their classmate and how he will look and feel when he returns.

This talk should include a question and answer session to clear up misconceptions and alleviate fears. All children, especially teenagers, should be involved in deciding what information should be discussed with classmates.

- Encourage your child's classmates to keep in touch. The class can make a card or banner or send a group photo. Individual students can call on the phone or send notes, e-mails, text messages, or pictures.

> We used Skype® and had a weekly time set up so that Patrik could see his classmates, and they could see him. If an oral presentation was due, he heard a few of theirs, and presented his. If nothing shareable was due, they just traded jokes or did a show and tell of something that had happened that week. Both Patrik and his classmates enjoyed collecting jokes all year. If he was not feeling well or was hospitalized, it was cancelled for that week. It sure helped make him feel still a part of his class, and the teacher said it really helped his classmates to see he was still okay, and still himself. He wasn't allowed to attend school at all for frontline treatment (almost 10 months).

> Patrik started the first day of 5th grade this year, having had his first treatment of long-term maintenance the day before. He was able to walk in the building, feel welcome, and step right back into his friendships. No problems at all with that. The teachers say he is well liked by all kids—boys, girls, and members of all the varying cliques that are starting to really gel in middle school. I really thank his teacher last year for keeping him a part of his class despite not being in school. I do think this was really important as all this chemo is tough enough without adding any social pressures!

> $\bullet \quad \bullet \quad \bullet \quad \bullet \quad \bullet$

> Communication was the key. I wrote weekly updates and made copies for each teacher, put their names on them, and delivered them to school. I learned that a single copy of a letter didn't get passed around to everyone. (Joel was in high school.) Some classes used a tape recorder; they all kept a record of what he'd missed. His math teacher got together with the librarian and arranged to videotape his math classes. They did so much on the board, on overheads, and with discussion in that class that an audiotape would not have helped. All teachers were willing to meet with him after or before school to essentially reteach the concepts that he had missed.

> I also told his teachers it was okay to discuss Joel, his leukemia, and his treatment with the other kids in his classes. They would never have done it without my okay. I knew that in the absence of information, there would be rumors flying. This might not work for everyone, but it served us well.

- If your child is old enough, allow him to establish a page on Facebook, MySpace, or another social network site, so he can communicate privately with his friends, express his feelings and thoughts, post photos, and keep up with his friends' lives.

Keeping up with schoolwork

As treatment progresses, your child will probably return to school full-time, but extended absences due to infections or complications from treatment are common. A child who is out of school longer than 2 weeks for any medical reason is entitled by law to instruction at home or in the hospital. It is a good idea to request off-site education as soon as you find out your child may be out of school for longer than 2 weeks. The school will require a letter from the physician stating the reason and expected length of time this service will be needed.

> My daughter Julia was diagnosed with T-cell ALL (acute lymphoblastic leukemia) when she was in second grade. We had her tutored at home by a district-sponsored, certified teacher and it was a great experience. She received the tutoring right through the end of the school year. (She started around mid-January with the tutoring, and it continued through June.) The teacher we had was fabulous, and Julia stayed caught up with (and even ahead of) her class. Our school district has everything in place for kids who, for medical reasons, need to be tutored at home. I think it was much less stressful than trying to get into school for a day or two at a time and not being able to keep track of homework. Plus, we didn't have to worry about all the germs floating around. It was hard being home all those months (I took a leave of absence from work), but we managed. Actually, I believe our relationship really deepened during the time home. I now have a closeness with Julia that is really special. When Julia went back to school last year, she had no adjustment problems and did very well.

If the child is in the hospital, the school district in which the hospital is located must provide the teacher. If the child is at home, the home school district provides the teacher. The teacher is responsible for gathering materials from the school and judging how much schoolwork the child is capable of handling. Joanne Holt, a high school director of special education, suggests:

> If children are having difficulty remaining interested in school work due to fatigue and not feeling well, it may be useful to consider alternative learning activities. In such circumstances, a parent and child might identify an area of special interest or curiosity (e.g., dinosaurs, space, animals, nature, the Wild West, etc.). Children may find it more interesting to develop reading skills, learn math concepts, develop writing skills, and learn research and study principles in the context of a high-interest area. Play is a significant part of such activities and can often spark imaginative activities. It is important that the school be aware of and supportive of such an approach; most often they are and, in fact, may be valuable resources for ideas and activities. The goal is to encourage confidence and prepare the child for the least disruptive reentry to school routines.

Helping siblings

The diagnosis of cancer affects all members of the family. Siblings can be overlooked when the parents are spending most of their time caring for the ill child at the hospital, clinic, or in the home. Many siblings feel frustrated, angry, frightened, neglected, or guilty, but they may try to keep their feelings bottled up to prevent placing additional burdens on their parents. Often, the place where these complicated feelings emerge is at school. It is common for siblings to cry easily, fall behind in classwork, do poorly on tests, cut classes, challenge teachers, withdraw from friends or school activities, or disrupt the classroom.

To help prevent these problems from developing, you can send a letter to each sibling's school principal that requests teachers, counselors, and nurses be informed of the cancer diagnosis in the family and that asks for their help with and support for the siblings.

> *Lindsey was in kindergarten when Jesse was first diagnosed. Because we heard nothing from the kindergarten teacher, we assumed that things were going well. At the end of the year, the teacher told us that Lindsey frequently spent part of each day hiding under her desk. When I asked why we had never been told, the teacher said she thought that we already had enough to worry about dealing with Jesse's illness and treatment. She was wrong to make decisions for us, but I wish we had been more attentive. Lindsey needed help.*

If possible, try to include the siblings' teachers in some of the school discussions concerning the ill child. If the siblings' teachers are in different schools, or if the siblings have several teachers (e.g., in middle school and high school), ask the principal to send a school representative. Teachers of siblings need to be aware that the stresses facing the family may cause the siblings' feelings to bubble to the surface during class. Parents must advocate just as strongly for their healthy children's emotional and educational needs as they do for their sick child's needs. Chapter 14, "Siblings," deals exclusively with siblings and contains suggestions about how to help them cope.

Returning to school

Parents may not even think about school during the early efforts to save their child's life, but a quick return to school helps children regain a sense of normalcy and provides a lifeline of hope for the future. Preparation is the key to a successful school reentry. You or the liaison may want to prepare a written package that covers the following information and concerns:

- A physician's statement that addresses your child's health status; ability to safely return to the school environment; physical restrictions, including any limits to physical education or recess; and probable attendance disruptions.

- Whether your child will attend full or half days.

- A description of any changes in her physical appearance, such as weight gain or hair loss, and suggestions about how to help the other children handle it appropriately.

- Whether the school administration is willing to bend the rules pertaining to head coverings so your bald child can wear a wig, hat, or scarf to school.

- Your child's feelings about returning to school.

- Any anticipated behavioral changes resulting from medication or treatment.

- The possible effect of medications on academic performance.

- Any medications or other health services that will need to be given at school.

- A reminder that no medication should ever be given without parental permission.

- Any special considerations, such as extra snacks, rest periods, extra time to get from class to class, use of the nearest restroom (even if it is the staff restroom), and the need to leave for the restroom without permission.

- Concerns about exposure to communicable diseases.

- A list of signs and symptoms requiring parent notification (e.g., fever, nausea, vomiting, pain, swelling, bruising, or nosebleeds) and, if parents are divorced, what notification procedures should be followed.

- An assurance that the teacher is not expected to handle any medical issues beyond notifying the parents or school nurse about any signs, symptoms, or problems she notices.

- A request to schedule a meeting, which includes parents, the liaison, teachers, administrators, the school nurse, the school counselor and psychologist, and special education service providers, to answer any questions and to share additional information that may help with your child's reentry to school.

At the requested meeting, you may wish to distribute booklets about children with cancer in the classroom, as well as age-appropriate information to share with the classmates. You can formulate a communicable disease notification strategy if necessary, discuss the ongoing need for appropriate discipline, and do your best to establish a rapport with the entire staff. Take this opportunity to express appreciation for the school's help and your hopes for a close collaboration in the future to create a supportive climate for your child.

> I still feel unbelievable gratitude when I think of the school principal and my daughter's kindergarten teacher that first year. The principal's eyes filled with tears when I told her what was happening, and she said, "You tell us what you need and I'll move the earth to get it for you." She hand-picked a wonderful teacher for her, made sure that a chicken pox notification plan was in place, and kept in touch with

me for feedback. She recently retired, and I sent her a glowing letter, which I copied to the school superintendent and school board. Words can't express how wonderful they were.

• • • • •

Jeremy's kindergarten teacher was the pits. Jeremy was on chemotherapy, and she told Jeremy not to wash his hands, as it took too long. I was disappointed that even after the nurse came to class and gave a presentation, the kids still teased my son. They would say things like, "You've got Jeremy germs; you are going to catch cancer," and "You can't get rid of cancer; you always die." During his kindergarten year, Jeremy needed to have heart surgery. I called the teacher to let her know, but my son did not hear from anyone in his class, not one card or phone call, even from the teacher. She didn't even tell the class why Jeremy was absent.

The following are parent suggestions about how to prevent problems through preparation and communication:

- Keep the school informed and involved from the beginning to foster a spirit that "we're all in this together."

- Reassure other children that leukemia is not contagious.

- Arrange for places that your child can rest if she is too exhausted to participate in class.

  > *The school librarian had a bed set up in the library for ailing students to use. I found out that sometimes Preston would spend the whole day there, because he was just too exhausted to attend class. It was very important to him and his sense of well-being to be at school. He would just drag himself in there in order to be with the other kids. Fortunately, all of his classmates were always nice to him.*

  > • • • • •

  > *There was a beanbag chair in the back of Brent's class, and he just curled up in it and went to sleep when he needed to.*

- Bring the pediatric oncology nurse into the class to talk about cancer and answer questions whenever necessary. If treatment is lengthy, this should be done at the beginning of each new school year to prepare the new classmates. Because the sick child may be given special privileges that could cause other students to feel upset or jealous, the nurse should also explain the reasons for different rules or privileges.

  > *My 16-year-old son was allowed to leave each textbook in his various classrooms. This prevented him from having to carry a heavy backpack all day. They also let him out of class a few minutes early, because he was slower moving from room to room.*

- For elementary school children, enlist the aid of the liaison or school counselor to help select the teacher for the upcoming year. You have no legal right to request a particular teacher, but you are entitled to write to the administration to discuss your child's particular needs and request that these needs be considered when making assignments for the upcoming year.

> Because my son has had such a hard third-grade year, I have really researched the fourth-grade teachers. I sat in class and observed three teachers. I sent a letter to the principal, outlining the issues, and requested a specific teacher. The principal called me and was very upset. He said, "You can't just request who you want. What would happen if all the parents did that? You'll have to give me three choices just like everybody else." I said, "My son has had 3 years of chemotherapy, has a seizure disorder, behavior problems, and learning disabilities. Can you think of a child who has a greater need for special consideration?" My husband and I then requested a meeting with him, and at the meeting he finally agreed to honor our teacher request.

- Prepare the teacher(s) and your child for the upcoming year.

> I asked for a spring conference with the teacher selected for the next fall and explained what my child was going through, what his learning style was, and what type of classroom situation seemed to work best. Then, I brought my son in to meet the teacher several times, and let him explore the classroom where he would be the next year. This helped my son and the future teacher get to know to one another.

- A mental health therapist can talk with your child about emotions and the child's life both inside and outside of school.

> My daughter went to a psychotherapist for the years of treatment. It provided a safe haven for frank discussions of what was happening, and also provided a place to practice social skills, which was a big problem for her at school.

- Recognize that children's responses to treatment varies.

> Chemotherapy can really zap some kids, leaving them a pale, tired version of themselves. Other children can have chemo and still have lots of energy to participate in school. Some children have always gotten every little bug they are exposed to—others are never sick. We were some of the lucky ones. Robby continued to attend school, do karate, and play baseball. He had few hospitalizations and rarely even had a cold. Cancer was pretty much just a reason he had to go to the doctor every once in a while. We didn't dwell on it, but we also didn't deny it. He still had to make his bed every morning and do his homework and behave in an acceptable manner.

- Realize that teachers and other school staff can be frightened, overwhelmed, and discouraged by having a child in their classroom with a life-threatening illness. Accurate information and words of appreciation can provide much-needed support.

Avoiding communicable diseases

The dangers of communicable diseases to immunosuppressed children are discussed in Chapter 10, "Common Side Effects of Chemotherapy." To prevent exposure, parents need to work closely with the school to develop a chicken pox, shingles, measles, and flu outbreak plan if the school does not already have a disease notification plan in place. Parents need to be notified immediately if their child has been exposed to chicken pox so that the child can receive the varicella zoster immune globulin (VZIG) injection within 72 hours of exposure.

Several methods can be used to ensure prompt reporting of outbreaks. Some parents notify all the classmates' parents by letter to ask them for prompt reports of illness. If the parents have a good rapport with the teacher, they can ask the teacher to report any cases of disease.

My daughter's preschool was very concerned and organized about the chicken pox reporting. They noted on each child's folder whether he or she had already contracted chicken pox. They told each parent individually about the dangers to Katy, and then frequently reminded everyone in the monthly newsletters. The parents were absolutely great, and we always had time to keep her out of school until there were no new cases. With the help of these parents, teachers, our neighbors, and friends, Katy dodged exposure for almost 3 years. She caught chicken pox 7 months after treatment ended and had a perfectly normal case.

· · · · ·

My son was diagnosed at age 14. He was starting ninth grade, the last year of junior high. He missed about a third of that year. He was able to keep up, thanks to some terrific teachers and a very cooperative administration, not to mention being a really motivated kid. He hated missing school and would go even when he didn't feel very good, just to say he'd been to school that day, even if only for two periods. Our oncologists gave him the okay to be in school, saying that infection in kids his age was usually from bacteria they were already carrying around, so other kids were not a big threat, provided they weren't sick.

Other parents enlist the help of the office workers who answer the phone calls from parents of absent children.

We asked the two ladies in the office to write down the illness of any child in Mrs. Williams' class. That way the teacher could check daily and call me if any of the kids in her class came down with chicken pox.

What about preschoolers?

A large number of children diagnosed with leukemia are preschoolers. Parents face the dilemma of having their child attend preschool through treatment, risking exposure to all the usual childhood illnesses, or holding their child out, which denies the child the opportunity for social growth and development. The decision is a purely personal one that should be made after considering the following issues:

• Has your child already had chicken pox or received the chicken pox vaccine?

• Is your child already enrolled and comfortable in a preschool program?

• Are your child's social needs being met by siblings and/or neighbors?

• Is preschool an option, given medical considerations?

• Does your child need special services, such as early childhood intervention (e.g., physical, occupational, and speech therapy), which are available through the school system?

> *Elizabeth was in preschool at the time of her diagnosis. The manager did a wonderful job of integrating her back into the fold. All of the other children at the school were taught what was happening to Elizabeth and what would be happening (such as hair loss). They learned that they had to be gentle with her when playing. The manager was a former home health nurse, so I was very confident that she would be able to take care of my daughter in the event of an emergency. She was already familiar with central lines and side effects from chemotherapy. She was a gem!*

U.S. federal law mandates early intervention services for disabled infants, toddlers, and preschoolers, and, in some cases, children at risk for developmental delays. Infants, toddlers, or preschoolers with leukemia may be eligible for these services in order to avoid developmental delays caused by the cancer or treatments. These services are administered either by the school system or the state health department. You can find out which agency to contact by asking the hospital social worker or by calling the special education director for your school district.

The law requires services not only for the eligible infant, toddler, or preschooler, but for the family, as well. Therefore, an Individualized Family Service Plan (IFSP) is developed. This plan includes:

• A description of the child's physical, cognitive, language, speech, psychosocial, and other developmental levels.

- Goals and objectives for the family and child.

- The description, frequency, and delivery of services needed, such as speech, vision, occupational, and physical therapy; health and medical services; and family training and counseling.

- A caseworker who locates and coordinates all necessary services.

- Steps to support transition to other programs and services.

> *We have had an excellent experience with the school district throughout preschool and now in kindergarten. We went to them with the first neuropsychological results, which were dismal. They retested him and suggested a special developmental preschool and occupational therapy. Both helped him enormously. He had an evaluation for special education services done and now has a full-time aide in kindergarten. He is getting the help he needs.*

Your legal rights (United States)

The cornerstone of all federal special education legislation in the United States is the Individuals with Disabilities Education Improvement Act (IDEA). This law, first passed in 1990, has been amended several times, most recently in 2004. The major provisions of this legislation are the following:

- All children, regardless of disability, are entitled to a free and appropriate public education (FAPE) and necessary related services in the least restrictive environment.

- Children will receive fair testing to determine if they need special education services.

- Parents can challenge the decisions of the school system, and disputes will be resolved by an impartial third party.

- Parents of a child with disabilities participate in the planning and decision-making for their child's special education.

Of course, each school district has different interpretations of the requirements of the law, and implementation varies, so you should contact the school superintendent, director of special education, or special education advisory committee in your school district to obtain a copy of the school system's procedures for special education. Depending on the district, this document may range from two to several hundred pages. Also write to your state Superintendent of Public Instruction to obtain a copy of the state special education regulations. To get the address, ask the school principal, a reference librarian, or look it up online.

The "referral for services" process has a required time line, although it varies by state. Some school districts take advantage of parents who do not know the state regulations, and they drag out the process. Your state's special education regulations will explain the time requirements for your state's referral process.

Another law, called the Federal Rehabilitation Act (Section 504), provides for rehabilitative support for individuals with disabilities. Some children, whether on or off treatment, may be eligible for services under Section 504 of the Rehabilitation Act. This Act applies when a child does not meet the eligibility requirements for an Individualized Education Program (IEP) but still needs accommodations to perform successfully in school. For example, a child undergoing chemotherapy might need some special accommodations temporarily, such as:

- Permission to use the staff bathroom.
- Different behavior management on prednisone days.
- Permission to keep a water bottle on the desk.
- Reduced homework when ill or hospitalized.
- Exemption from regular attendance/tardy policies.

> *Robby was diagnosed in January of his kindergarten year. He returned to kindergarten the same day he got out of the hospital. His teacher was wonderful. She moved the desks around in the classroom so that if Robby got tired, she would go get his cot and put it in the center of the classroom so he could lay down and still listen. If a child had a cold, she would move him/her to the other side of the classroom. The kids washed their hands at least four times a day. The teacher's aide would sit in the rocking chair holding Robby if he was sad (prednisone days). Also on prednisone days, Robby was allowed to have his lunch box, which weighed at least 10 pounds a day, at his desk, and he could eat all day.*

The list and story above describe accommodations made during treatment. However, Section 504 is also frequently used when a child off treatment has cognitive impairments that do not meet the IDEA requirements. In this situation, a child might use Section 504 to obtain necessary accommodations, such as elimination of timed tests or more time to finish written assignments. For dozens of other accommodations used by survivors and children on treatment, call Candlelighters for a free copy of the book *Educating the Child with Cancer,* listed in Appendix C, "Books, Websites, and Videotapes."

Numerous online sources provide reliable information about learning styles and parents' rights under special education law, but one that many parents find especially useful is Wrightslaw at *www.wrightslaw.com*. The U.S. Department of Education's Office of Special Education website about IDEA can be viewed at *http://idea.ed.gov/explore/home*.

Identifying cognitive late effects

State-of-the-art treatment for childhood cancer has resulted in greater numbers of long-term survivors, but not without cost. Some survivors suffer neurotoxic effects, which cause changes in their learning style and abilities, as well as social behavior. Parents and educators need to remain vigilant for potential learning problems so intervention can occur quickly. The signs of possible learning disabilities include problems with:

- Handwriting.

- Spelling.

- Reading or reading comprehension.

- Understanding math concepts, remembering math facts, comprehending math symbols, sequencing, and working with columns and graphs.

- Using calculators or computers.

- Auditory or visual language processing, which includes trouble with vocabulary, blending sounds, and syntax.

- Attention deficits. Some children become either inattentive or hyperactive, or both. Short-term memory and information retrieval may also be affected.

- Planning and organizational skills.

- Social maturity and social skills.

You should also suspect learning difficulties if:

- Your child was an A student prior to cancer, and she is working just as hard now and getting Cs.

- Your child takes 3 hours to do homework that used to take 1 hour.

- Your child reads a story and then has trouble explaining the plot.

- Your child frequently comes home from school frustrated, saying he just doesn't understand things as well as the other kids.

- Your child's teacher complains that she "just doesn't pay attention" or "just needs to work harder."

If any of the above situations are occurring, take action to begin the evaluation process for educational intervention before your child's self-esteem plummets. It is often hard to take this first step because children affected by radiation and/or chemotherapy may reason well, think clearly, and be above average academically in several areas. They may fall behind their classmates, however, on tasks that require fast processing skills, short-term memory, sequential operations, and organizational ability (especially visual). Once identified, these differences can be addressed by strategies such as eliminating timed tests, improving organizational skills, and providing extra help in mathematics, spelling, reading, and speech.

> *When she entered adolescence, my daughter became very angry about her learning disabilities. She used to be gifted, and now does very well, but it is a struggle for her. We honestly explained that the choices were life with the possibility of some academic problems versus death, and we chose life.*

Referral for services

The first step to get your child educational support is called "referral for services." The next steps in the special education process are evaluation, eligibility, individualized education plan (IEP) development, annual review, and 3-year assessments. You will need to become an advocate for your child as your family goes through the necessary steps to determine what placement, modifications, and services will be used to help your child learn.

> *My son had problems as soon as he entered kindergarten while on treatment. He couldn't hold a pencil, and he developed difficulties with math and reading. By second grade, I was asking the school for extra help, and they tested him. They did an IEP and gave him special attention in small remedial groups. The school system also provided weekly physical therapy, which really helped him.*

To make a "referral for services," a parent or the child's teacher writes to the school principal specifically requesting special education testing and stating that the child is "health impaired" due to treatment for cancer. Do not ask them verbally; you must request testing and services in writing. Obtain written notification of the date the school received the letter, as school staff have a legally mandated period of time in which to respond.

Evaluation

Once the referral is made, an evaluation is necessary to find out if the school district agrees that the child needs additional help, and if so, what types of help would be most beneficial. Usually a multidisciplinary team composed of the teacher, school nurse, district psychologist, speech and language therapist, resource specialist, medical advocate (whoever is serving as the hospital liaison with the school), and social worker meet to administer and evaluate the testing. Parents should request that the 504 coordinator be present at the IEP meetings. Areas usually considered in the evaluation process include educational, medical, social, and psychological. An excellent article about getting the best results from the IEP meeting is available at *www.wrightslaw.com/advoc/articles/iep.bollero.hearts.htm.*

> *This past week we found out Tori's testing from kindergarten. Although she missed more than a third of the school year, she is ready for first grade; except for math, she*

was above the 50th percentile for all the other testing. She was in the 95th percentile for visual (identifying patterns). For math she was in the 5th percentile. We had really been working on visual stuff, and obviously it paid off. I am not going to worry much about math yet, as we just didn't work on things besides counting. My mom (a recently retired first grade teacher) was thrilled with the results, which were much better than expected. Tori was able to do practically all the beginning and ending sounds (identification) and got all the blends! Not bad considering we were also working on things like potty retraining and relearning how to eat when she started school in the fall.

Children with a history of chemotherapy and/or radiation to the brain require thorough neuropsychological testing, which is best administered by neuropsychologists experienced in testing children with cancer. Most large children's hospitals have such personnel, but it sometimes takes very assertive parents to get the school system to use findings from these evaluations for the IEP. Your written consent is required prior to your child's evaluation, and you have the right to obtain an independent evaluation if you believe the school's evaluation is biased or flawed in any way. However, you are responsible for the cost unless the district agrees to use the outside expert or you follow the required procedures for your state for prior approval. For a thorough description of neuropsychological testing, visit the following website *www.candlelighters.org/ Information/neuropsychtesting/tabid/328/Default.aspx.*

Initially, the school was reluctant to test Gina because they thought she was too young (6 years old). But she had been getting occupational therapy at the hospital for 2 years, and I wanted the school to take over. I brought in articles from Candlelighters Childhood Cancer Foundation and spoke to the teacher, principal, nurse, and counselor. Gina had a dynamite teacher who really listened, and she helped get permission to have Gina tested. Her tests showed her to be very strong in some areas, and very weak in others. Together, we put together an IEP, which we have updated every spring. Originally, she received weekly occupational therapy and daily help from the special education teacher. She's now in fourth grade and is doing so well that she no longer needs occupational therapy; she only gets extra help during study hall. They even recommended her for the student council, which has been a tremendous boost for her self-confidence.

Parents should come to IEP meetings prepared. Bring (or send ahead of time if possible) copies of all current testing and recommendations by specialists that will help support your requests for services. It is best to create a positive relationship with the school so you can work together to promote your child's well-being. After the evaluation, a conference (including the parents and often the child or teen) is held to discuss the results and make a determination whether your child is eligible for services.

Eligibility for special education

There are 13 eligibility categories for special education under the federal law:

- Autism
- Deaf/blindness
- Deafness
- Hearing impairment
- Cognitive disability
- Multiple disabilities
- Orthopedic impairment
- Other health impairment (OHI)
- Serious emotional disturbance
- Specific learning disability
- Speech or language impairment
- Traumatic brain injury (TBI)
- Visual impairment.

Most children with late effects from treatment for leukemia tend to fall under the category of OHI. Some school districts instead use TBI as an eligibility category for these children. Participants at the IEP meeting in which test results are discussed will decide on the most appropriate category if your child meets eligibility requirements for special education.

Individual education program (IEP)

After eligibility is determined, an IEP that describes the special education program and any other related services specifically designed to meet the individual needs of your child will be developed. The IEP is developed as a collaboration between parents and professional educators to determine what the student will be taught, how and when the school will teach it, and any educational accommodations that will be made for the child. Students with disabilities need to learn the same things as other students: reading, writing, mathematics, history, and other subjects that help them prepare for college or vocational training. The difference is that, with an IEP in place, many specialized services, such as small classes, speech therapy, physical therapy, counseling, and instruction by special education teachers, are used.

The IEP has five parts:

1. **A description of the child.** Includes present level of social, behavioral, and physical functioning, academic performance, learning style, and medical history.

2. **Goals and objectives.** Lists skills and behaviors that your child can be expected to master in a specific time period. These goals should not be vague like "John will learn to cooperate," but rather, "John will prepare and present an oral book report with two regular education students by May 1." Each goal should answer the following questions: Who? What? How? Where? When? How often? When will the service start and end?

3. **Related services.** Many specialized services can be mandated by the IEP that will be provided at no cost to the family, including:

   - Speech therapy

   - Social skills training

   - Mental health services

   - Occupational therapy

   - Assistive technology assessment

   - Psychological and neuropsychological testing

   - Behavioral plans and functional behavior assessment

   - Physical therapy and adaptive physical education

   - Parent counseling and training

   - Transportation to and from school and therapy sessions.

For each of these services, the IEP should list the frequency, duration, start date, and end date, for example, "Jane will receive physical therapy twice a week, for 60 minutes a session, from September until December, when her needs will be reevaluated."

4. **Placement.** Describes the least restrictive setting in which the above goals and objectives can be met. For example, one student may be in the regular classroom all day with an aide present, while another might leave the classroom for part of each day to receive specialized instruction in the resource room or physical therapy room. The IEP should state the percent of time the child will be in the regular education program and the frequency and duration of any special services.

5. **Evaluating the IEP.** A meeting with all members of your child's IEP team is held periodically to review your child's progress toward attaining the short- and long-term goals and objectives of the IEP. In order to ensure the IEP is working for your child, make sure her IEP is reviewed at least once a year, and more frequently if needed, to address parent or teacher concerns. Some states have limits on the number of IEP meetings per year.

If at any time, communication deteriorates and you feel your child's IEP is inadequate or not being followed, here are several facts you need to know:

- Changes to the IEP cannot be made without parental consent.

- If parents disagree about the content of the IEP, they can withdraw consent and request (in writing) a meeting to draft a new IEP; or they can consent only to the portions of the IEP with which they agree.

- Parents can request to have the disagreement settled by an independent mediator and hearing officer.

> This year (third grade) has been a nightmare. My son has an IEP that focuses on problems with short-term memory, concentration, writing, and reading comprehension. The teacher, even though she is special-ed qualified, has been rigid and used lots of timed tests. She told me in one conference that she thought my son's behavior problems were because he was "spoiled." We asked her at the beginning of the year to please send a note home with my son if he has a seizure, and she has never done it. She even questions him when he tells her that he had a seizure at recess. I began communicating directly with the principal, and I finally received a written notice that he had a seizure. I learned that the IEP is only as valuable as the teacher who is applying it.

More about placement and modifications

IDEA intentionally falls short on detailing specific types of educational placement, modifications, and related services. Because options are open, your child's IEP should reflect those programs and services uniquely appropriate for his needs. Advocates, disability organizations, and your child's medical team, teachers, and therapists can assist you in determining which options best suit your child, although ultimately you know your child best.

Possible accommodations available through a 504 plan or IEP include:

- Preferential seating

- Instruction of student in preferred learning mode

- Study groups with discussion for learning/memory

- Taping of classes for reinforcement

- Reduction in reading load

- Books on tape

- Copy of peer notes to increase listening in class and reduce writing

- Copy of teacher's planning notes prior to instruction

- Reduction in writing load
- Computer for written assignments
- Keyboard training (kindergartners are not too young to learn)
- Use of planning organizers
- Calculator use permitted after mastery of concepts demonstrated
- Extended time for tests
- Travel between classes with adult/responsible peer
- Locker placement consideration
- Assignment check-off system
- Breakdown of large assignments into steps.

Transition services

Transition planning should begin in the early years of middle school, when the student's peers are beginning to gain work skills and prepare for high school graduation. The law states that transition services must begin no later than age 14. Special education students have the right to be prepared for graduation, higher education, and employment in ways that fit their needs. For some cancer survivors, extra support is needed to help ease the transition from high school to adulthood. For more information, visit *www.wrightslaw. com/idea/art/defs.transition.htm*.

Your legal rights (Canada)

Canada has no federal education agency or nationalized standards of education. Each province and territory has its own ministry or department of education and establishes its own laws, policies, procedures, and budgets pertaining to educational requirements and services. The Council of Ministers of Education operates on a voluntary basis to advocate for educational services, establish common goals, and improve the quality of education across the country. One of the shared goals of this group in recent years has been to improve the delivery of special education services to children across Canada.

Most provinces and territories have a neurobehavioral evaluation process similar to the one used in the United States. Canada also employs a similar IEP process, although the specific rules vary by province. Canadian parents of leukemia survivors may find help and support from the Learning Disabilities Association of Canada (*www.ldac-taac.ca*).

Accepting disabilities

Many of the disabilities of childhood cancer survivors are invisible. The children look the same as the did before treatment, but their intellectual abilities have changed. To help children and teens reach their true potential, changes in intellectual functioning and social skills must be diagnosed and addressed early. Students whose style of learning has changed as a result of treatment need their parents and teachers to explore the many excellent methods that can enhance their ability to learn.

It is also important to remember that although some survivors of leukemia develop learning problems, their innate intelligence usually remains intact. Their situation is analogous to an office staffed by extremely bright individuals whose filing system is a mess. They can think and act perfectly well, it just sometimes takes them a longer time than average to access the information they know. Children who were gifted before treatment usually remain so; children with average abilities retain them. Their performance may be slower, and they may require extra instruction in memory enhancement and organizational skills, but they can still do well in school and the workplace.

Record-keeping

Other than medical record-keeping, no records are more important to keep than those concerning your child's special education. Many parents recommend keeping a yearly file that includes the name of the teacher, principal, and district psychologist, copy of the IEP, all test results, all correspondence, a current copy of the local and state regulations, and all of your child's report cards. You should also include in the file a list of medications taken by your child during the year. Do not throw these records out—give them to your child when she reaches age 18—as they can be crucial for college testing and accommodations.

The thought of keeping all of these records may seem overwhelming, but try to think of it this way: appropriate schooling is what will enable your child to overcome the cancer experience and become a productive adult, and your child needs your help to secure that future.

The terminally ill child and school

In the sad event that the child's health continues to deteriorate and all possible treatments have been exhausted, it is time for the students and staff to discuss ways to be supportive during a child's final days. Students need timely information about their ill classmate so they can deal with his declining health and prepare for his death. The possibility of death from cancer should have been sensitively raised in the initial class presentation before the child's return to school, but additional information is needed if the child's health declines. The following are suggestions about how to prepare classmates and school personnel for the death of a student:

- The school staff needs to be in close communication with parents and the hospital. They need to be reassured that death will not suddenly occur at school; rather, the child will either die at home or in the hospital.

- Staff needs to be aware that participation at school is vital to a sick child's well-being. School staff members should welcome and support the child's need to attend school as long as possible.

- Staff can design flexible programs for the ill student, for example, part-time school attendance coupled with part-time home tutoring (if appropriate) for a child who is too weak to attend school all day.

    Jody was lucky because he went to a private school, and there were only 16 children in his class. Whenever he could come to school, they made him welcome. Because children worked at their own pace, he never had the feeling that he was getting behind in his classwork. He really felt like he belonged there. Sometimes he could only manage to stay an hour, but he loved to go. Toward the end when he was in a wheelchair, the kids would fight over whose turn it was to push him. The teacher was wonderful, and the kids really helped him and supported him until the end.

- Staff can designate a "safe person" and "safe haven" in the school building so the student can retreat if she is physically or emotionally overwhelmed.

- The hospital advocate should meet with school personnel and the student's class to answer questions about the student's health status and to address fears and misconceptions about death.

- It is helpful to provide reading materials about death and dying for the ill child's classmates, siblings' classmates, teachers, and staff.

- Extraordinary efforts should be made to keep in touch when the child can no longer attend school. Cards, banners, tapes, texts, e-mails, telephone calls, Webcam, or conference calls (on the principal's speaker phone) from the entire class or individual classmates are good ways to share thoughts and best wishes.

- Visits to the hospital or child's home should be made, if appropriate. If the child is too sick to entertain visitors, the class can come wave at the front window and drop off cards or gifts.

- The class can send a books, video games, an iTunes® gift card, or a basket of small gifts and cards to the hospital or home.

- The class can decorate the family's front door, mailbox, and yard when the child is returning home from the hospital.

All of the above activities encourage empathy and concern in classmates, as well as help them adjust to the decline and imminent death of their friend. The activities also help the sick child know she has not been forgotten by her teachers, friends, and classmates, even if she cannot attend school.

When the child dies, a memorial service at school gives students a chance to grieve. School counselors or psychologists should talk to the classmates to allow them to express their feelings. Parents may appreciate receiving stories or poems about their departed child from classmates, and having some of the children attend the funeral helps support the grieving family.

The following passage was written by Brigit Tuxen and is reprinted with permission from *Candlelighters Youth Newsletter*:

> *My diagnosis of high-risk ALL gave me a 50 percent chance of survival. Cranial radiation and 3 years of blood tests, IVs, chemotherapy, bone marrows, and spinal taps were my prescription. A positive outlook pushed me through the bad times. Somehow I understood that all the hurt was for a good reason, and that it would make me well.*
>
> *Call it a miracle, luck, or determination to live—I survived! But I would soon realize that I would never be like all the other kids. The radiation that destroyed cancer cells also harmed some of my brain cells. For the past 5 years, I have had slight difficulty with math and science courses at school, but with the help of a tutor I've managed to pull through challenging honors classes with As and Bs. However, I am often the last to finish class assignments or tests. It is very frustrating and often embarrassing. The SAT has become my ultimate challenge. Despite this minor disability, I continue to set high standards for myself. I feel extremely lucky to have beaten this disease, and I want to do anything I can to help those who are fighting cancer or some other hardship.*

Chapter 16

Sources of Support

> *The effort to "put up a front" is draining, isolating, and counterproductive. Support groups can be a powerful way of letting down these fronts a bit at a time among people who understand and feel the same conflicting pressure— to act as though everything is all right when it is not.*
>
> — David Spiegel, MD
> *Living Beyond Limits*

THE DIAGNOSIS OF CANCER CAN BE a frightening and isolating experience. Every parent of a child with cancer has a story to tell of lost or strained friendships. Yet we are social creatures, reliant on a web of support from family, friends, neighbors, and churches. We need the presence of people who not only care for us, but who sincerely try to understand what we are feeling. Many parents experience deep loneliness after the first rush of visits, cards, and phone calls ends—when the rest of the world goes back to normal life.

Members of families struck by childhood cancer—parents, the child with cancer, and siblings—are increasingly turning to support groups and various other forms of psychological help. Families join support groups to dispel isolation, share suggestions for dealing with the illness and its side effects, and talk to others who are living through the same crisis. Individual and family counseling can help address shifting responsibilities within the family, explore methods to improve communication, and help find ways to channel strong feelings constructively.

This chapter offers resources that can help families regain a sense of control over their lives and find wonderful new friends who understand what they are going through.

Candlelighters

Candlelighters Childhood Cancer Foundation is an excellent resource for families facing childhood cancer. Candlelighters provides access to information about available treatments, clinical trials, support, and other resources. It also advocates for and directly supports research and legislation to protect the rights of children and families affected by cancer. The national organization is headquartered in Kensington, MD, but there are more than 40 local affiliates across the country. For more information about Candlelighters, to find an affiliate group, or to start one yourself, go to its website at *www.candlelighters.org* or call (800) 366-2223.

Hospital social workers

Although the need for skilled pediatric social workers is widely recognized, shrinking hospital budgets often prevent adequate staffing. If your child is treated at a children's hospital well staffed with social workers, child life specialists, and psychologists, consider yourself lucky. Sadly, millions of dollars are spent on technology, while programs that help people cope emotionally are often the first to be discarded. If your pediatric center offers no emotional support, get help through some of the other methods described in this chapter.

Pediatric social workers usually have a master's degree in social work, with additional training in oncology and pediatrics. They serve as guides through unfamiliar territory by mediating between staff and families, helping with emotional or financial problems, locating resources, and easing the young patient back into school. Many social workers form close, long-lasting bonds with families and continue to answer questions and provide support long after treatment ends.

> On the day of Carl's diagnosis, we were introduced to a team whom we worked with for the next several years. The team included a primary nurse, a primary oncologist, a first-year resident, a second-year resident, a third-year resident, and our social worker. I remember that first day the social worker told us she was there to help us with anything we needed, such as hospital problems, billing, insurance, emotional issues, or behavior issues. She said her job was to be there for us, and she was, whenever we needed her.

• • • • •

> We went to a children's hospital that was renowned in the pediatric cancer field. The medical treatment was excellent, but psychosocial support was nonexistent. The day after diagnosis, we were interviewed for 20 minutes by a psychiatric resident, and that was it. I never met a social worker, and the physicians were so busy they never asked anything other than medical questions. If I started crying, they usually left the room. I didn't know Candlelighters existed; I didn't know there was a local support group; I didn't know there was a summer camp for the kids. I felt totally isolated.

In addition to social workers, some hospitals have child life specialists, psychiatric nurses, psychiatrists, psychiatric residents, and psychologists on staff who can help you deal with problems while your child is an inpatient.

After Meagan's first bone marrow aspiration, which did not go well and was very painful for her, she stopped talking and she wouldn't even look at us. We couldn't comfort her in any of the normal ways; she didn't want to be held, read to, talked to, sung to. At the time, this was more devastating than the leukemia. Any time somebody would come to the door, she would start shaking. Days into this, we asked, "Isn't there anybody here who helps kids who are feeling this way?" So they sent up a psychiatric nurse, who came once and really worked wonders. However, she never came back, so we made arrangements to see her occasionally on an out-patient basis. When we started getting Meagan anesthesia for her procedures, the withdrawal stopped, and she's a healthy and happy first-grader now.

Support groups for parents

Support groups offer a special perspective for parents of children with cancer and fill the void left by the withdrawal or misunderstanding of family and friends. Parents in similar circumstances can share practical information learned through personal experience, provide emotional support, give hope for the future, and truly listen and empathize.

Coping with a life-threatening illness requires a unique perspective—the ability to focus on the grave situation at hand while balancing other aspects of daily life. In support groups, many families find this frame of reference and are better able to find emotional balance, for there are always those with more severe problems than yours, as well as those whose children have completed treatment and are thriving. Just meeting people who have lived through the same situation is profoundly reassuring.

The group was a real lifeline for us, especially when Justin was so sick. We looked forward to the meetings and were there for every one. It was a real escape; it was a place to go where people were rooting for us. People from the group would always swing by to see us whenever they were bringing their own kids in for treatment. They always stopped by to visit and chat. We amassed a tremendous library of children's books that the group members would drop off. The support was wonderful.

• • • • •

I felt like I was always putting up a front for my family and friends. I acted like I was strong and in control. This act was draining and counterproductive. With the other parents, though, I really felt free to laugh as well as cry. I felt like I could tell them how bad things were without causing them any pain. I just couldn't do that with my family. If I told them what was really going on, they just looked stricken, because they didn't know what to do. But the other parents did.

• • • • •

Our Tuesday gatherings were an anchor for us. It was a time to meet with parents who truly understood what living with cancer meant. These parents had been in the trenches. They knew the midnight terrors, the frustrations of dealing with the medical establishment; after all, it was an alien world to most of us. They knew about chemo, hair loss, friend loss, and they knew the bittersweet side of cherishing a child more than one thought one could cherish anyone. We gathered to cry, to laugh, to whine, to comfort one another, to share shelter from a frightening world. It was a haven.

Cancer can be a very isolating experience. For the parents of a child with cancer, the issues that other parents in their social circles are dealing with seem light years away. But the moms and dads in the kitchen at a Ronald McDonald House or the ped-onc lounge can just look at a child on prednisone wolfing down a complete second dinner and tell the new parents how fast the appetite goes when the prednisone is tapered. They understand each other's feelings and emotions, because they are sharing the same experience. It is a bond that cuts across all social, economic, cultural, and racial barriers.

My 2-year-old daughter was diagnosed 1 week after I gave birth to a new baby girl. I remember early in her treatment, I was sitting with Gina on my lap, and my husband sat next to me, holding the new baby. The doctor breezed in and said in a cheerful voice, "How are you feeling?" I burst into sobs and could not stop. He said "Just a minute" and dashed out. A few minutes later a woman came in with her 8-year-old daughter who had finished treatment and looked great. She put her arms around me and talked to me. She told me that everyone feels horrible in the beginning; and it might be hard to believe, but treatment would soon become a way of life for us. She was a great comfort, and of course, she was right.

Dozens of different types of support groups exist, ranging from those with hundreds of members and formal bylaws to a group of three moms who meet for coffee once a week. Some groups deal only with the emotional aspects of the disease, while others may focus on education, advocacy, social opportunities, or crisis intervention. Some groups are facilitated by trained mental health practitioners, while others are self-help groups only for parents. And, naturally, as older members drop out and new families join, the needs and interests of the group may shift.

We have found that it is hard to keep people coming to monthly meetings, even though we have a large membership. We have a 15-member board, which meets every month and plans parties and informational meetings with speakers. We have parties for Christmas, Easter, and Halloween, as well as trips to amusement parks and picnics. Our motto is, "If there's food, families will come." We are also lucky to have a full-time staff person who takes care of information, advertising our services, correspondence, and connecting parents with similar needs.

• • • • •

Our group is very informal. We do have two social workers who are considered the facilitators and are there as resource persons. We just talk about whatever anyone

*wants to discuss. Occasionally we have invited speakers in. I remember having
a psychiatrist discuss stress management, and we also had a talk on therapeutic
massage. We have formed close friendships from the group, and we still go twice a
month, even though our daughter is a year off treatment and doing great. I think our
presence comforts the new families.*

It is important to remember, however, that support group members are not infallible. One person may say something thoughtless or hurtful. Someone else may provide incorrect information. It is best to accept the support in the spirit in which it is given, but to always take any concerns or questions you have to your physician or nurse practitioner.

Online support

Parents from small, isolated communities may have a difficult time finding a support group in their area that fits their needs, as may single parents, parents who aren't able to attend support group meetings, or parents who prefer some anonymity. For these parents and families, finding emotional support is possible via the Internet. Many online discussion groups exist for families dealing with childhood cancer. Such groups can provide parents with the understanding that only another parent of a child with cancer can give. Topics might include coping skills that have been effective for other families or helpful medical information you can use in your fight against childhood cancer.

*The support I have gained through online discussion groups is priceless. I have
received a great deal of comfort from my participation in these groups. They have
enabled me to connect with families from all over the world, many of whom are
fighting the exact same disease. I have often come to my computer in the middle of
the night, when everyone else in the house was asleep. I can express my fears at 3:00
a.m. and know someone will always be there to reassure me with the knowledge that
they have felt these things, too. That's one of the most beautiful things about these
groups. Someone is always there, even in the middle of the night.*

• • • • •

*How ironic that we subscribed to this list in a moment of panic, with a black cloud
lined with despair lingering above. But now we can say we have lassoed cyberspace,
and here, among new friends, we have found and we have shared love, hope, support,
disparity, informative information, mutual stories, mutual questions, thoughtful and
sincere answers, honesty, disagreement, pain, inspiration, fundraising, friendship,
humor, and enjoyment, as well as understanding. This list reflects the roller coaster
of life. Activity on this list enables individuals to place that initial black cloud in
their back pocket, hold sunshine in their hand, and watch hope dance above.*

A well-respected host of more than 150 online support groups for people facing cancer is the Association of Cancer Online Resources at *www.acor.org*. Appendix C, "Books, Websites, and Videotapes" has more information about Internet support groups.

Support groups for children with cancer

Many pediatric hospitals have ongoing support groups for children with cancer. Often these groups are run by experienced pediatric social workers who know how to balance fun with sharing feelings. For many children, these groups are the only place where they feel completely accepted, and where most of the other kids are bald and have to take lots of medicine. The group is a place where children or adolescents can say how they really feel, without worrying that they are causing their parents more pain. Many children form wonderful and lasting friendships in peer groups.

> *I went to Junior Candlelighters, which was very helpful. The gal who facilitated the group was a survivor of osteosarcoma and had had her leg amputated. Yet, she skied, she drove, she did everything. I always thought, "If Patty can do it, I can, too. If she can live so well without a leg, I should be able to put up with having a cancer in my blood."*

· · · · ·

> *All four of my kids have been going to the support groups for over 7 years now. We have one group for the kids with cancer, which is run by a social worker. The siblings group is run by a woman who specializes in early childhood development. Both groups do a lot of art therapy, relaxation therapy, playing, and talking. They meet twice a month, and I will continue to take them until they ask to stop. I think it has really helped all of them. We also have two teen nights out a year. All of the teenagers with cancer get together for an activity such as watching a hockey game or basketball game, or going bowling, to the movies, or out for pizza. They also see each other at our local camp for children surviving cancer (Camp Watcha-Wanna-Do) each year.*

· · · · ·

> *Kristin goes to the kids' support group while my wife and I attend the parents' group downstairs. She doesn't talk much about what goes on, but the facilitator keeps the parents apprised of how things are going. One very vocal 9-year-old boy has recently broken the ice with the kids. He really likes to talk about his feelings about having leukemia, and it has prompted the other children to begin to share their thoughts and reactions about the things that have happened to them. They also have lots of fun.*

For children who are too ill or shy to join a group, there are alternatives. Thousands of kids use computers to contact and chat with other kids in similar situations. Use Appendix C to locate some of the available computer groups.

Support groups for siblings

Many hospitals have responded to the growing awareness of siblings' natural concerns and worries by creating hospital visiting days for them. This allows both one-on-one parent time for the siblings and the opportunity for them to explore and become familiar with the hospital environment. Sibling days allow interaction with other siblings and with staff, and a time to have questions answered and concerns addressed. Some hospital staffs have expanded these 1-day programs into ongoing support groups to improve communication, education, and support for siblings.

> *Both of Shawn's brothers went to the sibling group for years. It seemed to really help them. I don't really know what they did in that room upstairs, but they always came down happy.*

• • • • •

> *Annie went to Club Goodtimes long after her brother stopped going and attended camp as many years as they would allow. She intends to be on the staff at camp next summer.*

Parent-to-parent programs

Some pediatric hospitals, in conjunction with parent support groups such as Candlelighters, have developed parent-to-parent visitation programs. The purpose of these visits is for veteran parents to provide one-on-one support to parents of newly diagnosed children. The services provided by the veteran parent can be informational, emotional, or logistical. The visiting parent can:

- Empathize with the parents

- Help notify family and friends

- Ease feelings of isolation

- Provide hospital tours

- Write down parents' questions for the medical team

- Offer advice about sources of financial aid

- Explain unfamiliar medical terms

- Be available by phone for any problems that arise

- Supply lots of smiles and hugs, and most of all, hope.

Families of newly diagnosed children can ask if the hospital has a parent-to-parent program. If not, ask to speak to the parent leader of the local support group. Often, this person will ask a parent to visit you at the hospital. Many, many parents are more than willing to visit, as they know only too well what those first weeks in the hospital are like. They are often accompanied by their child who has completed therapy and is rosy-cheeked and full of energy—a living beacon of hope.

> *I am the parent consultant for our region. Among the services I provide are: meet with all newly diagnosed families; give a packet of information to each child or teen with cancer; continue to visit the families whenever they return to the hospital; educate families about the various local resources; provide moral support; stay with children during painful procedures if the parents can't; organize and present all of the school programs; liaison with schools for school reentry; organize and send out monthly reminders for Candlelighters meetings, child support group meetings, and sibling group meetings; send out birthday cards to kids on treatment; serve as activities director at the summer camp; and generally try to help out each family in any way possible. My job is a part-time, paid position funded through the local independent agency, Cancer Services of Allen County, Inc.*

Hospital resource rooms

Hospital resource rooms are now becoming more widely available, and they exist specifically to help patients and their families find information—electronic or print—about specific conditions. Make a point during your next doctor visit to ask if your facility has one. You can also check with your hospital's medical library to see if they allow families to do research on site.

> *I think I first learned from a medical librarian about www.nih.gov and Medline, where you can find current research on chemotherapy and other treatments. If your local hospital is a teaching facility, they often have all the major medical journals, so we were able to get full-text versions of papers that we needed. Until we had our own home access to the Internet, most of our research was done through our local hospital's medical library.*

· · · · ·

> *Patient resource rooms are wonderful places. They usually have basic information on your child's illness, listings of agencies and cancer organizations, online access, and a person available to answer questions and help get you started if you're unfamiliar with doing Internet searches. It should be one of the first places families are directed to.*

Clergy and religious community

Religion is a source of strength for many people. Some parents and children find that their faith is strengthened by the cancer ordeal, while some begin to question their beliefs. Others, who have not relied on religion in the past, may now turn to it for solace and strength.

Most hospitals have staff chaplains who are available for counseling, religious services, prayer, and other types of spiritual guidance. The chaplain often visits families soon after diagnosis and is available on an on-call basis. As with any mental health encounter, approaches that work well with one family may not be helpful for others.

The day after my daughter was diagnosed, a chaplain started coming to the room every day. She was very nice, but I felt like she wanted me to talk about the cancer, and I just couldn't. I clearly remember feeling as if my body parts were being held together by the weakest of threads. I felt if I started talking, or even said the word leukemia, that those threads holding me together would break and I would fly apart into a million pieces. So we chatted about inconsequential things until one day I thanked her for coming, but said I felt strong enough to start talking to my family and friends.

· · · · ·

When Shawn was first diagnosed, Father Ron came in, and we all just really bonded with him. Shawn was in the hospital most of the first year, so we had a chance to become very close. Often Shawn would ask for Father Ron before he had to have a painful procedure. Father Ron would talk to him, give him a little stuffed animal and a big hug, and then Shawn would feel better.

When Shawn was very ill, I began to worry about the fact that he had never been baptized, and I asked Father Ron to baptize him in the chapel. We ended up going to his own little church nearby, and we had a private service with just godparents and family, because Shawn's counts were so low. It was a wonderful, special service; I'll never forget it.

Parents who were members of a church, synagogue, or mosque prior to the diagnosis of their child's cancer may derive great comfort from the clergy and members of their home religious base. Members of the congregation usually rally around the family, providing meals, babysitting, prayers, and support. Regular visits from clergy provide spiritual sustenance throughout the initial crisis and subsequent years of treatment.

We belong to a religious study group that has met weekly for 8 years. In our group, during that time, there have been three cancer diagnoses and one of multiple sclerosis. We have all become an incredibly supportive family, and we share the burdens. I cannot begin to list the many wonderful things these people have done for us. They consistently put their lives on hold to help. They fill the freezer, clean the house, support us financially, parent our children. They do the laundry covered with vomit. They quietly appear, help, then disappear. I can call any one of them at 3:00 a.m. in the depths of despair and find comfort.

Individual and family counseling

Cancer is a major crisis for even the strongest of families. Many find it helpful to seek out sensitive, objective mental health care professionals to explore the difficult feelings—fear, anger, depression, anxiety, resentment, guilt—that cancer arouses.

Family dynamics undergo profound changes when a child is diagnosed with leukemia. Seeking professional counseling for ways to adjust and manage is a sign of strength. When a child has cancer, problems may be too complex and family members may be too tired to manage on their own. Seeking professional help sends children a message that the parents care about what is happening to them and want to help face it together.

One of the first questions that arises is, "Who should we talk to?" There are numerous resource people in the cancer community who can make referrals and valuable recommendations, including:

- Other parents who have sought counseling

- Pediatricians

- Oncologists

- Nurse practitioners

- Clinic social workers

- School psychologists or counselors

- Health department social workers.

You can ask the people listed above for a short list of mental health professionals who have experience working with your issues, for example, traumatized children, marital problems, stress reduction, or family therapy. Generally, the names of the most well-respected clinicians in the community will appear on several of the lists.

> Choosing to get therapy isn't easy. And going to a psychologist isn't easy. The only way to really work through the emotional pain is to look closely at it. Sometimes they ask hard questions. But it has been very beneficial for me. The best part about therapy is the person you are talking to is impartial. She isn't related to you, doesn't go to church with you, doesn't live with you, and has no connection to you or your situation. A totally unbiased perspective can be helpful when it feels like you are at the bottom of the pit, with no handholds, no ladder, but a shovel right beside you to help you dig deeper.
>
> If you decide to begin therapy, do your research. I called and asked for references from a cancer helpline and the social worker at the clinic. Then I talked to a couple of therapists before I decided which one to go with. She was willing to work with me on a payment schedule.

In making your decision, it helps to understand the various types of mental health care professionals and their different levels of education and liscensure. The following disciplines train individuals to offer psychological services:

- **Psychology (EdD, MA, PhD, PsyD).** Marriage and family psychotherapists have a master's degree; clinical and research psychologists have a doctorate.

- **Social work (MSW, DSW, PhD).** Clinical social workers have either a master's degree or a doctorate in a clinically emphasized program.

- **Pastoral care (MA, MDiv, DMin, PhD, DDiv).** These are laymen or clergy who receive specialized training in counseling.

- **Medicine (MD, RN).** Psychiatrists are medical doctors who completed a residency in psychiatry (they are the only mental health professionals who can prescribe medications). In addition, some nurses obtain postgraduate training in psychotherapy.

- **Counseling (MA).** In most states, individuals must have a master's degree and a year of internship before they can work as counselors.

You may hear all of the above professionals referred to as "counselors" or "therapists." The designations LCSW (Licensed Clinical Social Worker), LSW (Licensed Social Worker), LMFCC (Licensed Marriage, Family, Child Counselor), LPC (Licensed Professional Counselor), and LMFT (Licensed Marriage and Family Therapist) refer to licensure by state professional boards, not academic degrees. These initials usually follow others that indicate an academic degree (e.g., PhD); if they don't, inquire about the therapist's academic training. Most states require licensure or certification in order for professionals to practice independently; unlicensed professionals are allowed to practice only under the supervision of a licensed professional (typically as an "intern" or "assistant" in a clinic or licensed professional's private practice).

When you are seeking a mental health professional, ask the professional how long she has been in practice. A licensed marriage and family therapist who has been seeing patients for 10 years may be a better clinician for your needs than a licensed psychologist or psychiatrist in his first year of practice.

Another method for finding a suitable counselor is to contact the American Association for Marriage and Family Therapy in Alexandria, VA, at (703) 838-9808, or online at *www.aamft.org*. This is a national professional organization of licensed/certified marriage and family therapists. It has more than 24,000 members in the United States and Canada, and its membership also includes licensed clinical social workers, pastoral counselors (who are MFCC/LMFTs), psychologists, and psychiatrists.

A psychiatrist who is the mother of a child with cancer offers a few thoughts:

> *Counseling helps, preferably from someone who regularly deals with parents of seriously ill children. This therapy is almost always short—although there may be*

some pre-cancer problems complicating the cancer issues that need to be hammered out.

Antidepressants definitely have a role in the "so your child has cancer" coping strategy. They cannot make the diagnosis go away. They can improve concentration, energy, sleep, appetite, ability to get pleasure in life, and hope for the future—all of which you, your child with cancer, your spouse, and your other kids need you to have! They are not a magic bullet. They take 2 to 8 weeks to work, and you may need to change once before you get the right medication, but it can make all the difference.

Also, nurture yourself. Take bubble baths. Buy flowers. Let people pamper you. Say yes when people offer to help. Redefine normal so things can be good again. Make time for yourself. Spend time with your spouse (even an hour to walk and talk and hold hands). Find time for your non-cancer kids, reveling in their accomplishments. Celebrate what is good about your life.

Pick out things that you feel are important to keep up with and do them. (For me it was laundry.) Ignore things that don't matter for the time being. (For me it was tidy rooms and cooking.) Make peace with your decisions and follow them.

To find a therapist, a good first step is to call two or three therapists who appear on several of your lists of recommendations. Following are some suggested questions to ask during your telephone interview:

- Are you accepting new clients?

- Do you charge for an initial consultation?

- What training and experience do you have working with ill or traumatized children?

- How many years have you been working with families?

- What is your approach to resolving the problems families develop from trauma? Do you use a brief or long-term approach?

- What evaluation and assessment procedures will be used to define the problem?

- How and when will treatment goals be set?

- What are your fees? Do you bill the insurance company directly? Do you accept my insurance?

The next step is to make an appointment with one or two of the therapists you think might best address your needs. Be honest about the fact that you are interviewing several therapists prior to making a decision. The purpose of the introductory meeting is to see if you feel comfortable with the therapist. After all, credentials do not guarantee that a given therapist is a good fit for you. Compatibility, trust, and a feeling of genuine caring are essential. It is worth the effort to continue your search until you find a good match.

I called several therapists out of desperation about my daughter's withdrawal and violent tantrums. I made appointments with two. The first I just didn't feel comfortable with at all, but the second felt like an old friend after 1 hour. I have been to see her dozens of times over the years, and she has always helped me. I wasn't interested in theory; I wanted practical suggestions about how to deal with the behavior problems. My 8-year-old daughter asked why I was going to see the therapist, and I said that Hilda was a doctor, but instead of taking care of my body, she helped care for my feelings. She asked to go to the "feelings" doctor, but was concerned about whether her conversations would be private. I asked the counselor to explain about the limits of confidentiality. So that began a very helpful course of therapy for my daughter.

· · · · ·

We went to family counseling because I was concerned that my son seemed to be increasingly withdrawn and depressed. It was a disaster. The kids clammed up, I talked too much, and my husband was offended by some of the remarks the counselor made. She was not a good choice for our family. It's a hard decision to change counselors when you know you need help, but it's better to make a move than to stay in an uncomfortable situation.

· · · · ·

We went into family therapy because every member of my family experienced misdirected anger. When they were angry, they aimed it at me—the nice person who took care of them and loved them no matter what. But I was dissolving. I needed to learn to say "ouch," and they needed to learn other ways to handle their angry feelings.

Children need to be prepared for psychological interventions, just as they do for any unknown procedure. Following are several parents' suggestions about how to prepare your child:

- Explain who the therapist is and what you hope to accomplish. If you are bringing your child in for therapy, explain why you think talking to an objective person might benefit him.

- Older children should be involved in the process of choosing a counselor. Younger children's likes and dislikes should be respected. If your young child does not get along well with one counselor, change.

- Make the experience positive rather than threatening (e.g., call him or her "the talking doctor").

- Reassure young children that the visit is for talking, drawing, or playing games, not for anything that is physically painful.

  In the beginning of treatment, my son had terrible problems with going to sleep and then having nightmares, primarily about snakes. We took him to a counselor, who worked with him for several weeks and completely resolved the problem. The counselor had him befriend the snake, talk to it, and explain that it was keeping him awake. He would tell the snake, "I want you to stop bothering me because I need to go to sleep." The snake never returned.

- Ask the therapist to explain the rules of confidentiality to both you and your child. Do not quiz your child after a visit to the therapist.

    David had a very difficult time dealing with his brother's cancer. Realizing that we were unable to provide him with the help he needed, we sought professional help for him. I think the reason he feels so comfortable with his therapist is that he is aware of the rules of confidentiality. After his sessions, I'll always ask him how it went. Sometimes he'll just grin and say it was fine, and other times he might share a little of his conversation with me. I never push or question him about it. If it is something he needs to discuss, I wait until he decides to broach the subject.

- Make sure your child does not think she is being punished; assure her that therapists help both adults and children understand and deal with feelings.
- Go yourself for individual or family counseling or to support group meetings.

Some other types of therapy used to help children with cancer or their siblings are music therapy (*www.musictherapy.org*), art therapy (*www.arttherapy.org*), and dance therapy (*www.ADTA.org*).

In *Armfuls of Time*, psychologist Barbara Sourkes quotes Jonathan, a boy with cancer, who told her, "Thank you for giving me aliveness." She discusses the importance of psychotherapy for children with a life-threatening illness:

Even when life itself cannot be guaranteed, psychotherapy can at least "give aliveness" to the child for however long that life may last. Through the extraordinary challenges posed by life-threatening illness, a precocious inner wisdom of life and its fragility emerges. Yet even in the struggle for survival, the spirit of childhood shines through.

Camps

Summer camps for children with cancer, and often their siblings, are becoming increasingly popular. These camps provide an opportunity for children with cancer and their siblings to have fun, meet friends, and talk with others in the same situation. Counselors are usually cancer survivors and siblings of children with cancer, or sometimes oncology nurses and residents. At these camps, children can have their concerns addressed in a safe, supportive environment that is supervised by experts. These camps provide a carefree time away from the sadness and stress at home or from the all-too-frequent hospital visits.

Of all the ways to get support, I think the camp really helps the most. You are all there together for enough time to break down the barriers. Although camp does not focus on cancer, many times we really got down to talking about how we really felt. I have been a counselor at the camp for eight summers now. Most of the campers know that I relapsed three times and I'm doing great many years later. They see the many other long-term survivors who are counselors, and it gives them what they need the most—hope. The best support is meeting survivors, because nobody else truly understands.

• • • • •

When we went to pick up 7½-year-old Kristin from camp, she told us how wonderful it had been and exclaimed, "I want to come back every year until I am old enough to be a counselor." That said it all to me.

• • • • •

Caitlin went to camp, and this was a dream come true for her. As we pulled into the parking lot, she exhaled a deep breath and said, "I made it. I am finally normal!"

Some camps are set up to accommodate not only the child who has undergone treatment, but also their siblings and parents. Many other camps offer separate weeklong camping experiences just for siblings. Appendix B, "Resource Organizations," contains a short list of camps with contact information. To view a comprehensive list, visit *www. acor.org/ped-onc/cfissues/camps.html.*

It's like your psyche has been hit by a truck. Some days the pain is worse than others. Some days your threshold is stronger than others, but allow yourself the help that is available to get back to stable. Take it from me; it is next to impossible to pull on a dry well. So unlike children, we can't temper tantrum ourselves out of our feelings, we can't rant and scream and stomp our feet at the unfairness of it all. We can't just sit in momma's arms and have a hug and feel better. We have to handle it with an attitude and the responsibility that is expected of being adult. And we have to be a nurse, teacher, mom, emotional measuring stick for our kids, care for the marriage, pay the bills, and, oh yeah, don't forget about ourselves—all at the same time. It's just far too much. Say "Yes" to yourself, and your needs—get help when you need it. Other things that I found helpful were:

- *Saying "no," "no, thank you," and "I'll take that into consideration when I make my decision."*

- *Saying "yes," "yes, please, that would be a great help," and "sure, if you could drop off a lasagna or pick up some milk on your way over that would be great."*

- *Writing in a journal.*

- *Taking a retreat weekend.*

- *Playing cards with the girls.*

- *Counseling (on occasion with priest, psychologist, social worker).*

- *Having movie night with my sisters (usually a comedy—you are allowed to laugh).*

- *Treating myself to an inside-and-out car wash.*

- *Allowing myself to "cry in my cornflakes," then getting up, splashing some cold water on my face and getting on with the day.*

- *Enjoying a glass of wine, a candle, and Andrea Boccelli.*

- *Gardening.*

- *Having coffee with a friend.*

- *Helping someone else who was in worse shape than I was.*

- *Talking with other cancer kid moms about cancer kid family stuff.*

- *Talking with other non-cancer kid moms about non-cancer family stuff (the kids bickering, too much housework, the latest magazine, and what the women in it are wearing).*

- *Declaring the next 5 minutes was "get the crazies out" time, and tickling, dancing silly, and playing "make me laugh" (you know you're losing it when you do this, and no one else is home).*

- *Being an online (www.acor.org) listserv member.*

- *Going out with my husband. (Even if I had to drag him, we always enjoyed the evening in spite of ourselves.)*

And anything else I deemed necessary to help me get through it.

Chapter 17

Nutrition

*Let your food be your medicine and
your medicine be your food.*

— Hippocrates (fifth century B.C.)

NOW, MORE THAN EVER, it is important for your sick child to eat balanced, healthful, and energy-packed meals. Yet, the reality is that the eating habits of children with leukemia go haywire. Although, your child's body needs added energy to metabolize medications and repair the damage to healthy cells caused by chemotherapy and radiation, those same treatments can wreak havoc on your child's appetite and taste sensations. This chapter discusses eating problems, explains good nutrition, suggests ways to pack extra calories into small servings, and offers tips about how to make food more appealing to children.

How treatment affects eating

Eating is tremendously affected by most types of chemotherapy. Listed below are several common side effects of treatment that conspire to prevent good eating. Other side effects that affect eating—nausea, vomiting, diarrhea, constipation, and mouth and throat sores—are covered in detail in Chapter 10, "Common Side Effects of Chemotherapy."

Loss of appetite

Loss of appetite is one of the most common problems associated with the treatment of cancer. Children suffering from nausea and vomiting, diarrhea or constipation, altered sense of smell and taste, mouth sores, and other unpleasant side effects understandably do not feel hungry. Loss of appetite is most pronounced during the intensive periods of treatment, such as induction, consolidation, and delayed intensification. If your child loses more than 10 to 15 percent of her body weight, she may need to be fed intravenously or by nasogastric tube. Sometimes this can be avoided if parents learn how to increase calories in small amounts of food.

My son looked like a skeleton several months into his protocol for high-risk ALL. I used to dress him in "camouflage" clothes—several layers thick. This kept him warm and prevented stares.

In addition to simple loss of appetite, your child may experience a side effect of chemotherapy called early filling. This means the child has a sense of being full after only a few bites of food. If the child is suffering from early filling and only eats when hungry, she may begin losing weight and become malnourished. This chapter provides dozens of creative ways to encourage your child to eat more.

Increased appetite and weight gain

When children are given high doses of steroids such as prednisone or dexamethasone, they develop voracious appetites. They are hungry all the time, develop food obsessions, and frequently wake parents up during the night begging for another meal.

Early in her treatment, when Carrie Beth was taking dexamethasone, she would start hitting me in the face in the middle of the night demanding food. I learned to have a bag of snacks and a bottle sitting next to the bed, so I could just hand them over and go back to sleep.

Most parents become very concerned if their child consumes huge quantities of food and gains weight. A moon face with chubby cheeks and a rotund belly are classic features of a child on high-dose steroids. Much of the extra weight is fluid, which steroids cause the body to retain. There are two important points for parents to remember about treatment with steroids. First, when the steroids stop, the extra fluid is excreted and weight drops. Second, the child's appetite may go from voracious to poor after the steroids stop, so it is unwise to limit food when your child is taking steroids. Instead, try to make the most of this brief time of good appetite to encourage consumption of a variety of nutritious foods. A well-balanced diet now will help your child withstand the rigors of the treatments ahead.

My daughter didn't sleep when she was on steroids for weeks, and she gained a lot of weight. She'd sit in bed and demand, all day and all night long, "toast with butter spread on it like icing on a cake." So, I gave it to her. When she was off the steroids, she'd rapidly lose the weight and she'd look skeletal. Both extremes were really hard on all of us emotionally.

If you are concerned about the weight gain, consult your child's oncologist. If the fluid retention is extreme, the doctor may have you restrict your child's salt intake; in some cases, children are given drugs called diuretics to rid the body of excess fluid.

Lactose intolerance

Lactose intolerance is when the body can't absorb the sugar (lactose) contained in milk and other dairy products. Both antibiotics and chemotherapy can cause lactose intolerance in some individuals. The part of children's intestines that breaks down lactose stops functioning properly, resulting in gas, abdominal pain, bloating, cramping, and diarrhea. If your child develops lactose intolerance, it is important to talk to a nutritionist to learn about low-lactose diets and alternate sources of protein. The following are suggestions for parents of lactose-intolerant children:

- Add special enzyme tablets or drops to dairy products to make them more digestible for children with an intolerance to lactose. Some of these products are over-the-counter additives, but others require a prescription. Discuss these additives with the oncologist before giving them to your child.

- Children who cannot tolerate the lactose in cow's milk often can manage acidophilus milk, soy milk, or lactose-free milk. These are easier to digest and come in a variety of flavors.

- Always be sure dairy products are pasteurized, not raw.

- Remember that milk is a common ingredient in other foods, such as bread, candy, processed meats, and salad dressings. Read ingredient lists carefully.

- If your child can't tolerate any dairy products, add calcium to her diet by serving canned salmon, sardines, spinach, or calcium-fortified fruit juices. Consult your child's oncologist and nutritionist about calcium supplements. Many children like the taste of a chewy calcium supplement called Viactiv®, which is available at most drug stores.

Altered taste and smell

One common reason children on treatment do not eat is because, for them, food has no taste or tastes bad. If food tastes bland to your child, try serving spicy cuisines, such as Italian, Mexican, or Greek foods.

Chemotherapy often causes foods, particularly red meats, to taste bitter and metallic. If that happens, avoid using metal pots, pans, and utensils, which can magnify the metallic taste. Serve your child's food with plastic knives, forks, and spoons. You can also replace red meat with tofu, pork, chicken, turkey, eggs, and dairy products.

For some children, taste returns to normal when maintenance starts; for others, it returns after treatment ends. And for a few children, it is years before some foods taste pleasant again.

What kids should eat

A good diet includes sufficient calories to ensure a normal rate of growth; fuels the body's efforts to repair and replace healthy cells; and provides the energy the body needs to break down the various chemotherapy drugs given and excrete their by-products. Research shows that well-nourished children can tolerate more treatment with fewer side effects, recover faster from treatment, and maintain weight better.

When the body becomes malnourished, body fat and muscle decrease. This leads to weakness, lack of energy, weight loss, a decreased ability to digest food, and a diminished ability to fight infection and recover from injury. These health issues often require a reduction in the dose of chemotherapeutic drugs.

To keep your child's body well-nourished, foods from all six basic food groups are needed. The groups are (1) bread, cereal, rice, pasta; (2) fruits; (3) vegetables; (4) milk, yogurt, cheese; (5) meat, poultry, fish, dry beans, eggs, nuts; and (6) fats, oils, sweets. Children on chemotherapy also benefit from a higher than average intake of fats, to add calories.

Examples of foods contained in each group are listed below, with a small child's serving size in parentheses beside each food. Consult a nutritionist to determine the serving size appropriate for your child.

Meat and meat substitutes (two or three servings per day)

Meat (1 ounce)	Eggs (1)
Fish (1 ounce)	Peanut butter (2 tbsp.)
Poultry (1 ounce)	Dried beans, cooked ($\frac{1}{2}$ cup)
Cheese (1 ounce)	Dried peas, cooked ($\frac{1}{2}$ cup)

These foods provide protein, which helps build and maintain body tissues, supply energy, and form enzymes, hormones, and antibodies. Some typical 1-ounce servings of meat and meat substitutes are: a meatball 1 inch in diameter, a 1-inch cube of meat, one slice of bologna, a 1-inch cube of cheese, or one slice of processed cheese.

Dairy products (two or three servings per day)

Milk ($\frac{1}{2}$ cup)	Tofu ($\frac{1}{2}$ cup)
Cheese (1 ounce)	Custard ($\frac{1}{2}$ cup)
Ice cream ($\frac{1}{2}$ cup)	Yogurt ($\frac{1}{2}$ cup)

Dairy products provide calcium, vitamin D, and protein. Steroids can weaken bones, so calcium and vitamin D (both necessary for bone growth and strength) are very important.

Breads and cereals (six to 11 servings per day)

Bread ($^1/_2$ slice)	Dry cereal ($^1/_2$ cup)
Oatmeal ($^1/_2$ cup)	Granola ($^1/_2$ cup)
Cream of wheat ($^1/_2$ cup)	Cooked pasta ($^1/_2$ cup)
Graham crackers (1 square)	Saltines (3 squares)
Rice ($^1/_2$ cup)	Potatoes (1 baked)

Breads and cereals supply vitamins, minerals, fiber, and carbohydrates. Try to use only products made with whole wheat flour and limited sugar to get more nutrients per serving. One sandwich made with two slices of bread provides four servings of this food group.

Fruits (two to four servings per day)

Fresh fruit (1 medium piece)	Dried fruits ($^1/_4$ cup)
Canned fruit ($^1/_4$ cup)	Fruit juice ($^1/_2$ cup)

Fruits provide vitamins, minerals, and fiber. Fruits can be camouflaged by puréeing them with ice cream or sherbet in the blender to make a tasty milkshake or smoothie, or by adding them to cookie and muffin recipes.

Vegetables (three to five servings per day)

Raw vegetables ($^1/_4$ cup)	Cooked vegetables ($^1/_4$ cup)

Vegetables, like fruit, are excellent sources of vitamins, minerals, and fiber. If your child does not want vegetables, they can be grated or puréed and added to soups or spaghetti sauce. If you own a juicer, add a vegetable to fruits being juiced. There are also many brownie, cake, bread, and muffin recipes that use vegetables that cannot be tasted, such as zucchini bread, brownies with spinach, carrot cake, and veggie muffins.

Sweets and fats (several servings a day)

Butter or margarine	Nuts
Mayonnaise	Whipped cream
Peanut butter	Avocado
Meat fat (in gravy)	Olives
Ice cream	Chocolate

Although the food pyramid calls for fats to be used sparingly, higher consumption of fats is needed for children being treated for cancer. Experiment to find the fats your child enjoys eating and serve them frequently.

What kids really eat

This chapter lists ideas for increasing calories and making food more appealing. It also describes the wild cravings kids get while taking steroids, usually for foods that are spicy, fatty, salty, or all three. What follows are accounts of what several kids really ate while on chemotherapy. You'll notice how varied the list is, so experiment to see what your child finds palatable. Remember that children's tastes and aversions may change throughout treatment.

> Judd craved chicken chow mein and fried rice takeout from a Chinese restaurant. He also loved Spaghetti-Os® and hot dogs.

· · · · ·

> I let Preston eat whatever tasted good to him, which was usually lots of potatoes and eggs. He liked spicy food (especially Mexican) while on prednisone.

· · · · ·

> Katy typically only ate one food for days or weeks at a stretch. One time, she ate pesto sauce (made from olive oil, garlic, Parmesan cheese, and basil leaves) on pasta for every meal for weeks. She also went through a spicy barbecue sauce phase, in which she wouldn't eat any food unless it was completely immersed in sauce. She ate no fruits, vegetables (except potatoes), or meat for the entire period of treatment. She ate mostly cereal and beans when she was feeling well, and mostly puréed baby food when she was really sick.

· · · · ·

> In the beginning, when Meagan lost so much weight, we snuck Polycose® (a powdered nutritional supplement) into everything. She finally got stuck on cans of mixed nuts. They are high calorie and were instrumental in putting back on the weight. She also craved capers and would eat them by the tablespoonful.

· · · · ·

> All Brent asks for are "peanut butter and jelly sandwiches, cut in fours, no crusts, with Fritos®." The only fruit he has eaten for 3 years is an occasional banana, and he eats no vegetables. He always ate everything before his diagnosis at age 6.

· · · · ·

> The doctor told me to keep Kim on a low-salt, low-folic-acid diet. She wouldn't eat anything, so he eventually said he didn't care what she ate, as long as she ate. She liked Spaghetti-Os®, Chick-fil-A® nuggets, Chick-fil-A® soup, and McDonald's® sausage and pancakes.

All Carl ate was dry cereal, dry waffles, oatmeal, and bacon. He ate no other meat or vegetables throughout treatment, but did drink milk. I thought that he would never be healthy, but he's 15 now (diagnosed when 2), eats little junk food, never gets sick, and looks great.

. . . . .

While Shawn was on prednisone I felt like I could never get out of the kitchen because he ate nonstop. The rest of the time he ate almost nothing. He survived on bagels, dry cereal, french fries, popcorn, and burritos.

. . . . .

Stephan's appetite went back to normal on maintenance. But after he relapsed and had cranial and spinal radiation, things have never been the same. He only wants junk food such as hot dogs and chicken nuggets. Most meats make him sick, and he's having problems with smells making food unappetizing.

. . . . .

John (14 months old) craved creamed corn and pork and beans. I would just sit him on a potty chair at the table and let him eat, and it would go in one end and out the other. When on prednisone, he would sit at the table almost all day. He also drank a gallon of apple juice a day. He rarely eats meat to this day (2 years off treatment).

. . . . .

On prednisone, Rachel ate only hot dogs, bologna, scrambled eggs with cheese, and potato chips. She would eat until she literally threw up. Now, 2 years off treatment, she is gradually expanding her repertoire. She only drinks milk (no water, juice, or soda), eats no sweets, and prefers all salty foods. I really have no idea whether it is learned behavior or a result of the cancer treatment.

. . . . .

I guess Carrie Beth is the exception that proves the rule. She is on maintenance and has an excellent appetite. She eats fruits, vegetables, and lots of meat.

Making eating fun and nutritious

In some homes, mealtimes turn into battlegrounds, with worried parents resorting to threats or bribery to get their child to eat. Parents rarely win these battles: Eventually they give in, exhausted and frustrated, and serve the sick child whatever she will eat (often to the dismay of the siblings who still have to eat their vegetables). The next several sections are full of methods used successfully by many parents to make mealtimes both fun and nutritious.

How to make eating more appealing

Many children are finicky eaters at the best of times. Cancer and its treatment can make eating especially difficult. Here are some general suggestions for making eating more enjoyable for your child:

- Give your child small portions throughout the day rather than three large meals. Feed your child whenever she is hungry.

- Remember that your child knows best which foods he can tolerate.

> In the beginning of treatment, we decided that my son had to eat what the rest of the family was having. If he didn't eat that, he got no more food. He usually just didn't eat. Some mornings, I had trouble waking him up. He was limp and would have his eyes rolled back in his head. He was tested and diagnosed with hypoglycemia (low blood sugar). The doctor told us to make sure he ate something right before bed, even if it was ice cream or cookies and milk. Since he has been off chemotherapy, he has not had any problems.

- Explain clearly to your child that eating a balanced diet will help him fight the cancer.

- Make mealtimes pleasant and leisurely.

- Rearrange eating schedules to serve the main meal at the time of day when your child feels best. If she wakes up feeling well most days, make a high-protein, high-calorie breakfast.

- Don't punish your child for not eating.

- Set a good example by eating a large variety of nutritious foods.

- Have nutritious snacks available at all times. Carry them in the car, to all appointments, and in backpacks for school.

- Serve fluids between meals, rather than with meals, to keep your child from feeling full after only a few bites of food.

- Limit the amount of less nutritious foods in the house. Potato chips, corn chips, soda, and sweets with large amounts of sugar may fill your child up with empty calories.

- If your child is interested, include him in making a grocery list, shopping for favorite foods, and food preparation.

Make mealtime fun

Here are some suggestions for making mealtime more fun:

- Try to take the emphasis off the need to eat food "because it's good for you;" focus instead on enjoying each other's company while sharing a meal. Encourage good conversation, tell stories and jokes, and perhaps light some candles.

- Make one night a week "restaurant night." Use a nice tablecloth and candles, allow the children to order from a menu, and pretend the family is out for a night on the town.

- Because any change in setting can encourage eating, consider having a picnic on the floor occasionally. Order pizza or other takeout, spread a tablecloth on the floor, and have an in-home picnic. One parent even sent lunch out to the treehouse.

   My son enjoyed eating in different places around the house and seemed to eat more when he was having fun. I sometimes fed the kids on their own picnic table outdoors in good weather, and at the same picnic table in the garage during the winter. They were thrilled to wear their coats and hats to eat. Occasionally I would let them eat off TV trays while watching a favorite program or tape.

- Some families have theme meals, such as Mexican, Hawaiian, or Chinese. They use decorations, wear costumes, and cook foods with exotic spices.

- Some children seem to eat better if food is attractively arranged on the plate or is decorated in humorous ways. Preschoolers enjoy putting a smiley face on a casserole using strips of cheese, nuts, or raisins. Sandwiches can be cut into funny shapes using knives or cookie cutters.

   My daughter liked to have food decorated. For example, we would make pancakes look like a clown face by using blueberries for eyes, a strawberry for a nose, orange slices for ears, etc. She also enjoyed eating brightly colored food, so we would add a drop of food coloring to applesauce, yogurt, or whatever appealed to her.

How to serve more protein

Because many children cannot tolerate eating meat while on chemotherapy, below are suggestions for increasing protein consumption:

- Add 1 cup of dried milk powder to a quart of whole milk, then blend and chill. Use this extra-strength milk for drinking and cooking.

- Use extra-strength milk (above), whole milk, evaporated milk, or cream instead of water to make hot cereal, cocoa, soup, gravy, custards, or puddings.

- Add powdered milk to casseroles, meat loaf, cream soups, custards, and puddings.

- Add chopped meat to scrambled eggs, soups, and vegetables.

- Add chopped, hard-boiled eggs to soups, salads, sauces, and casseroles.

- Add grated cheese to pizza, vegetables, salads, sauces, omelets, mashed potatoes, meat loaf, and casseroles.

- Serve bagels, English muffins, hamburgers, or hot dogs with a slice of cheese melted on top.

- Spread peanut butter on toast, crackers, and sandwiches. Dip fruit or raw vegetables into peanut butter for a quick snack.

- Spread peanut butter or cream cheese onto celery sticks or carrots.

- Serve nuts for snacks, and mix nuts into salads and soups.

- Serve yogurt and granola bars for extra protein. Top pies, pudding, or fruit with ice cream or whipped cream.

- Use dried beans and peas to make soups, dips, and casseroles.

- Use tofu (bean curd) in stir-fried vegetable dishes.

- Add wheat germ to hamburgers, meat loaf, breads, muffins, pancakes, waffles, and vegetables, and use it as a topping for casseroles.

Guidelines for boosting calories

Parents need to change their perceptions about what constitutes healthy food when they are struggling to feed a child who is on chemotherapy. Many parents have ingrained habits about serving only low-fat meals and snacks. While your child is on chemotherapy, it is necessary to reverse that focus: Your mission is to find ways to add as many calories as possible to your child's food. Here are some suggestions:

- Add butter or margarine to hot cereal, eggs, pasta, rice, cooked vegetables, mashed potatoes, and soups.

- Use melted butter as a dip for raw vegetables and cooked seafood such as shrimp, crab, and lobster.

- Use sour cream to top meats, baked potatoes, and soups.

- Use mayonnaise instead of salad dressing on salads, sandwiches, and hard-boiled eggs.

- Add mayonnaise or sour cream when making hamburgers or meat loaf.

- Use cream instead of milk over cereal, pudding, Jell-O®, and fruit.

- Make milkshakes, puddings, and custards with cream instead of milk.

- Serve your child whole milk (not 2 percent or skim milk).

- Sauté vegetables in butter.

- Serve bread hot so it will absorb more butter.

- Spread bagels, muffins, or crackers with cream cheese and jelly or honey.

- Make hot chocolate with cream and add marshmallows.

- Add granola to cookie, bread, and muffin batters. Sprinkle granola on ice cream, pudding, and yogurt.

- Serve meat and vegetables with sauces made with cream and pan drippings.
- Combine cooked vegetables with dried fruit.
- Add dried fruits to recipes for cookies, breads, and muffins.

Nutritious snacks

Try to always bring a bag of nutritious snacks whenever you leave home with your child. This allows you to feed her whenever she is hungry and avoid stopping for non-nutritious junk food. Examples of healthful snacks include:

- Apples or applesauce
- Baby foods
- Breakfast bars
- Burritos made from beans or meat
- Buttered popcorn
- Celery sticks stuffed with cheese or peanut butter
- Cookies made with wheat germ, oatmeal, granola, fruits, or nuts
- Cereal
- Cheese
- Cheesecake
- Chocolate milk
- Cottage cheese
- Crackers with cheese, peanut butter, or tuna salad
- Custards made with extra eggs and cream
- Dips made with cheese, avocado, butter, beans, or sour cream
- Dried fruit such as apples, raisins, apricots, or prunes
- Fresh fruit
- Granola mixed with dried fruit and nuts
- Hard-boiled and deviled eggs
- Ice cream made with real cream
- Juice made from 100 percent fruit
- Milkshakes made with whole milk or cream
- Fruit smoothies made with frozen fruit, sherbet or ice cream, and ice

- Muffins

- Nuts

- Peanut butter on crackers or whole wheat bread

- Pizza

- Puddings

- Protein bars

- Sandwiches with real mayonnaise or butter

- Vegetables such as carrot sticks or broccoli florets

- Yogurt, regular or frozen.

Vitamin supplements

The nutritional needs of kids with cancer are higher than other children's, yet kids on treatment often eat less food. Most children and teens with cancer are unable or unwilling to eat the variety of foods necessary for good health. In addition, damage to the digestive system from chemotherapy alters the body's ability to absorb the nutrients contained in the food your child does manage to eat. As a result, vitamin supplements are usually necessary.

Vitamin supplementation should only be done after consultation with your child's oncologist and nutritionist. Oversupplementation of some vitamins, folic acid for example, can make your child's chemotherapy less effective. But providing other vitamins can make the difference between a pale and listless child and one with bright eyes and a positive attitude. Vitamin supplements should be individually tailored for your child in consultation with the oncologist and nutritionist.

Halfway through maintenance, my daughter just looked awful. Her new hair began to thin out and break easily and her skin felt papery. I had been giving her a multivitamin and mineral tablet every day because her appetite was so poor, but it didn't seem to be enough. I talked to her doctor, then began to give her more of the antioxidant vitamins: betacarotene, E, and C. I bought the C in powder form, which effervesced when mixed with juice. She really liked her "bubble drinks." The betacarotene and E she swallowed along with the rest of her pills. Within a few weeks her hair stopped falling out, her skin stopped peeling, and she felt better.

• • • • •

I gave my teenage daughter supplements of vitamins and some minerals. I also increased her vitamin intake by using the juicer every day. She always drank a big glass of fruit or vegetable juice, and I really think it helped her do as well as she has.

Nutritionists and dieticians

It can be very helpful to consult with the hospital nutritionist to obtain more information and ideas about how to add more protein, calories, and vitamins/minerals to your child's diet. You can also consult with a private nutritionist who has experience with both children's nutritional needs and those of cancer patients. The American Dietetic Association (ADA) is the country's largest group representing registered nutrition professionals. It awards the Registered Dietician (R.D.) credential to those who pass an exam after completing academic coursework and a supervised internship. You can consult the ADA's website at *www.eatright.org* for a list of nutritionists near you.

> *I had two quite different experiences with hospital nutritionists. At the children's hospital, I couldn't get the doctors concerned about my daughter's dramatic weight loss. She was so weak she couldn't stand, and her muscles seemed to be wasting away. I finally asked them to please send in a nutritionist. A very young woman came in and talked to me about the major food groups. I felt my cheeks begin to flush, and my eyes glistened as I said, "I know what she is supposed to eat; I need to know how I can make her want to eat." I must have sounded a bit crazy, because she just handed me a booklet and backed out the door.*

> *The next week when my daughter began her radiation, the radiation nurse took one look at her and called the nutritionist right down. This nutritionist was very warm and caring. She helped me understand that I needed to think fat, protein, and calories, and she gave me lots of practical suggestions on how to boost calories. I think that she probably saved my daughter from tube feedings.*

Advice from parents

Several parents whose children have completed therapy offer the following suggestions about how to handle the inevitable eating problems of children on therapy.

> *Doctors sometimes reassure parents by saying, "His appetite will return to normal." Don't be surprised if this does not happen until long after the most intensive parts of treatment are completed.*

· · · · ·

> *Let the child control what type of food and how much he wants. In the beginning, any food is good food.*

· · · · ·

> *Buy a juicer and use it every day. This was the only way we got any fruits or vegetables into our daughter. Make apple juice and sneak in a carrot. Sometimes we would make the juice, then blend it in the blender with ice cubes to make an iced drink, which we would serve with a straw.*

I solved my daughter's salt cravings by buying sea salt and letting her dip french fries in it once a week. For some reason, that satisfied her and stopped her from begging for regular table salt at every meal.

One magic word: butter, butter, butter. We would make Maddie peanut butter and jelly sandwiches with a layer of butter on each side of the bread first. Milkshakes are great and Häagen Dazs® ice cream has the highest fat content. We also went to an "eat when she's hungry" mode. It was definitely more relaxing.

When your child is on prednisone, don't try to restrict his food intake. It can be hard to watch these rotund little ones just shovel the food in, but once they get off the prednisone, they stop eating and quickly lose the weight. Then you have the opposite problem: how to get them to eat anything!

If you only keep good food in the house, and don't buy junk food, your child will eat more nutritious food.

Take good care of yourself by eating well. We are all under tremendous stress and need good nutrition. I gave my daughter healthy foods and glasses of juiced fresh fruits and vegetables while I was living on lattés (a coffee drink). I now have breast cancer and wish that I had eaten well during my daughter's treatment.

There is reason for hope. My daughter ate almost nothing while on treatment. After treatment ended, she ate more food, but still no variety. She didn't turn the corner until a year off treatment, but now she is gradually trying new foods, including fruits and vegetables again. I'm glad I never made an issue of it.

Commercial nutritional supplements

Many children cannot tolerate solid food or can only eat small amounts each day. Liquid supplements can help provide the necessary calories. The following is a sampling of the variety of supplements that can be purchased at pharmacies or grocery stores. If you are unable to locate a particular brand, your pharmacist may be able to order it for you.

- **Sustacal®.** Lactose-free liquid. Flavors are chocolate, vanilla, eggnog, and strawberry. It also comes in a high-protein or extra-fiber formula. (Mead Johnson)

- **Sustacal Pudding®**. Sustacal in pudding form. Flavors are chocolate, vanilla, and butterscotch. (Mead Johnson)

- **Sustacal HC®**. Concentrated liquid. Flavors are vanilla, chocolate, strawberry, and eggnog. (Mead Johnson)

- **Ensure®**. Lactose-free liquid. Flavors are chocolate, vanilla, black walnut, coffee, butter pecan, banana, and strawberry. Other formulas have high protein or extra fiber. (Ross Laboratories)

- **Ensure Plus®**. Concentrated liquid. (Ross Laboratories)

- **Isocal®**. Lactose-free, vanilla-flavored liquid. (Mead Johnson)

- **Enrich®**. Lactose-free liquid with fiber. (Ross Laboratories)

- **Instant Breakfast®**. Powder that is added to milk. Variety of flavors. (Carnation)

- **Citrotein®**. Orange-flavored powder that is added to water or juice. (Doyle Pharmaceutical)

- **Polycose®**. Liquid or powder. Powder is added to milk, juice, gravy, or soups. Adds carbohydrates for extra calories. One tablespoon adds 30 calories. (Ross Laboratories)

- **Myoplex® Nutrition Shake.** A liquid that is added to water and a little ice and mixed in a blender. Flavors include orange, piña colada, banana cream pie, chocolate, strawberry, and vanilla. (EAS, Inc.)

- **Boost Kids Essential®**. High in calcium and formulated for kids aged 1 to 10. Flavors are chocolate, strawberry, and vanilla. (Nestle)

- **Nutren Junior®**. Vanilla-flavored liquid formulated for children aged 1 to 10 who need nutritional support. It comes with or without added fiber. It is 50 percent whey and 50 percent casein. (Nestle)

- **Kindercal®**. Lactose-free liquid in vanilla and chocolate flavors. Formulated for children. (Mead Johnson)

> We tried all the high-calorie drinks: Pediasure® in three flavors, Boost®, and Scandishake®. The one that Emily would drink is called Nutrashake® (tastes like melted ice cream and can also be eaten frozen). Of course Pediasure® and Boost® are available over the counter. We had to get Scandi-shake® (a powder that you mix with milk) at the hospital. I had to do some research to obtain the Nutrashake®. It comes frozen, and Kroger® grocery stores carry it. Since there were no Kroger® stores near us, I finally found an outfit called American Medical Supply that would ship it.

> • • • • •

> The home health agency I worked for did a study on the nutritional content of Ensure®, Sustacal®, and Carnation® Instant Breakfast. All were basically the same, with Carnation® being much more palatable. The other two have a bit of a medicinal smell and taste to them. You can add calories by throwing it in a blender with

ice cream, bananas, or strawberries. My other two non-cancer kids loved this stuff. Mandy would "sip" a tiny bit but would rather eat the spicy food: bologna, Polish sausage, or tomatoes drowning in Catalina dressing. Reese's® peanut butter cups were breakfast for a long time (7 grams of protein!).

Feeding by tube and IV

Sometimes, it becomes necessary to feed children intravenously or through a gastric or nasogastric tube. Although feeding by tube and IV may require additional hospitalization, it helps if parents understand the benefits clearly. If a child with cancer becomes malnourished, events are set in motion that can have grim consequences. As appetite and weight decrease, the child's ability to tolerate and recover from chemotherapy diminishes. The child becomes progressively weaker and his resistance to infection decreases. Infections and weakness may require interruptions in treatment. To prevent this scenario, most protocols require tube or IV feeding after 10 percent of body weight is lost. The two types of supplemental feeding are described below.

Total parenteral nutrition (TPN)

TPN, also known as hyperalimentation, is a form of intravenous feeding used to prevent or treat malnutrition in children who cannot eat enough to meet basic nutritional needs. Below are some of the many reasons why your child may require TPN:

- Severe mouth and throat sores that prevent swallowing

- Severe nausea and vomiting

- Severe diarrhea

- Inability to chew or swallow normally

- Loss of more than 10 percent of body weight.

TPN ensures that the child receives all the protein, carbohydrates, fats, vitamins, and minerals she needs. The TPN is administered through the central venous catheter, but children receiving TPN can also eat solids and drink fluids.

My daughter needed TPN for 2 weeks after her stem cell transplant. They told us ahead of time that it would be necessary, and they were right. She got terrible sores throughout her GI tract and couldn't drink or eat. They just hooked the bag up to her Broviac®. After a couple of weeks, she started gingerly sipping small amounts of water and apple juice. For some reason, I just didn't worry about her eating. I assumed that when she could eat, she would. She was a robust eater before her illness, so I thought that would help. Before we left for home, she asked for a hospital pizza (yuck!) and ate a few bites. Her eating at home quickly went back to normal, although it took some time to regain the weight she lost.

In most cases, TPN is started in the hospital. Each day the concentrations of glucose, protein, and fat will be increased in a step-wise fashion, and doctors will assess your child's tolerance for the mixture. Generally, TPN is given 8 to 12 hours per day, depending on your child's unique situation. The infusion may be delivered over the hours that work best for your family. If your child attends school, overnight infusions will probably work best. If your child is at home during the day, infusions during these hours will give the entire family a better night's sleep.

Be sure to request a small portable infusion pump and backpack from your home care company so your child can go about his daily activities as usual. Your child's oncologist may need to write a letter to your insurance company to verify your child's malnutrition so he can receive coverage for this therapy.

Enteral nutrition

The doctor may recommend enteral feeding if your child requires supplemental nutrition and her bowel and intestines are still functioning well. Enteral feedings are preferred over IV when possible. Enteral nutrition is feeding via a tube placed through the nose and into the stomach or small intestine (NG tube) or via a tube surgically placed directly into the stomach through the abdominal wall (G-tube). Nutritionally complete liquid formulas are fed through the tube. Your child's oncologist and nutritionist will determine the appropriate formula for your child. Infrequent side effects of enteral nutrition are irritated throat, nausea, diarrhea, or constipation.

> Rachel (age 14) was diagnosed in 1997. She used a backpack to carry a G-tube pump and her bag of Ensure® with her when she went out. When chemo was over, she worked for about a month with a psychiatrist who used hypnotherapy to get her to start eating normally again. After about 3 months, she was eating everything she used to. The tube was removed, and the hole closed on its own.

Enteral feedings are usually started in the hospital. If your child's malnutrition is profound, she may initially require continuous feeding at a slow rate. These feedings will be increased as tolerated, with the eventual goal being four to six feedings per day. Blood tests can help the oncologist determine whether your child is malnourished in spite of the obvious weight gain that results from steroid therapy.

> Nikhi found it almost impossible to eat. She said that apart from her stomach feeling sick, everything tasted bad, and she didn't want to put that food in her mouth because the taste made her feel worse. As an adult you can say to yourself, this is for my own good, and force yourself to eat, but not kids.

> When Nikhi had to get an NG tube after she'd lost a third of her body weight, I felt nearly as bad as when she was first diagnosed. I believed that because she wasn't eating she had given up the will to live. I was a mess! The ward social worker gently

pointed out to me that it was not Nikhi's choice about whether to eat or not—it was entirely the fault of the chemo. When she got the nasogastric tube, it was wonderful! She was able to get nutrition without forcing herself to eat when she really couldn't. And sure enough, once we got over the hurdle of that part of the treatment, she slowly regained her appetite again and we were able to wean her off the NG feeds. Four years later, she is still a very fussy eater—but I can live with that!

I feel good nutrition is very important to good health, but the reality of the situation with our child was that he hated anything nutritious when he was on chemotherapy. I could doctor it up, add the best toppings, make it look terrific, season it just right, and it would still be rejected. So I decided that since my son wasn't allowed to make any decisions in regard to the pills, treatments, tests, or hospital stays, he wouldn't be forced to eat everything nutritious if he didn't want to. Whether this was a right or wrong decision, I don't know. I just know that I served him a lot of processed foods during those years, and he's a healthy and happy boy 10 years later. After he was finished with chemotherapy, however, we did require that he eat healthier foods.

Chapter 18

Medical and Financial Record-keeping

Prosperity is not without many fears and distastes; and adversity is not without comfort and hopes.

— Francis Bacon

KEEPING TRACK OF voluminous paper work—both medical and financial—is a trial for every parent of a child with leukemia; but keeping accurate records prevents medical errors and reduces insurance over-billings. Checking results of tests allows parents to identify changes in lab reports that might otherwise go unnoticed and untreated. Having easy access to medical reports and proper organization of bills can also mean less time spent in conflicts with insurance companies and collection agencies. This chapter suggests a few basic systems for keeping both medical and financial records.

Keeping medical records

Think of yourself as someone with two sets of books, the hospital's and yours. If the hospital loses your child's chart or misplaces lab results, you will still have a copy. If your child's chart becomes a foot thick, you will still have your simple system that makes it easy to spot trends and retrieve dosage information. The following are suggested items that you should record:

- Dates and results of all lab work

- Dates of chemotherapy, drugs given, and doses

- All changes in dosages of medicine

- Any side effects from drugs

- Any fevers or illnesses

- Dates of all scheduled and unscheduled hospitalizations

- Dates of all medical appointments and name(s) of the doctor(s) seen

- Dates for any procedures performed (both surgical and non-surgical)
- Dates of radiation therapy, including total dose delivered and areas treated
- Dates of diagnosis, completion of therapy, and recurrences (if any)
- Child's sleeping patterns, appetite, and emotions.

Keeping daily records of your child's health for 2 or 3 years is hard work. But remember that your child will be seen by pediatricians, oncologists, residents, radiation therapists, lab technicians, nutritionists, psychologists, and social workers. Your records will help keep it all straight and help pull all the information together. Your records will help you remember questions to ask, prevent mistakes, and notice trends. In short, your records will help the entire team provide your child with the best possible care.

The following sections describe several record-keeping methods parents have used successfully.

Journal

Keeping a notebook works extremely well for people who like to write. Parents make entries every day about all pertinent medical information and often include personal information such as their own feelings or memorable things their child said or did. Journals are easy to carry back and forth to the clinic, and journal entries can be written while waiting for appointments. Journals have the advantage of unlimited space; but one disadvantage is that they can be misplaced.

> Stephan's oncologist is kind of hard to communicate with. I learned early on to keep a journal of Stephan's appointments, drugs given, side effects, and blood counts. That way if I ever had to call the doctor I would have it right in front of me. I also recorded Stephan's temperature when his counts were low to keep track of infections.

In *You Don't Have To Die*, Geralyn Gaes writes of the value of keeping a journal:

> Some days my entries consisted of only a few words: "Good day. No problems." Other times I had so many notes and questions to jot down that my handwriting spilled over into the next day's space. I must confess that I probably went overboard, documenting every minute detail of Jason's life down to what he ate for each meal. If he gets over this disease, I thought, maybe this information will be useful for cancer research.

> I'm not so sure I was wrong. Jason went two years without a blood transfusion, unusual for a child receiving such aggressive chemotherapy. Studying my journal, one of his physicians remarked, "This kid eats more oatmeal than anybody I've ever seen." Which was true. Jason wolfed it down for breakfast, after school, and before bedtime. The doctor speculated, "Maybe that's why Jason's blood is so rich in iron and builds back up so fast."

Many institutions give families a notebook that contains information about their child's cancer and treatment plan. Often, these notebooks have blank pages for recording blood counts.

Record-keeping—very important! My father came to the hospital soon after diagnosis and brought a three-ring binder and a three-hole punch. I would punch lab reports, protocols, consent forms, drug information sheets, etc., and keep them in my binder. A mother at the clinic showed me her weekly calendar book, and I adopted her idea for recording blood counts and medications. Frequently the clinic's records disagreed with mine as to medications and where we were on the protocol. I was very glad that I kept good records.

Calendar

Many parents report great success with the calendar system. They buy a new calendar each year and hang it in a convenient place, such as next to the telephone. You can record counts on the calendar while talking on the phone to the nurse or lab technician and take the calendar with you to all appointments.

Each year I purchase a new calendar with large spaces on it. I write all lab results, any symptoms or side effects, colds, fevers, and anything else that happens. I bring it with me to the clinic each visit, as it helps immensely when trying to relate some events or watch trends. I also use it like a mini-journal, recording our activities and quotes from Meagan. Now that she's off treatment, I'm superstitious enough to still bring it to our monthly checkups.

• • • • •

I wrote the counts on a calendar or on little pieces of paper that got lost. But, to be honest, I didn't keep the medical records very well. I'm upset with myself when I think of it now.

• • • • •

For a long time I was unorganized, which is very unlike the way I usually am. I found that my usual excellent memory just wasn't working well. It all seemed to run together, and I began to forget if I had given her all of her pills. Then I began using a calendar for both counts and medications. I wrote every med on the correct days, then checked them off as I gave them.

Blood count charts

Many hospitals supply folders containing photocopied sheets for record-keeping. Typically, they have spaces for the date, white blood cell count, absolute neutrophil count, hematocrit, platelet level, chemotherapy given, and side effects.

My record-keeping system was given to me by the hospital on the first day. We were given a notebook with information about the illness and treatment. Also included were charts that we could use to keep all the information about my child's blood work, progress, reactions to drugs, etc. While we were at the hospital we were able to get the information off one of the computers on our floor each afternoon. My notebook holds records and notes for 3 years. Perhaps I was being compulsive with my record-keeping, but it made me feel that I was part of the team working on bringing my boy back to health.

Tape or digital recorder

For parents who keep track of more information than a calendar can hold, and who find writing in a journal too time consuming, using a voice recording device works well. Small machines are very inexpensive and can be carried in a pocket or purse. Digital devices can be downloaded to a flash drive or computer for storage.

I started keeping a journal in the hospital, but I was just too upset and exhausted to write in it faithfully. A good friend who was a writer by profession told me to use a tape recorder. It was a great idea and saved a lot of time. I could say everything that had happened in just a few minutes every day. I kept a separate notebook just for blood counts so I could check them at a glance.

Computer

For the computer literate, keeping all medical records on the computer is a good option. Parents can print out bar graphs of the blood counts in relation to chemotherapy and quickly spot trends. You can also keep a running narrative of your thoughts, feelings, and concerns during your child's treatment. As with all other computer records, keep a backup copy on a flash drive or external hard drive.

At our hospital, the summary of counts for a given child can be formatted to print out as a "trend review," with each date printed out on the left side of the page and the various lab values in columns down the page. The system permits printouts from the very first blood draw if that is desired. Periodically, on slow days, I'll ask if I can have a trend review. Then I can discard the associated single printouts (much less paper that way).

Keeping financial records

You will not need a calendar or journal for financial records, just a big, well- organized file cabinet. It is essential to keep track of bills and payments. Dealing with financial records is a major headache for many parents, but keeping good records can prevent financial catastrophe. Financial record-keeping is most important in countries such as the United States, where most individuals must purchase private medical insurance. In countries with standardized healthcare, such as Canada, parents never receive a bill for their child's cancer treatment. The following are ideas about how to organize financial records:

- Set up a file cabinet just for medical records.

- Have hanging files for hospital bills, doctor bills, all other medical bills, insurance explanation of benefits (EOB), prescription receipts, tax-deductible receipts (e.g., tolls, parking, motels, meals), and correspondence.

- Whenever you open an envelope related to your child's medical care, file the contents immediately. Don't leave it on the desk or throw it in a drawer.

- Keep a notebook with a running log of all tax-deductible medical expenses, including the service, charge, bill paid, date paid, and check number.

- Don't pay a bill unless you have checked over each item listed to make sure the charge is correct.

- Start new files every year.

> I bought an accordion-style file folder each year to hold everything to do with Stephan. It had a slot each for hospital bill printouts, insurance explanation of benefits, receipts for all prescriptions, all Candlelighters' newsletters, pediatrician bills, laboratory bills, and Leukemia Society information.

· · · · ·

> To be honest, the paper trail really gets me down. I can only deal with the stacks every few months. I open things and make sure the insurance company is doing its part, and then I try to sort through and pay our part.

· · · · ·

> I started out organized, and I'm glad I did because the hospital billing was confusing and full of errors. I cleared out a file cabinet and put in folders for each type of bill and insurance papers. I filed each bill chronologically so I could always find the one I needed. I made copies of all letters sent to the insurance company and hospital billing department. I wrote on the back of each EOB any phone calls I had to make about that bill. I wrote down the date of the call, the person's name who I spoke to, and what she said. It saved me a lot of grief.

Deductible medical expenses

It is estimated that families of children with cancer spend 25 percent or more of their income on items not covered by insurance. Examples of these expenses are gas, car repairs, motels, food away from home, health insurance deductibles, prescriptions, and dental work. Many of these items can be deducted from federal income tax. Often parents are too fatigued to go through stacks of bills at the end of the year to calculate their deductions. If a monthly total is kept in a notebook, then all that needs to be done at tax time is to add up the monthly totals.

The Internal Revenue Service (IRS) generally allows you to deduct any reasonable cost for procedures or expenses that are deemed by a doctor to be medically necessary. You may also deduct certain ancillary expenses with proper documentation. Some costs that are currently deductible include wheelchairs, wigs, acupuncture, psychotherapy and counseling, insurance premiums and HMO fees, special education or tutoring costs for sick children, meals at the hospital, parking at the hospital, and transportation and lodging costs while the child is in the hospital.

To find out what can be deducted legally for the years your child is undergoing treatment, get IRS Publication 502 for the relevant tax year. You can download this publication from the IRS website at *www.irs.gov* or make a copy from a master at your local library. The IRS discourages telephone calls, but if necessary you can contact an IRS representative at (800) 829-1040, Monday through Friday from 7 a.m. to 10 p.m. in your local time zone.

Canadian families are able to deduct many of the same medical expenses as U.S. families. To find out what can be legally deducted in Canada, you can visit the Revenue Canada website at *www.cra-arc.gc.ca* and type in the search term "deductible medical expenses," or call them at (800) 959-8281.

If you keep a calendar, an easy way to keep track of tax-deductible items is to glue an envelope to the inside cover. Whenever you incur an expense that may be tax deductible, put the receipt in the envelope and file it when you get home.

Dealing with hospital billing

Unfortunately, problems with billing are common for parents of children with leukemia. Here are two typical experiences:

> *Insurance was an absolute nightmare. It almost gave me a nervous breakdown. After all we go through with our children, to have to deal with the messed-up hospital billing was just too much—it was the worst part of the whole experience.*

> *We would stack the bills up and try to go through them every 2 or 3 months. Our insurance was supposed to pay 100 percent, but the billing was so confusing that they refused to cover some things because it wasn't clear what they were being billed for. The hospital frequently double billed, especially for prescriptions. We just stopped getting our prescriptions there.*

We would call them to try to get the mess straightened out, but the billing department was just as confused as we were. They kept sending our account to collections. We did everything in our power to get it straight, but we never did.

• • • • •

We had two distinctly different experiences at the two institutions we dealt with. The university hospital where my daughter received her radiation gave me a folder the first day. It included, among other things, a sheet from a financial counselor giving all the information needed for preventing and solving billing problems. I never needed to call her because the hospital billing was clear, prompt, and organized.

The children's hospital where my daughter was a frequent inpatient and clinic patient was another story altogether. They billed from three different departments, put charges from the same visit on different bills, frequently over-billed, continuously made errors, and constantly threatened to send the account to collections. I never spoke to the same billing clerk twice. It was a never-ending grind and a constant frustration.

It is impossible to prevent billing errors, but it is necessary to deal with them. Here are step-by-step suggestions for solving billing problems:

• Keep all records filed in an organized fashion.

• Check every bill from the hospital to make sure there are no charges for treatments not given or errors such as double billing.

> *During maintenance, my daughter went to the clinic every 3 months. She had identical treatments every visit—port accessed, vincristine given, physical exam, and intrathecal methotrexate given via spinal tap. Each bill was different, differing by hundreds of dollars, for identical visits! There were errors on each bill, including numerous charges for IV Benedryl® that she never received. I would get the errors removed, then they would reappear on the next bill.*

• Check to see if the hospital has financial counselors. If so, make contact early in your child's hospitalization. Counselors provide services in many areas, including help with understanding the hospital's billing system, billing insurance carriers, understanding explanations of benefits, managing hospital/insurance correspondence, dealing with Medicaid, working out a payment plan, designing a ledger system for tracking insurance claims, and resolving disputes.

• If you find a billing error, call the hospital immediately. Write down the date, the name of the person you talk to, and the plan of action.

> *I often couldn't even get through to the billing representative; I was just put on hold forever. Then I tried to discuss the problems with the director of billing, but she was never in. After about 20 phone calls, I finally said to her secretary, "You know, I have*

a desperately sick child here, and I have more important things to do than call your boss every day. I've been as patient and polite as I can. What else can I do?" She said, "Honey, get irate. It works every time." I told her to put me through to somebody, anybody, and I would. She connected me to the person who mediates disputes, I got irate, and we went through all the bills line by line.

- If the error is not corrected on your next bill, call and talk to the billing supervisor. Explain the steps you have already taken and how you would like the problem fixed.

    The hospital billing was so bad, and I had to call so often, that I developed a telephone relationship with the supervisor. I always tried to be upbeat, we laughed a lot, and it worked out. She stopped investigating every problem and would just delete the erroneous charge from the computer.

- If the problem is still not corrected, write a brief letter to the billing supervisor explaining the steps you have taken and requesting immediate action. Keep a copy of each letter that you write and all written responses.

- Every time you receive an EOB from your insurance company, compare it to the hospital bill. Track down discrepancies.

- If you are inundated with a constant stream of bills and there are major discrepancies between the hospital charges and what is being paid for by your insurance, ask both the hospital billing department and your insurance company, in writing, to audit the account. Insist on a line-by-line explanation for each charge.

    Within 5 months of my daughter's diagnosis, the billing was so messed up that I despaired of ever getting it straight. When the hospital threatened to send the account to a collection agency, I took action. I wrote letters to the hospital and the insurance company demanding an audit. When both audits arrived, they were $9,000 apart. I met with our insurance representative, and she called the hospital, and we had a three-way showdown. We straightened it out that time, but every bill that I received for the duration of treatment had one or more errors, always in the hospital's favor.

- If you are too tired or overwhelmed to deal with the bills, ask a family member or friend to help. He could come every other week, open and file all bills and insurance papers, make phone calls, and write all necessary letters. Your friends could even scan your records into your computer for storage.

- Don't let billing problems accumulate. Your account may end up at a collection agency, which can quickly become a nightmare.

    Our insurance was constantly months behind in paying our bills to the Children's Hospital. The hospital sent our account to collections, despite my assurances that I was doing everything I could to get the insurance to pay. We were hounded on the phone constantly by the collection people, often until we were in tears. We finally just took out a second mortgage and paid off the hospital, but now I don't know if we will be reimbursed by insurance.

• • • • •

I had a horrible run-in with the collection agency that works for the Children's Hospital. All of our bills are current, except one. Yesterday, a woman called me saying she is filing a subpoena against me and is having me arrested. She threatened to take away our house if that is what it takes to get this bill ($614) paid. She even tried to call my husband at work yesterday. Luckily, my brother-in-law called the company lawyer and was told that what she did was illegal. He said collection agencies have strict rules and this woman broke them all. They are not allowed to bother you at work. They can never threaten legal action. He said that medical bills cannot even go on your credit report. The attorney called the collection agency and he assured me they would never call again. He also gave me a name at the Consumer Protection Agency, and if she calls here again, I am to call them. (They already have the complaint on file and will take additional action if she calls again.) I also filed a written complaint with the hospital. I want them to know the people they have hired are harassing their patients. I was in tears.

Not all stories are so grim. People who are in a socialized healthcare system, some managed care systems, or on public assistance never even see bills. Many people with insurance encounter no problems throughout their child's treatment.

Our insurance paid 80 percent of everything, no questions asked, and always paid us within a month. People shouldn't have to worry about finances or their insurance program at a difficult time like this.

• • • • •

We have a low income, so we are on the state plan. They give us coupons for each child, and we just hand over a coupon at each visit. I have never seen a bill.

Coping with insurance

Finding one's way through the insurance maze can be a difficult task. However, understanding the benefits and claims procedures can help you get the bills paid without undue stress. The following sections outline some steps to help prevent problems with insurance.

Understand your policy

As soon as possible after diagnosis, read your entire insurance manual. Make a list of any questions you have about terms or benefits.

- Learn who the "participating providers" are under the plan and what happens if you see a non-participating provider. It is possible you will be penalized financially or your claims may be denied if you go outside the network.

- Determine if your physician needs to document specific requirements to obtain coverage for expensive or extended services.

    With our insurance, neuropsychological tests, outpatient occupational therapy, speech therapy, and physical therapy are covered, but the phrasing must be that it is a "medical necessity" due to diagnosis and treatments.

- Find out what your insurance co-pays are for different levels of service (e.g., office visit, outpatient surgery, outpatient testing).

- Find out what your outpatient prescription drug benefits are for generic and non-generic drugs.

- Find out what your deductible is.

- Find out if there is a point at which coverage increases to 100 percent.

- Determine if there is a lifetime limit on benefits.

- Find out when a second opinion is required.

- Learn when you have to pre-certify a hospitalization or specialty consultation. Many firms require pre-certification, even in emergencies.

    I realized that my daughter had been treated for over 4 months, and I had never called the insurance company. When I read the manual, I was horrified to find out that I had not pre-notified them about three scheduled hospitalizations. There was a $200 penalty for each lapse. I called in tears, and they only charged me for one mistake, not all three.

- Get a copy of every form you may need to submit—claim forms for inpatient care, outpatient care, or prescriptions. If your provider allows it, you can cut down on paperwork by filling in all the subscriber information on one of each type of form (except date and signature) and making many copies. Then you will have a form ready to send in with each bill.

- Determine whether your policy has benefits for counseling. If so, find out how many visits are covered, the payment structure, and the level of training required. Most health insurance policies offer very limited coverage for mental health services. For example, you may not be allowed to see certain kinds of providers or you may be limited to a certain number of visits per year.

- Find out the names of approved providers for home infusion supplies (e.g., IV medications, central venous catheter supplies, and home nutrition) and home nursing care. These are often separate companies. Determine policy coverage for these services.

We changed to a new pediatrician, and he asked me if I thought it would be easier on my son to have visiting nurses come to our home to do the chemotherapy injections and some blood work. Since he had very low counts, it made a lot of sense not to have to go out. It also lessened his fears to be able to stay at home and have the same nurse come to do the procedures. It was a pleasant surprise to find these services covered by our insurance.

Find a contact person

As soon as possible after diagnosis, call your insurance company and ask who will be handling your claims. Explain that there will be years of bills with frequent hospitalizations, and it would be helpful to deal with the same person each time. Insurers may be able to provide a contact person for claim review or special needs. Ask the contact person to answer any questions you have about benefits. Try to develop a cooperative relationship with your contact person, because she can really make your life easier. Some insurance companies may assign your child's account to a case manager, who will review your child's plan of care in detail and make suggestions designed to make proper use of your policy benefits. Also, your employer may have a benefits person who can operate as a liaison with the insurer.

My employee benefits representative was Bobbi. She was just wonderful. The hospital would send her copies of the bills at the same time they sent mine. Since I found so many errors, she would hold the bills a week until I called to tell her that they were correct before she paid them. She was very pleasant to deal with.

Negotiate

Don't be afraid to negotiate with the insurance company over benefits. Often, your contact person may be able to redefine a service your child needs to allow it to be covered.

Our insurance company covered 100 percent of maintenance drugs only if the patients needed them for the rest of their lives. Christine's drugs were only needed for 2 years but were extremely expensive. I asked my contact person for help, and she petitioned the decision-making board. They granted us an exemption and covered the entire cost of all her maintenance drugs.

• • • • •

My husband works for a small city that contracts out health insurance. A year into our child's treatment, the contract was being renegotiated. He brought home a copy of the proposed contract, and I was horrified to see that they had halved the benefit for transplants, from $200,000 to $100,000. I called the members of the committee negotiating the contract, the union representative, the city insurance liaison, and the city attorney. I was very polite, but I told them that if my child needed a bone marrow transplant, the new contract would bankrupt us. We would lose our home *and have to sell all of our belongings to pay our part of the procedure. Then I called two transplant centers, and had them fax me the estimated cost of a routine bone marrow transplant (about $220,000). I sent copies of the fax to everyone that I could think of, and followed it up with phone calls. They changed the new contract back to $200,000. One person can make a big difference.*

• • • • •

Some of us have employer-paid health insurance benefits. If we are not comfortable with the level of service that the insurance contractor is providing (particularly when it comes to not resolving a bill for months or even years), that's an employee satisfaction and compensation issue. Remember, those of us with employer-paid health insurance get this instead of additional cash. Non-cash compensation has significant advantages for the employer. Sometimes, with a little luck, the right presentation, and the facts, we can persuade our employer to help resolve the issue that is causing all the grief.

Challenging a claim

The key to obtaining the maximum benefit from your insurance policy is to keep accurate records and to challenge any denied claims, sometimes more than once. Some tips on good record-keeping follow:

- Make photocopies of everything you send to your insurance company, including claims, letters, and bills.

- Pay bills by check or credit card, and keep all your canceled checks and/or credit card monthly summaries of charges.

- Keep all correspondence you receive from billing companies and insurance.

- Write down the date, name of person contacted, and content of all phone calls concerning insurance.

- Keep accurate records of all medical expenses and claims submitted.

Policy holders have the right to appeal a claim denied by their insurance company. The following are suggested steps to contest a claim:

- Keep original documents in your files and send photocopies to the insurance company with a letter outlining why the claim should be covered. Make sure to request the reply in writing and keep a copy of the letter for your records.

  We were making inquiries into hospice care, feeling it was time to explore that option. I found out that the only pediatric hospice provider in the state of Georgia was not on the preferred provider list. Our insurance company would pay for benefits, but at a reduced rate; not a good thing since the lifetime maximum for hospice care was $7,500. With these benefits, we would get 78 days of hospice care. I felt like my only options were reduced pediatric care or full benefits using adult services.

I wrote a letter of appeal stating that medically and ethically, neither of these were good choices. Well, we got a better outcome than I asked for. Not only will they cover the pediatric provider, but they have waived the lifetime maximum!

- Contact your elected representative to the U.S. Congress. All Senators and members of the House of Representatives have staff that help constituents with problems. You may also contact your state insurance board with concerns and complaints.

When I ran into insurance company problems, I wrote a letter to the insurance company detailing the facts, the decisions the insurance company made, and a logical explanation about why the procedure needed to happen. I also noted on the letter that a copy was going to our state insurance commissioner, and sent both letters by certified mail. Within 2 days, the insurance company all of a sudden decided to cover the procedure. I later found out that the insurance commissioner's office started an investigation against them. Letters help, especially when sent by certified mail.

- If none of the above steps resolves the dispute, take your claim to small claims court (does not require you to hire an attorney), find an attorney who will represent you for free (called pro bono) or hire an attorney skilled in insurance matters to sue the insurance company.

It may not feel comfortable being so persistent, but sometimes it is necessary to ensure you get the support you and your child are entitled to.

When I finally got an advocate assigned for my child within our insurance company, I fretted to her one day that every single claim was initially rejected. She replied that the agents were trained to reject all claims the first two times they were submitted as a cost-saving strategy. She said, "Very few subscribers are tenacious enough to come back three times, so we save millions of dollars each year just because they give up."

Sources of financial assistance

Sources of financial assistance vary from state to state and town to town. To begin tracking down possible sources, ask the hospital social worker for assistance. In addition, some hospitals have community outreach nurses or case workers who may point out potential sources of assistance.

Hospital policy

If you are unable to pay your hospital bills, don't sell your house or let your account go to collections. Ask the social worker to set up an appointment for you with the appropriate person to discuss the hospital policy for financial assistance. Many hospitals write off a percentage of the cost of care if the patient is uninsured or underinsured. Be proactive and talk to the hospital about setting up a monthly payment plan.

Supplemental Security Income (SSI)

SSI is an entitlement program of the U.S. Government that is based on family income and administered by the Social Security Administration. Recipients must be blind or disabled and have a low family income and few assets. Children with cancer qualify as disabled for this program, making some of them eligible for monthly aid if the family income and assets are low enough. To find out if your child qualifies, contact your nearest field office to determine if your child is eligible for SSI.

Additionally, there is a professional organization of attorneys and paralegals called the National Organization for Social Security Claimants' Representatives (NOSSCR). NOSSCR can refer you to a member in your geographic location. You can contact NOSSCR by phone number at (800) 431-2804, or on the Internet at *www.NOSSCR.org*.

> *Our Katie was approved for SSI right away. It did take a large amount of preparation with the required paperwork. I researched, and when I found roadblocks, I asked the Social Security people what I needed to overcome these obstacles. In our case we had too much money in the bank, so we "spent down" by prepaying bills. I made sure I had all our birth certificates, that Katie's medical records were complete, etc. Since I found this so cumbersome, you can't imagine how happy I was when our income and Katie's health excluded us from SSI and we became self-sufficient again. That said, I sure was glad it was there when needed.*

Medicaid

Medicaid is administered by state governments in the United States, with the federal government providing a portion of the entitlement. Rules about eligibility vary, but families with private insurance sometimes are eligible if huge hospital bills are only partially covered. Call your local or county social service department to obtain the number for the Medicaid office in your area. If they tell you your child is ineligible, ask if the state has an "Aged, Blind, Disabled, Medically Needy" program.

Medicaid sometimes also pays transportation and prescription costs. Some states cover children under the age of 21 if they are hospitalized for more than 30 days, regardless of parental income. States are supposed to have Children's Medical Services programs to pay for medical treatment of physically disabled children: these programs allow a higher income level than Medicaid. Ask for a detailed list of benefits available in your state.

Free medicine programs

Many drug companies have programs to provide free medicines (including chemotherapy) to needy patients. Eligibility requirements vary, but most are available to those not covered by private or public insurance programs. To see if you are eligible for assistance, you can contact the Pharmaceutical Research and Manufacturers of America at *www.pparx.org* or by calling (888) 477-2669. Another website that lists different companies' assistance programs is *www.needymeds.com*. More information is available in the "Drug Reimbursement" section of Appendix B.

Although the cost of in-hospital treatment in Canada is covered by provincial governments, families have to pay for other medications at their own expense. For those without private insurance, this usually creates an extreme financial hardship. In many instances, the Department of Social Services can help pay for medications. The qualifications vary in each province and the decision is based on financial need. Canadian parents should contact their provincial Department of Social Services for further information.

State-sponsored supplemental insurance

Most states have supplemental insurance programs for families with children who are living with chronic conditions. These programs often help cover services, prescriptions, and co-payments that your primary insurance will not. You can get more information about the specific programs in your state from your medical team or hospital social worker, or by calling your state's department that regulates insurance (e.g., State Insurance Commission).

> *In Michigan, besides my husband's insurance, we also have what is called Children's Special Health Care Services (CSHCS). It is a secondary insurance that pays for what our primary insurance doesn't: Jake's co-pays and prescriptions, trips back and forth to the hospital, doctor appointment and prescription co-pays for my husband and me, our stay at the Ronald McDonald House. Any expenses related to treatment that our primary insurance won't cover, this will. The amount you pay for this coverage is based on family income. It has been a lifesaver for us.*

Service organizations

Numerous service organizations help families in need, providing aid such as transportation, wigs, special wheelchairs, and food. Often, all a family has to do is describe its plight, and good Samaritans appear. Some organizations that may exist in your community are: American Legion; Elks Club; fraternal organizations such as the Masons, Jaycees, Kiwanis Club, Knights of Columbus, Lions, and Rotary; United Way; Veterans of Foreign Wars; and churches of all denominations. In addition, local philanthropic organizations exist in many communities. To locate them, call your local health department, speak to a social worker, and ask for help.

Organized fund raising

Many communities rally around a child with cancer by organizing a fund. Help is given in various ways, ranging from donation jars in local stores to an organized drive using all the local media. There are many pitfalls to avoid in fund raising, and great care must be exercised to protect the sick child's privacy to the extent possible. Because there have been some unfortunate scams in which generous people were bilked out of contributions for sick children who did not exist, if you decide to try fundraising, it is best to obtain legal assistance and to establish a trust fund for the express purpose of paying the child's medical expenses.

If your child is on or seeking Social Security or Medicaid eligibility, funds must be held in a special needs trust and paid directly to providers. If the family receives the money, or the child's social security number is used to open the bank account, the child can lose funding from both Social Security and Medicaid.

Miscellaneous insurance issues

Loss of insurance coverage is every parent's worst nightmare. If you lose your job, change jobs, or move while your child is on treatment, speak to your employer's benefit manager promptly. It is advisable to continue your insurance coverage with your previous employer through the Consolidated Omnibus Budget Reconciliation Act (COBRA) plan until you are certain your new insurance coverage is in effect. Although this may impose some financial strain on your family for several months, it will ensure your child's coverage without interruption. Such expenditures are tax deductible.

Speak to your employer about whether participation in a Section 125 Plan is an option at your place of employment. These plans generally allow you to have your employer withhold pre-tax dollars from your pay for expenses such as childcare costs and non-reimbursed medical expenses. However, you will need to fill out reimbursement forms and submit them by year's end, or the money is lost. The amount you may withhold is determined by the size of the employee pool covered.

We had excellent insurance coverage, so we never experienced any major financial difficulties during my son's treatment. However, insurance company literature can be so complicated that I felt I almost needed an advanced degree in rocket science to decipher our coverage. Our hospital has a financial counselor available for families that need help. Given the enormous stress that parents are under, I think it's an invaluable service.

Chapter 19

End of Treatment
and Beyond

The best formula for longevity:
Have a chronic disease, and cure it.

— Oliver Wendell Holmes

THE LAST DAY OF TREATMENT is a time for both celebration and fear. Most families are thrilled that the days of pills and procedures have ended, but some fear a future without drugs to keep the disease away. Concerns about relapse are an almost universal parental response at the end of treatment; but for the majority of families, the months and years roll by without recurrence of leukemia. However, while many children and teens quickly return to excellent physical and mental health, others have lingering or permanent effects from the treatment. This chapter covers the emotional and physical aspects of ending treatment, the need for excellent medical follow-up, and employment and insurance issues.

Emotional issues

Many parents describe ending treatment as being almost as wrenching an experience as diagnosis. Families start experiencing the gamut of emotions—from elation to terror—months before the final day.

> *I had a lot of anticipatory worry—it started about 6 months before ending treatment. By the last day of treatment, I had been worrying for months, so it was just a relief to quit.*

• • • • •

> *I expected to feel a profound sense of relief when treatment ended. The 6 months prior to ending treatment I felt almost euphoric. But when she was finally finished, I began to be unexpectedly fearful. I just started to worry. I didn't really relax until she was a year off treatment. Now weeks go by without me thinking of relapse, although I still think of the years of leukemia treatment frequently.*

. . . . .

The last day was traumatic. It just wasn't a celebration because it felt exactly like every other day that we had to drive for hours, wait for hours, then have painful treatments. When it was over, he was just as physically exhausted and emotionally drained as on other clinic days. I just felt numb. But then, over time, there was a gradual awakening that it was really over.

. . . . .

We were thrilled when treatment ended. I knew many people who felt that celebrating would jinx them; they just didn't feel safe. Well, I felt that we had won a big battle—getting through treatment—and we were going to celebrate that. If, heaven forbid, in the future we had another battle to fight, we'd deal with it. But on the last day of treatment, we were delighted.

Parents should anticipate that after years spent watching their child go through the rigors of treatment, they will have lost the feeling of a "normal" life. They may experience relapse scares, and they may need to call the doctor to describe symptoms and be reassured everything is alright.

Several months after my son ended treatment, I was driving down the street, and I started to worry that he seemed excessively tired lately. I started to feel my throat constricting, and tears sprang to my eyes. I had to pull over because I literally couldn't breathe. I had to force myself to calm down, breathe slowly, and realize that I was just having a normal attack of being petrified that he would relapse.

. . . . .

We live in a cool climate, but went back east during a summer heat wave to visit relatives. My daughter was a year off treatment and doing extremely well. After a few days of 100-degree weather, she started waking up in bed soaked with sweat. I was terrified because she had done that at diagnosis. All of those horrible feelings washed over me, and I had to stand in the shower and sob. I called my doctor who was 3,000 miles away, and listed all the normal things: good appetite, good color, good energy level, no behavior problems, no bruising, but my voice shook when I described the sweats in an air-conditioned house. He reassured me that it was almost certainly the hot weather. He said if I was too worried to enjoy my visit, he would arrange for her to get a CBC (complete blood count), but otherwise, just to bring her by when we got back. I relaxed, didn't get the CBC, and the night sweats stopped when we got home.

With diagnosis came the awareness that life can be cruel and unpredictable. Many parents feel somewhat safe during treatment because they felt that therapy is keeping the cancer away. The end of treatment leaves some parents and children feeling exposed and vulnerable. When treatment ends, parents must find a way to live with uncertainty—to find a balance between hope and reasonable worry.

The first few weeks after Casey ended treatment, I was not worried at all. The sense of relief was so great! Finally our lives weren't controlled by the disease and fevers and meds. Only once a month are we bothered by doctor office visits. It is so nice.

I remember about 1 month after treatment ended, Casey ran a high fever. As I bathed him, I told him wasn't it nice we didn't have to rush off to the hospital; he could have a fever like a normal kid! We had decided to have his port taken out in August just for that simple reason—he can run a fever and we don't have to rule out infection in the port.

Now, as his counts start to rebound, my fear is growing. Up until now there was evidence that his body still retained the drugs—now he is on his own. I'm a nervous wreck. Every bruise stands out like a neon sign. I worry on his tired days. My paranoia is not healthy, and I'm working hard to reduce it. In the meantime, I've taken a step back, relying on the survival skills learned in the early days of treatment. Today he is well, and I have no control over tomorrow, so I try to relish the good health that he enjoys today. No energy I put into worrying will affect the outcome in the long run. So much easier said than done, isn't it?

Last day of treatment

Although individual cases vary, the last day of treatment for a child in remission from leukemia generally includes a diagnostic spinal tap, a bone marrow aspiration, a CBC and chemistry screen, a thorough physical exam, and a discussion with the oncologist. The oncologist should review the treatment, outline the schedule for future blood tests and exams, and sensitively discuss with the family the potential for long-term side effects. After the procedures, the family will usually wait to hear the preliminary report about the bone marrow aspiration, as true relief does not come until they know that no leukemic blasts are present.

One group of parents presented to physicians at a major children's hospital the following list of suggestions for the last day of treatment.

- Schedule enough time to have a conversation.
- Bring a sense of closure to the active phase of treatment.
- Express happiness that all has gone well.
- Be realistic but hopeful about the future.
- Praise the child for handling a very difficult time in her life with grace (or courage, or whatever word is appropriate).
- Praise the parents for all of their hard work.
- Allow time for the parents to give the physician feedback and thanks.

- Give a certificate of accomplishment to the child.

- Be aware that families are relieved but fearful of the future.

> *Our last day of treatment was horrible. The fellow was angry at me because I had arranged to have my daughter sedated. The fellow was signing the necessary forms muttering over and over, "This is ridiculous." When I asked her what was bothering her, she said that she was going on a business trip, which I was delaying, and her son had chicken pox and she was worried about it. She said another doctor was going to do the procedures because she was in a hurry. When I asked if I should wait for the results of the bone marrow, she said, "End-of-treatment bone marrows are at the bottom of the pathologist's priority list, emergencies come first, he'll get to it when he can, and the report won't be written for days." I thought that she was being heartless, but I didn't want to fight in front of my daughter. So I went across the hall and asked the director of the clinic if she would please call me that afternoon with the results of the bone marrow. She replied, "Absolutely." She called, told me it was clear, and we felt jubilant and relieved.*

• • • • •

> *The nurses at our clinic really made a big deal on the last day of treatment. They brought out a cake and balloons, and sang "Going off Chemo" to the tune of "Happy Birthday to You." They made Gina a banner and bought her a present. I sat in a corner and cried, because I was scared to death of the future. A nurse came over, hugged me, and said, "This must be so hard; we're taking away your security blanket." She was exactly right.*

Catheter removal

Children usually cannot wait for the catheter to be removed, as it symbolizes that treatment has truly ended. Physicians' opinions differ greatly about the best time to remove the catheter. Some doctors recommend removal when the child starts maintenance. Others suggest removing it when the child is sedated for the last bone marrow aspiration; and some doctors advise waiting several weeks or months after treatment ends. Ask the doctor for the reasons for her recommendation, and discuss it fully if you or your child have strong feelings about the timing.

Removal of an external catheter is usually an outpatient procedure. The child is given a mild sedative, then the oncologist gently pulls the catheter out of the child's body by hand.

> *Kristin's Broviac® removal wasn't too bad. They gave her fentanyl ahead of time, so she was fairly relaxed. I wish they had offered me a sedative as well! One of the nurses had her hand on Kristin's shoulder and quietly talked to her to try to keep her focused elsewhere. I held her legs, and my wife held her hand. The doctor put*

one hand on her chest, and pulled on the tubing with the other. It only took about 2 seconds to come out. There was little blood; they just put a Band-Aid on the site and sent us home.

Implanted catheters such as the PORT-A-CATH® are removed surgically in the operating room. Children are usually given general anesthesia, and the operation usually takes less than half an hour. Only one incision is made, generally just above the port at the same place as the scar from the implantation surgery. The sutures holding the port to the underlying muscle are cut, and the port with tubing is pulled out. The small incision is then stitched and bandaged. When the child begins to awaken, he is brought out to the parent(s). The family then waits until the surgeon approves their departure. Often, the wait is short, because as soon as the child is awake enough to take a small drink or eat a popsicle, he is released. However, if your child becomes nauseated from the anesthesia, the wait can be several hours; he won't be released until he is feeling better.

Brent had a very easy time with his port-removal surgery. We scheduled him to be the first patient early in the morning, so there was no delay getting in. Then the anesthesiologist asked him what flavor of gas he wanted, which he liked. They brought him out to us while he was still groggy, and he woke up feeling goofy and happy. We went home soon thereafter. It felt more like the ending than on the last day of treatment.

• • • • •

I remember when Andrew had his port out. As he was coming out of his anesthesia fog I leaned over to him and said rather tearfully, "Andrew, you did it; you're all done." He took his small hand and placed it at the site where that port sat for 2 years, felt its absence, and smiled. It was one of the best moments of my life.

Ceremonies

Some families enjoy having ceremonies to celebrate the end of cancer treatment. For younger children who have spent much of their lives taking pills and having procedures, ceremonies really help them grasp that treatment is truly over. Here are ideas from many families about how to commemorate this important occasion:

• Take "last day of treatment" pictures of the hospital and staff.

• Take a picture of your child taking his last pill.

• Give trophies to your child and siblings.

We had a big party during which my husband, Scott, stood up and called for everyone's attention. He gave a talk about how proud we were of Jeremy and handed him a big trophy. It had the victory angel on top and was engraved with "Jeremy, we are so proud of you and your victory. Love, Mom and Dad." We gave a plaque to his brother, Jason, for being the world's most supportive brother.

- Ask the clinic to present your child with a certificate.

- Throw a big party for friends and family.

  Erica ended treatment in December, and we threw a big party at the church. We called it a "Celebration of Life." We invited all of the families that we had become so close to through the support group. We especially wanted the families who had lost their children to cancer, and they all came. My normally even-tempered husband gave a talk about Club Goodtimes (the support group) and how it was a club that no one ever wanted to join. When he talked about the many wonderful people we met there, his voice shook with emotion. Then the preacher prayed for the children who weren't with us. We ate a huge cake, and the children were entertained by a clown. It was both moving and fun.

  · · · · ·

  We invited all of our friends and family to the park for "Tay's beating leukemia party." We had red and white balloons that we wrote on that said "Healthy red cells" and "Healthy white cells." We also had a round piñata that said "Leukemia" on it and one of the international symbols for "NO" drawn through it. The kids "beat" leukemia with a stick, and candy came pouring out. We all had a good time. We also had black balloons that were "bad cells" that the kids sat on and popped. It was a well-attended party. We grilled outside, drank sodas, ate watermelon, played a little volleyball, and just had a great time.

- Throw a big party at school.

  When Joseph finished treatment he was in kindergarten. The kids had gone through almost an entire year with him. They had known all about his treatments and frequent hospitalizations and had talked as a group about it when we made a presentation to the class, and at other times as well. It seemed appropriate to have an "all done with treatment" celebration. We even had his two best friends who go to different schools come over to join us; and his big brother, Nate, came down from his class to share in the fun.

  It was a very joyous occasion, and we made it as much like a birthday party as we could. I made cupcakes and juice and we played games. A friend who leads the story hour at our children's bookstore came and did some songs and stories with the kids; and I even sent each classmate home with a treat bag. At the end, right before time to go home, Joseph pulled out several cans of his favorite hospital discovery, and the kids took turns blasting a shower of Silly String® on everyone else! We all clapped and cheered, and Joseph's wonderful teacher and I had a chance to have a good celebratory cry while the kids put on their things to go home. Clean-up wasn't too darn bad, and it meant a lot to all of us.

There's still a tiny remnant of green Silly String® on one of the fluorescent light fixtures, and my big second-grader likes to go down and admire it when he visits his old kindergarten teacher.

- If your child has been seeing a counselor, schedule a visit to talk about the accomplishment.

- Have friends and family send congratulations cards.

- Ask the surgeon to give your child her port or external catheter line (if your child wants it).

    I know that this may sound odd, but my 6-year-old daughter hated her port and talked incessantly about getting it out. She even told me that she was going to slice it out herself with a knife. I told her it would be better to wait until the doctors put her to sleep; but I promised her she could have it after the operation to do with as she wished. That idea brought a smile to her face. She came out of the recovery room clutching a baggie with the port inside. Once we were home, she carried it around for weeks, jumped on it, hit it with a hammer, and finally cut it to pieces. That port really symbolized all of the painful things that had happened to her, and it made her feel better to hurt it back.

- If consistent with your beliefs, have a religious ceremony of thanksgiving.

    I preached the sermon at church after Kristin ended treatment. It was the first Sunday of Lent, and I related our experience to that. Other than that, we didn't celebrate, because it's still not over. We still have to go every month for blood work and need to be vigilant. Ending treatment was a big milestone, but it paled in comparison to having the line pulled. We all have so much more freedom: no more lines to flush, changing bandages, or wrapping up for baths and swimming.

- Go on a trip or vacation to celebrate.

    All of the parents of children with leukemia in our community have become very close. When 9-year-old Brent finished his treatment, I called to congratulate him. He was so excited telling me about it, but then his voice started to shake and he cried when he told me, "My two aunts gave me a card with money inside to go to a motel with a pool for the weekend. They gave it to me because I had leukemia. Can you believe that?"

Some parents do not feel comfortable celebrating the end of treatment. One mother described her feelings this way:

We did nothing, because we knew so many kids who relapsed. I didn't even throw away the pills for a year because I didn't trust that we were really done.

As you have read so often in this book, every child, brother, sister, parent, and relative reacts differently to treatment—and to the end of treatment. The differences do not matter. What is important is that you feel free to express your feelings, whatever they may be. You may feel joyful, relieved, fearful, or terrified, but end of treatment is emotionally charged for every member of the family.

What is normal?

After years of treatment, families grapple with the idea of returning to normal. Unfortunately, most parents don't really know what "normal" is any longer. Parents realize that returning to the carefree pre-cancer days is unrealistic, that life has changed. The constant interaction with medical personnel is ending, and a new phase is beginning in which routines do not revolve around caring for a sick child, giving medicines, and keeping clinic appointments. While it is true that the blissful ignorance of the days prior to cancer are gone forever, a different life—one often enriched by friends and experiences from the cancer years—begins.

> It just seems like I can't leave it behind. If he gets diarrhea, I worry that it's a tumor. He has a bad skin rash now, and I keep thinking it's cancer-related. My husband has terrible skin, so I know it's genetic, but there's a little part of my mind that keeps trying to connect it to leukemia. My son has been going to the playground; he's getting strong; he has rosy cheeks; he's just beautiful. When he has bruises on his legs, I automatically think his platelets are down. But when I look at the other kids, I realize that it's normal for active kids to have bruises on their knees. It's really hard to get used to. I still wake up at night, and the irrational side comes out. I'm just having a hard time letting go of it. I mean, I panicked when his feet were hurting, only to discover that his shoes were too small.

· · · · ·

> We're a year off treatment, and I really don't think about relapse very often. I do occasionally find myself studying her to see if she looks pale, or I worry when she seems tired or her behavior is bad. Usually, I'm feeling safer. But honestly, I don't think any of us will ever go back to the days when we just assumed that our kids would grow up, that the parents would die first—that sense of security is probably gone forever.

· · · · ·

> Shawn is 6 months off treatment, and he's just like a flower beginning to bloom. He's so happy, and I try to be happy with him. I try very hard to put worries about the future out of my mind, because I feel that those thoughts will rob me of just being able to enjoy Shawn.

• • • • •

Chemo is such a horrible thing for your child to endure, but at least you are actively fighting the beast; so when it ends you feel a bit like you're flying without a net. You get so used to this bizarre new "normal" of treatments and blood tests and doctor visits, and then suddenly you stop, but you don't get the old normal back.

I think it's probably best to approach the end of treatment as a chance to see your child get his healthy color and energy back, and an opportunity to create and explore a new "normal" for your family that is richer and more meaningful than the one you left behind. It's also really nice to finally have the chance to reconnect with your spouse (and other children) and heal all the relationships that have taken a beating during the stressful treatment period.

As for me, for perhaps a year after Joseph's treatment, I existed in a dazed mix of emotions and thoughts. I was fearful of relapse, thrilled that Joseph had survived the cancer and the treatment, concerned about what late effects lay around the corner, all tempered with a warm and thankful feeling that I knew I would never, EVER take my kids or my good life for granted anymore or sweat the small stuff the way I used to. There were days I felt like I didn't want to crawl out from under the bed, and other days I couldn't stop singing and being silly.

I think off treatment is a lot like on treatment—you just have to take it one day at a time.

Normal is a moving target—different for every person and family. No one can tell you what your normal will be. Normal is what keeps the family alive and planning and moving together to face their individual and collective futures.

Well, we finally did it. We took a deep breath, a heavy sigh, and we packed up the medical supplies. While this step may seem insignificant for some, those who have dealt with a chronic/life-threatening illness in their family know that the disposal of your arsenal of medical supplies is a symbolic rite of passage. It can only mean two things: your loved one has passed on, or you simply don't need the supplies anymore. We thank God every day that we ended up with the latter reason.

Katy's medical "tower" was stored in our hallway and included various bins and drawers full of central line supplies, a mini IV pump, masks and gloves, hypodermics, and sharps containers. It was very conspicuous. You simply couldn't miss it if you walked through the house. It was our constant reminder that we had a sick child, and was at times, for me, a crutch. I think I felt that as long as the tower was there and properly stocked and arranged, I was somehow in control of Katy's illness. I feared disposing of or putting anything away, thinking that if I did, she would most assuredly relapse and I'd need it again. No, of course that's not rational, but rationality has never been one of my strong points.

However, as the months passed, the tower gathered dust, and soon I couldn't remember the last time we'd even used any of the supplies. A few more months passed, and I began to realize what an eyesore this bunch of junk was! So, after my husband, David, brought some big boxes home from work, it was time. We did it together. Into the boxes went the tubing and syringes, masks, and dressing change kits for the kids' oncology camp. Into the garbage went everything else. It was so liberating! I can't imagine why we kept that stuff around for so long. It felt like the end of an era. And in a way it was.

For many people, helping others is a satisfying way to reach out or bring closure to the active phase of cancer treatment. Offering service can create something enormously meaningful out of personal challenges, which is why many parents and children like to give back to the cancer community in some way. Some examples of ways people have reached out include the following:

• I requested that the clinic and local pediatricians refer newly diagnosed families to me if the parents wanted someone to talk with. I remembered how impossible it was to go to meetings in the first few months, and how desperately I needed to talk to someone who had already traveled the same road.

• We started a Boy Scout project to keep the toy box full at the clinic.

• My children are counselors at the camp for kids with cancer.

• After my son died, I gave up my parish to begin work as a hospice chaplain.

• We organized a walk to raise funds for the Ronald McDonald House.

• We (a group of parents of children with leukemia) requested and were granted a conference with the oncology staff to share our thoughts about ways to improve pain management and communication between parents and staff. It was very well received.

• We circulated a petition among parents to request increased hospital funding for psychosocial support staff. We presented it to the director of the hematology/oncology service.

• I started a support group and organized meetings, conferences, and picnics; I also write a quarterly newsletter.

• We held a bone marrow donor drive.

• I give platelets and blood regularly.

• I took all of our leftover catheter line supplies to camp and gave them to a family who needed them.

The possibilities are endless. Parents and children can use whatever talents they have to help others—from designing head coverings to writing newsletters for families struggling with leukemia.

I am the administrator of several online support groups for parents of children with cancer. We have over 600 participants from 16 countries all over the world. Some of the members' children have been cured for years, some are newly diagnosed, and some of the children have died. We've become a family. It's important to me to remain involved in the fight against childhood cancer. There are so many others that are following behind in our footsteps. Perhaps showing that we've been there, too, yet we're still standing, might help another mom or dad.

An equally healthy response to ending cancer treatment is to put it behind you. Many families, after years of struggles, just want to move on. They don't want constant reminders of cancer and feel it's not good for children to be reminded of those hard times.

I realized that it was time to put it behind us when I watched my two children playing house one day. There was only one adult and one child in the family. I asked what happened to the rest of the family and they both said, "Cancer; they died." I didn't want them to have any more cancer in their lives. They had had enough. I know people who worry all the time about the leukemia returning, and it is not healthy for them or their children. I decided to get out of the cancer mode and back to being my usual upbeat self. I feel that we are finally back to normal, and it's a good place to be.

Parents and children need to talk to one another, examine their emotions, decide what course they want to chart, and work together toward creating a healthy life after cancer.

Follow-up care

Protocols for clinical trials require specific follow-up schedules to check for the recurrence of the disease. For instance, after treatment for average-risk acute lymphoblastic leukemia (ALL), your child may need monthly physical exams and a monthly CBC for the first year off treatment, and a less frequent schedule for the following years. Find out from the oncologist what the required schedule is, and where the appointments will be held. Make sure your child understands that after treatment ends, doctor appointments and blood draws will still be an occasional necessity. Follow-up care for possible late effects of treatment is usually a separate process.

Shawn is a year off treatment and I find myself letting go of the bad memories more and more. They are just fading away. What I am left with is awe, admiration, and amazement that my son handled all of the hardships of treatment and survived. He's very determined and strong-willed, and I'm so proud of him. When people say to me, "Oh, you were so strong to make it through that," I respond, "All I did was drive him to the appointments; he did the rest."

This experience has really changed me and my entire family. My marriage is much better, my other sons are stronger and closer to us, and Shawn has shown us all how tough a little kid can be. We take each precious day, one at a time, and try to get the most out of it. I so appreciate life and my family.

In the past, most survivors of leukemia were returned to their local doctors after follow-up for recurrence of disease ended. But as the population of long-term survivors grew, it became apparent that these young men and women often faced complex medical and psychosocial effects from their years of treatment. As a result, some institutions started late-effects clinics to provide a multidisciplinary team to monitor and support survivors. The nucleus of the team is usually a nursing coordinator, pediatric oncologist, pediatric nurse practitioner, social worker, and psychologist. The team also includes specialists such as endocrinologists and cardiologists.

Yearly appointments with follow-up programs usually include a review of treatments received, counseling regarding potential health risks (or lack thereof), and case-specific diagnostic tests (e.g., hormonal studies or testing for learning disabilities). Follow-up clinics not only provide comprehensive care for long-term survivors, they also participate in research projects that track the effectiveness of and side effects from various clinical trials. In addition, the follow-up clinics act as advocates for survivors with schools, insurance agencies, and employers.

As Grace Powers Monaco, one of the founders of Candlelighters Childhood Cancer Foundation, said:

Life is a hollow gift unless cancer survivors emerge from treatment as competent and worthy individuals, able to obtain insurance, equipped to earn a living, and prepared to participate in a medical surveillance program to "keep" the life they have won.

If your institution does not provide comprehensive, long-term, follow-up care, you can find a list of survivor programs at *www.acor.org/ped-onc/treatment/surclinics.html*. Many survivors travel to comprehensive programs for their yearly follow-up visits. Survivorship issues that should be addressed at the end of treatment are briefly described below.

Possible long-term side effects

Dr. Giulio J. D'Angio, MD, wrote, "Vigilance is essential if the blossoms of success in pediatric oncology are not to bear bitter fruit. Cure is not enough." At diagnosis, parents do not know what price their child will ultimately pay for reprieve from leukemia. For the majority of children with average-risk ALL, the price may be low. For children with high-risk ALL, acute myeloid leukemia (AML), chronic myelogenous leukemia (CML), juvenile myelomonocytic leukemia (JMML), or those who relapsed and required more intensive treatment, the price for life may be higher: subtle or pronounced learning disabilities, an impaired endocrine (glands that make hormones) system, growth difficulties, heart problems, and many other possible consequences.

The topic of late effects is too large for this book. To learn about the possible late effects your child might face, refer to *Childhood Cancer Survivors: A Practical Guide to the Future, 2nd ed.*, listed in Appendix C, "Books, Websites, and Videotapes."

Survivorship

An essential aspect of survivorship is making healthy choices. Good health habits and regular medical care help protect survivors' health and lessen the likelihood of late effects from cancer treatment. A sizable number of adult cancers are linked to lifestyle choices. Eating a healthy diet, staying physically active, using sunscreen, avoiding excessive alcohol consumption, maintaining a healthy weight, and not smoking all help keep survivors healthy and cancer-free. Wearing bike or motorcycle helmets, using seat belts, and calling a cab if the person driving has had too much to drink protect survivors from injury. Survivors have little or no control over their genetic make-up or the environment in which they live. But making healthy choices about how to live the rest of their lives gives them control over some of their future.

Immunizations

If your child was diagnosed before she received all her immunizations, ask the oncologist when you should resume the regular schedule for immunizations.

> *My doctor said to wait a year before beginning to catch up on shots. It was nice for her to get a long break before any more pokes.*

Risks of smoking

Teens need continuing counseling about problems associated with smoking (cigarettes or marijuana) or engaging in other high-risk behaviors. Most children and teens who received anthracycline therapy (Adriamycin®, daunomycin, or idarubicin) are at risk for damage to the heart muscle. Smoking not only damages the lungs, but it makes blood vessels hard, further decreasing the heart's ability to pump. The combination of heart damage from chemotherapy and smoking vastly increases the chance of heart disease; heart attack; congestive heart failure; stroke; cancer of the mouth, throat, and lungs; and death from sudden cardiac failure. An article about survivors and smoking in the Candlelighters youth newsletter ends with these words:

> *If you've had cancer and your friends haven't, they don't face the same risks from smoking that you do. You've fought hard for your life. Don't put it out in an ashtray.*

Safe sex

Every teen and young adult who has survived cancer should be counseled about safe sexual practices. Despite the prevalence of sexual messages in our culture, most teens and young adults are woefully underinformed about the facts. Many survivors think, erroneously, that if they are infertile, they do not have to be concerned about the use of condoms or other birth control methods. However, all sorts of diseases, some potentially fatal (hepatitis C, HIV/AIDS) and some not (genital herpes, genital warts, gonorrhea), can be transmitted through sexual intercourse. One nurse practitioner at a large follow-up clinic stated:

> I tell every teenager who comes through the door, regardless of their medical background, that I think he or she is too young to have sex, and I explain why. But then I say, in the event that you do choose to become sexually active, you always need to use a condom, and not just any condom. I tell them to only use a latex condom with a spermicide, which is the most barrier-protective. I explain that no sex is the only guarantee to avoid the many diseases out there, but a latex condom with spermicide offers the next best protection. And I really stress that this should be done whoever the partner is, and for whatever type of sex. So many teenagers think that diseases only happen to other kinds of kids.

Treatment summaries

Once treatment and follow-up for recurrence of disease are completed, many children and young adults will no longer be cared for by pediatric oncologists who are familiar with their history. A transition back to their community physician often occurs. Moreover, many primary care physicians—pediatricians, family practice doctors, internists, gynecologists—are not fully aware of all the different treatments used for the multitude of childhood cancers, or of the late effects they can cause.

Additionally, when treatment ends, patients and parents are not always given adequate information about the risks of developing late effects in the months, years, or decades after treatment ends. The risks of delayed effects are real, and it is imperative that survivors become informed advocates for their own health care. They need to be educated, in a supportive and responsible way, of the risk for future physical adversities; then if a problem does arise, it will be recognized early and receive prompt attention. Young adults who have survived childhood leukemia need to be fully cognizant of their unique medical history and be able to share this information with all doctors who care for them in the future.

A few months before the end of treatment, ask the oncologist to fill out the booklet in the back of this book. This health history will become an indispensable part of your child's medical records for the rest of her life. It should be kept in a safe place, and a copy should be given to each medical caregiver. When your child leaves home to begin her adult life, this booklet should go with her and a copy kept in a safe place.

If you do not have a copy of the health history booklet, write down the following important information that should be in your child's treatment summary:

- Name of disease
- Date of diagnosis and relapse, if any
- Place of treatment
- Dates of treatment
- Names of attending oncologist and primary nurse
- Name and number of clinical trial (if your child was treated on one)
- Names and total dosages of chemotherapeutic agents used
- Type and amount of radiation used and areas treated
- Name of radiation center
- Date(s) radiation received
- Dates and types of surgeries
- Date and type of stem cell transplant, if any
- Any major treatment complications
- Any persistent side effects of treatment
- Recommended medical follow-up for late effects
- Contact numbers for treating institutions.

If your child will not be examined periodically at a long-term follow-up clinic, write down this information and make sure your child has a copy to give to all doctors who treat her in the future.

Employment

The population of adults who have survived childhood cancer is growing at a rapid rate. It is estimated that one in every 250 young adults in the United States is a cancer survivor. Thousands of survivors are staying well, growing up, graduating from college, and successfully entering the workforce. Survivors of childhood leukemia are educators, sports figures, radio announcers, doctors, social workers, dancers, lawyers, and workers of all types.

Diane Komp, MD, in *A Child Shall Lead Them,* writes:

> *I lecture about long-term survivors to each new group of medical students that comes through pediatrics at Yale. I can see from their faces that most of them prefer memorizing the odds that someone will make it than tasting the sweetness of individual victories. "That's very nice, but how representative is that case?"*
>
> *Not all of them feel that way, though. I watch their faces and can now pick out from their ranks a special type of young person who is being seen in increasing numbers in medical classrooms. Although their classmates cannot tell who they are, I can spot a long-term survivor of childhood cancer 5 minutes into that lecture.*

Despite their numbers, some survivors still face job discrimination due to fears about cancer and its treatment. Under federal law and many state laws, an employer cannot treat a survivor differently from other employees because of a history of cancer. The Americans with Disabilities Act of 1990 (ADA) prohibits many types of job discrimination by employers, employment agencies, state and local governments, and labor unions. In addition, most states have laws that prohibit discrimination based on disabilities, although what these laws cover varies widely.

The ADA prohibits discrimination based on actual disability, perceived disability, or history of a disability. Any employer with 15 or more workers is covered by the ADA. The ADA requires the following:

- Employers may not make medical inquiries of an applicant, unless the applicant has a visible disability (e.g., uses a wheelchair), or the applicant has voluntarily disclosed her cancer history. Such questions must be limited to asking the applicant to describe or demonstrate how she would perform essential job functions. Medical inquiries are allowed after a job offer has been made or during a pre-employment medical exam.

- Employers must provide reasonable accommodations unless it causes undue hardship.

- Employers may not discriminate because of family illness.

The U.S. Equal Employment Opportunity Commission (EEOC) enforces Title 1 (employment) for the ADA. Visit *www.eeoc.gov* or call (800) 669-4000 for enforcement publications. Other sections are enforced or have their enforcement coordinated by the U.S. Department of Justice (Civil Rights Division, Public Access Section), which can be contacted online at *www.ada.gov* or by calling (800) 514-0301.

The Job Accommodation Network (JAN) is a service provided by the U.S. Department of Labor's Office of Disability Employment Policy (ODEP). The service supports the employment, including self-employment and small business ownership, of people with disabilities. JAN can be reached at *www.jan.wvu.edu* or by calling (800) 526-7234.

In Canada, the Canadian Human Rights Act provides essentially the same rights as the ADA. The act is administered by the Canadian Human Rights Commission. You can get more information by calling the national office at (888) 214-1090 or visiting its website at *www.chrc-ccdp.ca.*

If you feel you have been discriminated against due to your disability or a relative's disability, contact the EEOC or the Canadian Human Rights Commission promptly.

The military

Some survivors of childhood cancer wish to enlist in the military, or to apply for Reserve Officer Training Corps (ROTC) or the service academies. In an article in *Pediatric Clinics of North America,* Grace Ann Monaco, J.D. wrote:

> *The laws and regulations relating to admission to the armed services are permissive, not mandatory. This means that each of the armed services can enforce these laws and regulations if the service wishes to do so. Usually, taken on a case-by-case basis, survivors of childhood cancer who meet the requirements of the particular service and who are "otherwise physically fit for service" are eligible for a medical waiver to serve in the armed forces, reserves, and ROTC, and to obtain admission to service academies if the survivor is free of cancer and, generally, has completed therapy 5 years previously.*

Insurance

Job discrimination can spell economic catastrophe for cancer survivors because most health insurance is obtained through one's place of employment. As survivors mature, seek employment, and move away from home, many encounter barriers to obtaining health insurance, such as rejection of application based on cancer history, policy reductions, policy cancellation, pre-existing condition exclusions, increased premiums, or extended waiting periods.

> *I realize that I must do whatever is necessary to stay covered on my parents' insurance as long as possible. I don't particularly like that, but it is important. As long as I remain a full-time student, it will be okay.*

Most states offer high-risk individuals, such as cancer survivors, access to comprehensive health insurance plans (CHIPS). CHIPS, also called "high-risk pools," are a means for individuals to obtain insurance regardless of their physical condition or medical history. For more information about CHIPS, call (877) 543-7669 (877-KIDS-NOW) or visit *www.insurekidsnow.gov.*

Although neither the states nor the federal government mandate a legal right to insurance, there are some legal remedies for insurance discrimination.

- **COBRA.** The Comprehensive Omnibus Budget Reconciliation Act (COBRA) is a federal law that requires public and private companies employing more than 20 workers to provide continuation of group coverage to employees if they quit, are fired, or work reduced hours. Coverage must extend to surviving, divorced, or separated spouses, and to dependent children. You must pay for your continued coverage, but it must not exceed by more than 2 percent the rate set for the company's full-time employees. By being allowed to purchase continued coverage, you have time to seek other long-term coverage. The U.S. Department of Labor provides a COBRA fact sheet at *www.dol.gov/ ebsa/faqs/faq_consumer_cobra.html*.

- **ERISA.** The Employee Retirement and Income Security Act (ERISA) is a federal law that protects workers from being fired because of the cancer history of the employee or beneficiaries (spouse and children). ERISA also prohibits employers from encouraging a person with a cancer history to retire as a "disabled" employee. ERISA does not apply to job discrimination (denial of new job due to cancer history), discrimination that does not affect benefits, or to employees whose compensation does not include benefits.

- **Health Insurance Portability and Accountability Act of 1996 (HIPAA).** This law allows individuals to change employers without losing coverage, if they have been insured for at least 12 months. It prevents group health plans from denying coverage based on medical history, genetic information, or claims history, although insurers can still exclude those with specific diseases or conditions. It also increases portability if you change from a group to an individual plan. For additional information, a HIPAA fact sheet with frequently asked questions is available by visiting *www.dol.gov/ebsa/ faqs/faq_consumer_hipaa.html*.

Appendix B, "Resource Organizations," lists organizations that can help if you or your child faces job discrimination or problems with insurance due to treatment for cancer.

On November 19, 1998, we arrived by ambulance at the Children's Hospital where we were given the devastating news. Words that silenced time; that paralyzed my being. "Tommy has leukemia . . . and it's not good."

Tommy (17 years old) was diagnosed with T-cell ALL. His white count had risen to over 90,000 and the disease had also spread to his central nervous system (CNS). Chemotherapy had to start immediately . . . and it had to work. He began an intense protocol for the treatment of his cancer that included radiation and chemotherapy.

Through the next 3½ years we had many ups and many downs, too many to discuss. But during his illness, when he could, Tommy consumed his days with reading. On one chilly day in Pennsylvania, he asked me to drive him to the public library. He covered his bald head with a wool beanie and his once athletic physique was frail and weakened from the intense early months of chemotherapy and radiation. I pulled up to the front of the library, and I asked if he wanted me to go along to help. He said, "No thanks Mom, I can do it." After 20 minutes or so, Tommy exited with a HUGE stack of books—all medical books! Tommy had found his passion for life—his true love of medicine.

One of our biggest obstacles was Tommy's diagnosis of avascular necrosis (AVN) in his hips, shoulders, and knees. The AVN caused him excruciating pain, and he could only walk with the help of crutches. A partial hip replacement was done to preserve as much of the hip as possible and core decompressions were done on his shoulder and knee. Tommy's main concern was to get all the surgeries over quickly so he would not get behind in his studies, be able to take finals, and be able to walk without pain. And all the while he was still undergoing chemotherapy treatments for the leukemia. After the surgeries and much rehabilitation, I saw my 19-year-old son take his first steps without crutches for the first time in 9 months. It was more emotional and exciting than when he was 10 months old taking his first steps!

Tommy graduated from college in the Spring of 2004 with a major in biology and a minor in biochemistry and molecular biology. He spent 2 years at the National Institutes of Health/National Cancer Institute as a research fellow, and then he started his first year in medical school. He looks forward to graduating from medical school this year, getting married, and moving on to his residency in pediatrics with a future fellowship in pediatric hematology/oncology. His health is good, although he still suffers from pain due to the AVN. Because of the damage to his joints from this disease, future surgeries are inevitable.

Tommy has lived his life with enormous strength, determination, and grace. He never, ever let his illness dictate his life. With all his compassion and fortitude, I can only imagine what his future holds as a phenomenal doctor and human being. And those lives he touches along the way will only be richer for having crossed his path.

Chapter 20

Relapse

Hold fast to dreams
For if dreams die
Life is a broken winged bird
That cannot fly.

— Langston Hughes

PARENTS FREQUENTLY DESCRIBE the return of their child's leukemia as more devastating than the original diagnosis. They feel betrayed, guilty, and/or angry—they did everything the doctors told them to do, but the cancer came back anyway. They worry that if the first battery of treatments didn't work, what will? Mostly, they are afraid. And their unspoken but most crushing fear is: What if my child dies?

If your child has relapsed, it is worth remembering that you now have several strengths you didn't have before. You have already done this. You know the language, and you have a relationship with the medical team. You probably have friendships with other parents of children with cancer and you know they will be there for you. You know that something that seems insurmountable can be endured, one day at a time.

This chapter explains how doctors determine if a relapse has occurred, what emotional responses you might expect, and how to decide on a treatment plan. In addition, several parents and patients share their stories about how they managed to cope after a diagnosis of leukemia relapse.

Signs and symptoms

Although relapse can happen years after treatment ends, it most commonly occurs during treatment or in the first year off treatment. In fact, most treatment centers do not consider children to be long-term survivors of leukemia until they have been off treatment for at least 2 years or are 5 years past diagnosis.

The signs and symptoms of leukemia relapse can be the same telltale warnings that occurred prior to diagnosis:

• Fatigue

- Fevers

- Night sweats

- Nosebleeds

- Bruises and/or petechiae

- Pale skin

- Back, leg, or joint pain

- Loss of appetite

- Enlarged lymph nodes in the neck or groin

- Enlarged abdomen caused by a large spleen or liver

- Changes in behavior, such as excessive irritability

- Dizziness

- Headaches.

Normal childhood illnesses can cause most of these symptoms, and a tired day here or a bruise there is probably no cause for alarm. However, if your child has a persistent loss of appetite, if he is often fatigued, or if his symptoms escalate, it might be wise to call your oncologist. In some cases, parents have no warning. After they bring their child in for a routine bone marrow aspiration or spinal tap, they receive a totally unexpected telephone call from the doctor with the news.

> I am a long-term survivor (30 years old), who first was diagnosed with ALL at age 8 and subsequently relapsed three times, at ages 13, 15, and 16. The first relapse was by far the worst to deal with emotionally. It had been 5 years since my diagnosis, so I went in for my last spinal tap and bone marrow. I had been off treatment with good counts for 2 years. My mother and I didn't even wait for the test results; we went out to lunch and went shopping. Later that day, I called the clinic, and my doctor told me the bone marrow was fine, but she needed to talk to my mother. I heard my mother say, "No, no, oh no," and she started to cry. I just stood there feeling numb, knowing the news was bad. The cancer had returned to my central nervous system. We held each other and cried.

The three most likely sites for leukemia relapse are the bone marrow, the central nervous system (CNS), and the testes. Bone marrow relapse is the most common form of leukemia recurrence. Since the use of CNS prophylaxis—intrathecal (IT) methotrexate and sometimes radiation—was initiated, the likelihood of CNS relapse has dramatically decreased. Currently, CNS relapse occurs in less than 10 percent of young patients. Relapse in the testicles is also uncommon, occurring in less than 5 percent of boys.

The primary symptom of testicular relapse is a painless, enlarged testicle. Leukemia occasionally recurs at other sites, such as the ovaries or eyes.

> Right before Stephan went to camp, he went in for his maintenance spinal tap. I got a bill from a different specialist, and when I asked the oncologist about it, he said that Stephan had a few white cells in his fluid that he wanted to get another opinion on. He assured me that everything was okay, but I just had that feeling that something was about to go wrong. At his next spinal, his count was 88 in the cerebrospinal fluid. A central nervous system relapse.

· · · · ·

> Jody was complaining about pain and a feeling of pressure in his leg bones. I kept bringing him back to the oncologist, saying that something was wrong, that he was in great pain, but the doctor kept insisting that it was just growing pains. He didn't even examine his legs for a month. When he did, he could feel parts of the bone radiating heat. The bone scan showed the cancer in the exact spots Jody had pointed out.

· · · · ·

> My son relapsed in the left optic nerve, which is considered a posterior relapse. His first symptom, his only symptom, was some mild pain with extreme gaze (looking all the way down, up, or to the side). After a couple weeks of this, a family practice doctor looked at him and saw nothing. An optometrist saw some swelling of the optic disc (connected with the optic nerve). That sent us to an ophthalmologist, to a radiologist for a CAT scan, and back to the oncologist. So, his only symptoms were some mild pain and some swelling in the back of the eye that was hard to see. Further tests of the marrow and the cerebrospinal fluid showed no leukemia cells, so we were forced to do an optic nerve sheath biopsy, which was the only place ALL cells were found.

Emotional responses

Parents who have children with leukemia in remission think or speak of relapse with an almost palpable dread. Just the thought can cause an eruption of the same emotions that surged in them at diagnosis. The depth of the emotions generated by relapse is extremely hard for parents and survivors to relive and describe. As one survivor of relapse said in a shaky voice while being interviewed, "It's been 11 years since I finished treatment, but talking about it shows that you scratch the surface and those overwhelming feelings are still right there."

Parents and their child may feel a wide array of emotions at relapse: numbness, guilt, dread, anger, fear, confusion, denial, and grief.

I found that relapse was far worse than the original diagnosis. At diagnosis, after a certain period of adjustment, you think that treatment has a beginning, a middle, and an end. But relapse creates a bigger burden to accept. You begin to feel that maybe the disease is more powerful than the medicine. I found that for a while I just stopped functioning and thinking rationally. I felt that all the hell of treatment had been just a waste of time. I felt guilt and a tremendous sense of loss of control. I felt like I was on a runaway freight train, hurtling toward an end that didn't look so good anymore. This is the point at which people are willing to use any type of unconventional therapies, because they are desperate. I know one mom in our support group who was even willing to try coffee enemas. She looks back on it now and says, "I just went crazy."

Physical symptoms such as dizziness, nausea, fainting, and shortness of breath are common. Parents wonder how they can ask their child to endure treatment again. They wonder how they will survive it themselves. They may oscillate between optimism and panic.

My first relapse was the worst emotionally. Neither my parents nor I ever thought that after 5 years it would be back. I also had been so young when I was first treated that I didn't really think of leukemia as cancer and didn't understand that I could die from it. But at 13, I remembered clearly what I had been through, and all I could think was that it hadn't worked. I told my parents that I wouldn't do it again. My father sat me down and gave me a reality check. He explained that I would die if I didn't get treatment. He said, "If you don't do it for yourself, please do it for me and your mom." The next morning I went into the clinic and started all over again.

Goal setting and treatment planning

A difficult but necessary step in making plans is discussing and deciding on your and your child's goals. A first relapse in a child 2 years off treatment is very different than a fourth relapse in a child on treatment. Health Canada's publication, *This Battle Which I Must Fight: Cancer in Canada's Children and Teenagers* (*www.phac-aspc.gc.ca/publicat/ tbwimf-mcplv*), states:

This [relapse] is a time of crisis and ambivalence. The decision to be made is whether to continue to try to achieve a remission or to replace this hope with the hope for comfort for the child and a special time together. Each parent, and the child who is old enough to understand, requires differing amounts of time to reach a decision about how to proceed. Careful and frequent discussions with the medical team, as well as with trusted friends and relatives, may help clarify issues and bring some peace of mind.

In the Spring 1995 issue of the Candlelighters newsletter, Arthur Ablin, MD, (Director Emeritus of Pediatric Clinical Oncology at the University of California, San Francisco), writes of the importance of goal setting in the decision-making process after relapse:

Before determining which treatment is to be chosen, a decision must be made to determine the goal of treatment—in other words, what is it that we are trying to achieve. This crucial first step is the basis upon which any decision concerning treatment must be made. But it is too often omitted from consideration and/or discussion, even by the most experienced. The frustrations accompanying the previous failure of treatment, the fear of the loss of the hope for cure, the pressure of urgency to find solutions, the new awareness of the possibility or probability of death, lead us all to want to consider treatments first rather than these more difficult considerations involved in establishing goals. These also force us to deal with reality earlier, which could mean the almost intolerable confrontation with the death of a very-much-loved child, a tragedy to be avoided at all costs.

After discussion of goals, your family may decide on palliative care or aggressive treatment. If you decide to treat, there may be more than one option available. Treatment plans for a first relapse may be specified in the standard treatment or clinical trial protocol document, or your physician may suggest a different approach. Suggestions for treatment may include stem cell transplantion; radiation to the head, spine, testes, or other relapse site; more intensive chemotherapy; or a clinical trial.

Do not rush into treatment if you or your family feel uncomfortable about the plan. There is always time to obtain answers to all of your questions and to get a second opinion. Physicians make recommendations based on knowledge, experience, and consultations with other experts in the field. Do not hesitate to ask your physician why she has suggested a certain treatment approach to your child's relapse. Ask your doctor about treatment goals, methods, and possible side effects. Also ask if she has consulted with others in the decision-making process, and if so, with whom. Be certain older children and teens are involved in decisions regarding their care and treatment choices.

JaNette was diagnosed with AML with the Philadelphia chromosome. Four months into treatment, after a routine bone marrow aspiration, I got a phone call from the doctor saying she had relapsed. I remember going to the hospital where they did another bone marrow aspiration. At exactly 4 o'clock in the afternoon, they gave me a relapse protocol to read. I was sitting on the floor in the hallway reading it, and it was so horrible because I knew what it meant! I understood what we were in for, and I started to bawl and couldn't stop.

Treatment for ALL relapse

Relapsed acute lymphoblastic leukemia (ALL) is treated more aggressively than newly diagnosed ALL. Treatment will include chemotherapy (and often radiation) and sometimes stem cell transplantation. A stem cell transplant is the process of replacing diseased or damaged stem cells (primitive blood forming cells) of a child with relapsed leukemia with healthy stem cells (see Chapter 21, "Stem Cell Transplantation" for more information). There are three types of stem cell transplantion, depending on where the stem cells are collected from:

- Bone marrow transplant (stem cells from the bone marrow)
- Peripheral blood stem cell transplant (stem cells from the blood stream)
- Cord blood transplant (stem cells from the umbilical cord blood of newborns).

The regimen suggested depends on the characteristics of the relapse and, to some extent, the opinions of the doctors you consult. The determining characteristics of the relapse are time (early or late) and location:

- Bone marrow
- Extramedullary (meaning in the cerebrospinal fluid, testes, or elsewhere outside of the bone marrow)
- Combination of both.

Most pediatric oncology teams agree that early isolated bone marrow relapse should be treated with a stem cell transplant, while late extramedullary relapse should be treated with chemotherapy. Treatment choices in other situations, for instance, a combined late relapse, are not as clear cut. Because there may not be a consensus about the best treatment plan, parents often face difficult choices.

In non-clear cut cases, some oncology teams use sophisticated technology to measure the level of residual leukemia to help determine the best treatment plan for a child. For example, if the minimal residual disease (MRD) is high despite the absence of overt leukemia in the bone marrow, a decision may be made for the child to be treated with a stem cell transplant. On the other hand, if the MRD in the child is low or there is no residual leukemia left after relapse induction therapy, then the oncology team may decide that chemotherapy may be the best option for the child.

Bone marrow relapse

Initial treatment of bone marrow relapse starts with induction therapy to achieve a remission. Relapse induction regimens may include high doses of drugs used at initial treatment such as prednisone or dexamethasone, vincristine, asparaginase, and anthracyclines (daunorubicin or doxorubicin). Additional drugs are often used, alone or in combination (e.g., cytarabine in combination with teniposide or high-dose ifosfamide). A number of new drugs were also recently approved for treatment of relapsed or refractory ALL:

- Nelarabine (T-cell ALL)
- Clofarabine

- Imatinib (Philadelphia chromosome ALL)

- Desatinib (Philadelphia chromosome ALL).

If the child has a good response to induction, treatment usually continues with an intense multi-drug consolidation that lasts from 1 to 4 months, followed by maintenance therapy. CNS prophylaxis is also necessary. In cases in which a child previously had cranial radiation, intrathecal chemotherapy (containing one to three drugs) is given.

When children do not achieve remission from induction therapy or are at very high risk of another relapse (e.g., early bone marrow relapse), stem cell transplants are often recommended if a suitable donor can be found. As the chance of cure is low if remission is not achieved prior to transplant, most oncology teams will attempt to get the child into remission before proceeding to transplant by using different combinations of chemotherapy, or they may consider the use of experimental drugs.

Transplants of stem cells from the bone marrow of closely matched donors (allogeneic bone marrow transplants) have been the mainstay of transplant therapy for two decades. In recent years, however, doctors have achieved increasingly good results with cord blood transplants. If there is no closely matched donor, an autologous transplant, which uses the child's own bone marrow, can be performed. Autologous transplants have fewer side effects than allogeneic transplants; but the success rate is lower, because it is difficult to ensure that every diseased cell has been removed from the child's marrow. (See Chapter 21, "Stem Cell Transplantation" for more information.)

Extramedullary relapse

Children who have CNS relapse must receive aggressive treatment that includes IT chemotherapy, cranial/spinal radiation, or both. Treatment for CNS relapse often begins with an induction that includes systemic chemotherapy and IT methotrexate, followed by cranial and spinal radiation. Next comes a maintenance phase that includes systemic chemotherapy and more IT methotrexate. Some protocols use a triple IT therapy consisting of methotrexate, cytarabine, and hydrocortisone.

Occasionally, children relapse in the testes, ovaries, eyes, or other sites. Treatment in these cases usually consists of site-specific radiation and high-dose, multi-drug chemotherapy. To view the National Cancer Institute's descriptions of the most recent standards of care for different types of ALL relapse, *visit www.cancer.gov/cancertopics/pdq/ treatment/childALL/healthprofessional,* then click on "recurrent childhood acute lymphoblastic leukemia" on the left sidebar.

Questions to ask

You may want to ask your doctor some of the following questions about the relapse and suggested treatment plan. Also see the questions in the last section of this chapter, entitled "Making a decision about treatment."

- What kind of relapse is it? Bone marrow, extramedullary, or a combination?

- Is it considered an early or late relapse?

- What are the cytogenetics/molecular characteristics of the relapsed leukemia? Is the relapse showing the same cytogenetics as the initial diagnosis? If different, what does that mean for treatment?

- Will levels of MRD be measured during treatment, and will they affect the treatment plan? Will the levels direct the treatment plan? Will we be given the results of MRD testing?

- If testicular relapse is diagnosed, is it necessary to have testicular radiation? If so, at what dosage?

- If CNS relapse is diagnosed, is it necessary to have craniospinal radiation? If so, at what dosage?

Additional questions suggested by parents of children who relapsed can be found at *www.all-kids.org/relapsequestions.html*. Another source of real-time information can be obtained by joining the well-moderated discussion groups at *www.acor.org*, particularly the ALL-KIDS-RELAPSED group.

> *Making the decision as to what treatment to choose was much more difficult when my son relapsed. The stakes were higher. While I had faith in the skills and judgment of my son's oncologists, I could not rest easy unless I had educated myself on the options available for relapse treatment. His relapse had been suspected for weeks, so I had time to investigate possible treatment choices. His relapse site was rare, which made the usual channels less effective in our case. I started with the online NCI-PDQ and a PubMed search. I asked friends to search for me. From there I contacted a physician from the other leading children's oncology research group and asked what type of treatment protocol they had to offer for my son's type of relapse. I learned that the options were few in terms of protocols addressing my son's type of relapse. At this point I contacted an ombudsman program offered by a national cancer organization. This program sent the details of my son's situation to several pediatric oncologists for their anonymous opinions.*
>
> *When we sat down with the ped oncologists, I already had some background and knew what was available in terms of treatment. When they presented their choice of protocol, I asked for and was given a copy of the protocol. Reading the rationale and background of the study they were proposing helped me to understand why this pro- tocol was suggested. As a result, I was able to make a difficult decision and enroll my*

son in a protocol with confidence that he was getting the best treatment available. Since it was a very difficult and intense treatment protocol, it also helped my teenage son to understand why this was the path we were following. Once begun, neither of us had any serious doubts that we'd made the best choice. Now, almost 3 years later, I am still very pleased that I was able to make a fully informed decision. My son is now a healthy young man away at college. He completed relapse treatment over a year ago and is doing great. His concerns these days are about the dorm food, his next midterm, and when he can see his girlfriend.

Treatment for AML relapse

Most acute myeloid leukemia (AML) relapses occur in the bone marrow. Nearly all AML relapse treatment begins with an intensive induction regimen that commonly includes high-dose cytarabine (ARA-C) combined with some or all of the following: daunorubicin, mitoxantrone, fludarabine, idarubicin, etoposide, 2-chlorodeoxyadenosine, and asparaginase. A hormone to stimulate cell growth, called G-CSF, is often added to the mix. Some very high-risk patients have responded well to a complex induction consisting of the anti-CD33 monoclonal antibody, coupled with gemtuzumab ozogamicin (Mylotarg®), and either mitoxantrone plus cytarabine or high-dose cytarabine plus asparaginase. Several additional drugs are being evaluated in clinical trials.

Treatment for children with a CNS relapse of AML includes aggressive IT therapy (methotrexate and/or ARA-C) and intensive chemotherapy. Many of these children also receive a stem cell transplant and sometimes craniospinal radiation.

After induction, the remainder of the treatment depends upon the child's individual risk factors, as well as prior treatment. To view the National Cancer Institute's descriptions of the most recent standards of care for different types of AML relapse, visit *www.cancer.gov/cancertopics/pdq/treatment/childAML/healthprofessional*, then click on "recurrent childhood acute myeloid leukemia and other myeloid malignancies" on the left sidebar.

Questions to ask

You may want to ask your doctor the following questions about the relapse and suggested treatment plan. Also see the questions in the last section of this chapter, entitled "Making a decision about treatment."

- What kind of relapse is it? Bone marrow, extramedullary, or a combination?

- Is it considered an early or late relapse?

- What are the cytogenetics/molecular characteristics of the relapsed leukemia? Is the relapse showing the same cytogenetics as the initial diagnosis? If different, what does that mean for treatment?

- Will levels of minimum residual disease (MRD) be measured during treatment, and will they affect the treatment plan? Will the levels direct the treatment plan? Will we be given the results of MRD testing?

- If CNS relapse is diagnosed, is it necessary to have craniospinal radiation? If so, at what dosage?

Treatment for APL relapse

Children with recurrent acute promylocytic leukemia (APL) are often given treatments that include arsenic trioxide, all-trans retinoic acid, or both. Children treated with arsenic must be closely monitored and supported to prevent damage to the heart. Both allogeneic and autologous stem cell transplants have been used successfully in recent years. To view the National Cancer Institute's descriptions of the most recent standards of care for different types of APL relapse, visit *www.cancer.gov/cancertopics/pdq/treatment/childAML/healthprofessional*, then click on "recurrent childhood acute myeloid leukemia and other myeloid malignancies" on the left sidebar.

Making a decision about treatment

Pediatric cancer treatment is evolving quickly. The information gleaned from second opinions or your own research may reinforce what your doctor recommended, or it might provide you with additional treatment options. Either way, the information may increase your comfort level during the treatment planning process. You might want to ask your doctor the following questions about the relapse and suggested treatment plan:

- Why do you think this treatment is the best option? What are the other choices, and why are you recommending this one?

- Have you consulted with other physicians? If so, with whom? Did you all agree on this treatment or were several choices suggested?

- How many other facilities use this relapse/transplant protocol/study?

- Is there a standard treatment for this type of relapse? What is it?

- What clinical trials are available for this type of relapse? (You can also check *http://clinicaltrials.gov*, where you can search for open clinical trials by disease and location.)

- What are the potential benefits and possible side effects of the suggested treatment?

- How long is the proposed relapse treatment?

- If transplant is recommended, what is the timing strategy for the transplant?

- If radiation is to be included, what are the age parameters suggested at this facility?

- What are the known or potential risks of the treatment?

- Is any neurocognitive testing done prior to treatment/transplant and what kind of follow-up is there post treatment/transplant?

- What is the 5-year survival rate for this protocol?

- How often will my child need to be hospitalized?

- If the treatment is investigational, is there scientific evidence that it works for leukemia?

- Does insurance cover this type of treatment?

- What supportive services for associated health services are available? How do we contact the people responsible for these services? (Contacts might include a hospital school coordinator, social worker, psychologist, and physical therapist.)

- What is the goal of this treatment? Is it likely to cure my child, or is it to provide comfort?

Some of the questions above were printed in the Candlelighters Childhood Cancer Foundation's Newsletter (Spring/Summer 2007) and are reprinted with permission.

> *After his CNS relapse while on maintenance, Stephan (8 years old) received cranial and spinal radiation and went through another induction, and they started to give him spinals with ARA-C, methotrexate, and hydrocortisone. Even with ondansetron, it's bad. He's very sick to his stomach and just feels queasy all of the time. After the reinduction, he went back on his maintenance schedule and will finish at the expected time. But it's much harder for him now. His ankle bones ache, he's limping, and he can't run. Six days after vincristine, he gets severe back pain, like someone is pounding on his back hard. If he is bumped or jarred, he cries out in pain. He creeps along looking like an old man.*

· · · · ·

> *When Greg relapsed, they threw his protocol in the trash can, and our oncologist started making phone calls to other doctors in the Children's Cancer Group network to decide on a plan. Greg was put successively on three different relapse protocols in an attempt to keep him in remission. When his counts went down, the blasts would temporarily disappear, but when his counts rose, the blasts would creep back. His CNS relapse was followed by a bone marrow relapse, and the only option left was a bone marrow transplant; but we didn't know if he would be strong enough to survive it.*

· · · · ·

> *After another relapse, they wanted to try a chemotherapy with limited possible results, and we really didn't want our 11-year-old Caitlin to go through any more.*

But she talked it over with the doctor and concluded, "Of course I have to do it. I'm a fighting Irish."

If your child is old enough, it is a good idea to thoroughly discuss the options with her so you understand her wishes (e.g., if she wants to pursue additional treatment, or if she wants to stop treatment and get comfort care). Children have a radar for parents' feelings and they will know if you are uncertain about proceeding. If older children and parents disagree, use the hospital social worker or psychologist to help you negotiate a joint decision. These discussions will help clarify each family member's thoughts and feelings, and they will allow the child's emotional and physical well-being to be part of the equation.

> *Jesse relapsed four times, and in some ways it got harder and in other ways it got easier. We knew each time that her chances for survival were fading, and that was hard. But each time we grieved and worked through the feelings, and our skills at handling relapse improved. I turned to God for comfort, and I think that helped me feel that I was standing on a rock out in the ocean, rather than thrashing around in the water. My faith gave me solace. Jesse handled the relapses better than anyone else in the family. She would calmly listen to the doctors' explanations, then she would say, "Okay, what do we have to do?" She was never angry. She was sometimes sad, but mostly accepting.*

After you have set goals, received answers to all of your questions, obtained a second opinion if desired, and decided on comfort care or a treatment plan, it is time to proceed. Your knowledge and experience may prove to be a double-edged sword. You have no illusions about the difficulties ahead because you've done it before, but you also will be strengthened by your ties with the cancer community, your familiarity with your physicians and hospital routines, and your ability to work the system to get what your child needs. Many parents shared how their child took the lead with relapse treatment. While the parents agonized, their child said simply, "Let's just do it." And they did.

> *I encourage people to try to keep things in perspective. Attitude is a big part of survival. As difficult as it is, try to maintain a good attitude and keep focused on the future. I always thought, "I have cancer, this is a bad thing, but I am going to beat it." My analogy was a boxing match. When I relapsed, I was knocked down. But I always got up and kept fighting.*

> *I had a total of three relapses, two of which were on treatment. Every time we relapse, statistics say our chances of survival are less likely. But I survived those three relapses, and now I live a life as normal as if cancer never touched it. After cancer, I finished high school and went to college. I gave birth to a beautiful, healthy baby girl. My daughter (still beautiful) is now 7 years old. For me, life does go on after cancer.*

Chapter 21

Stem Cell Transplantation

The courage of life is often a less dramatic spectacle than the courage of the final moment; but it is no less a magnificent mixture of triumph and tragedy.

— John Fitzgerald Kennedy
Profiles in Courage

STEM CELL TRANSPLANTATION (SCT) is a complicated procedure used to treat leukemia, other cancers, and some blood diseases that were once considered incurable. Stem cells are the cells from which all blood cells develop. Three sources of stem cells—peripheral (circulating) blood, bone marrow, or cord blood—are used to restore stem cells destroyed by high-dose chemotherapy and sometimes radiation. During SCT, normal stem cells are infused into the child's veins. The stem cells migrate to the cavities inside the bones where new, healthy blood cells are then produced.

Transplants, although frequently life-saving, are expensive, technically complex, and potentially life-threatening. Understanding the procedure and its ramifications at a time of crisis can be tremendously difficult. To help with your decisions, this chapter presents the basics of SCT and shares the experiences of several families.

If SCT has been recommended for your child, see Appendix C, "Books, Websites, and Videotapes," which lists several publications and websites that provide more in-depth coverage of the subject.

When are transplants necessary?

In some children, leukemia cannot be cured with conventional doses of chemotherapy and/or radiation. SCT allows the delivery of high-dose therapy to kill the cancer cells, followed by an infusion of normal stem cells to rescue bone marrow function.

SCTs are sometimes recommended for children with chronic myelogenous leukemia (CML) in the chronic phase, juvenile myelomonocytic leukemia (JMML) with rapid progression, or acute myelogenous leukemia (AML) in first or second remission. Transplant from a matched related donor (MRD) is recommended for some children with very high-risk types of acute lymphoblastic leukemia (ALL) such as Ph+ in first remission and sometimes for infants with 11q23 rearrangements. Guidelines change over time as new information becomes available, and practices vary among institutions.

If SCT has been recommended for your child or teenager, you may want to get a second opinion before proceeding. Chapter 6, "Forming a Partnership with the Medical Team," gives several methods for obtaining an educated second opinion. In addition, to fully understand the procedure and its possible side effects, you may want to ask the oncologist some or all of the following questions:

- What are all the treatment options?

- For my child's type of cancer, history, and physical condition, what chance for survival does he have with a transplant? With other treatments?

- What are the short-term and long-term risks from the proposed transplant? Explain the statistical chance of each risk.

- What will be my child's short-term and long-term quality of life after the transplant?

- What is the institution's procedure for this type of transplant?

- What portion of the procedure will be outpatient versus inpatient?

- How long will my child have to take medicines after the transplant?

- What are the side effects of these medicines?

- Is this transplant considered experimental, or is it accepted clinical practice?

> *My daughter was 6 years old when she was diagnosed with AML. When she relapsed 4 months into treatment, an allogeneic bone marrow transplant (BMT) was her only hope.*
>
> · · · · ·
>
> *After my son's second relapse from ALL, the doctors told us that a bone marrow transplant was his last option for a cure.*
>
> · · · · ·
>
> *The day my daughter was diagnosed with CML, they told us her only chance for a cure was a BMT.*

Types of transplants

It is important to understand the type of SCT being recommended so you can better evaluate what has been proposed for your child.

Human leukocyte antigens

Everyone has proteins, called human leukocyte antigens (HLA), on the surface of their cells. These proteins allow a person's immune system to distinguish the body's own cells from those of another person. There is a strong association of some HLA types with a person's ethnic background. Scientists look at six HLA antigens to determine a person's HLA type. Two people are considered to be a possible match if all six antigens are identical. Because of new genetic knowledge, molecular analysis (called high-resolution typing) is done to provide additional information about compatibility of donor cells with the recipient's immune system.

Half of a person's HLA genes are inherited from each parent. Because there are four possible combinations of parental genes, a child has one chance in four (a 25 percent chance) of being matched with a sibling who has the same biological parents. This pattern of inheritance explains why parents are only rarely (1 percent of the time) matched with their children. More distant relatives are even less likely to be a match, because they are more likely to have different HLA genes. The odds of obtaining a match from an unrelated person were once slim. However, due to the rapid expansion of people typed and listed on various national and international marrow registries, and the development of more accurate tissue typing methods, a complete or partial match can now be found for almost 90 percent of patients.

Allogeneic transplants

Allogeneic transplants are those in which the stem cells come from a person who is not the child's identical twin. Thus, the donor could be a sibling, parent, close relative, or an unrelated individual. Sometimes a matched unrelated donor (called MUD) can be located through the U.S. National Marrow Donor Program (NMDP) or similar donor registries in the United States and other countries. The risk of complications increases if the donor is not a full match.

> Adele's transplant was June 16, 1997. She was 5½ years old at the time. Donor marrow was harvested from Ben, 2½ at the time. Harvesting took approximately 1 hour, and after the marrow was prepared for infusion, Adele received it (about 45 minutes later). The actual infusion was very simple—just hanging an IV (intravenous) bag. The doctor and nurses were, understandably, extremely careful with it, and it was very dramatic!

One hour after completion, Adele could get up, and she and Ben immediately went running to the playroom! She had not crashed yet from the preparative chemotherapy, which had just been completed 2 days before. Just like her response to most of the treatment, however, this was not the norm. The nursing staff said they'd never seen a kid who felt well enough to do that following a BMT.

Adele first showed something above a zero ANC (absolute neutrophil count) on Day T+15 (15 days after transplant). From then on, she improved quickly and steadily. She was released about 6 weeks after transplant, and met her goal of being at home and better (at least not sick!) for her sixth birthday. She did so well that she was off all medication except for prophylactic Bactrim® by the end of October. Because Adele showed basically no signs of graft-versus-host disease, she was taken off almost all meds early. She returned to school in January.

The primary life-threatening complications of an allogeneic bone marrow transplant (BMT) are rejection, graft-versus-host disease (GVHD), and infection. The new stem cells must relocate and grow in their new body. If the patient's immune system has not been suppressed adequately, the new marrow may be rejected. Rejection is more frequent in mismatched or unrelated donor transplants. The donor's marrow also may not grow well if the patient has a significant infection. Fortunately, in children with leukemia, rejection occurs in less than 5 percent of allogeneic transplants.

GVHD affects approximately 30 to 50 percent of children who have undergone an allogeneic transplant. It affects a higher percentage of children whose transplants used mismatched marrow or marrow from an unrelated donor. GVHD is a reaction of the donor stem cells against the patient (host). It may be triggered by HLA antigen differences, by the chemotherapy and irradiation used to prepare the patient for transplantation, or by infections. While GVHD is a serious complication, it may in fact decrease the likelihood that the child will relapse; this not-well-understood phenomenon is called the graft-versus-leukemia (GVL) effect. GVHD is discussed in detail later in this chapter.

Transplant centers use a variety of methods to reduce the risk of infection. The most effective methods are single-room isolation; thorough hand washing; and using screened, filtered, and irradiated blood products. Other infection control methods—air filters; requirements to cap, gown, and wear masks before visiting the patient; and prohibiting live plants, fruits, and vegetables in the patient's room—remain unproven.

Autologous SCT

In an autologous SCT, the stem cells come from the child's own blood or bone marrow. Some transplant centers use various methods to try to purge (kill) any leukemic cells that may be in the autologous product. Ongoing studies are evaluating the risks and benefits of purged versus unpurged autologous transplants and to determine whether autologous transplantation is better than conventional chemotherapy.

After the marrow is harvested and treated, it is cryopreserved (frozen). The child then undergoes radiation and chemotherapy, or high-dose chemotherapy alone, to destroy any remaining leukemia. The frozen marrow is then thawed and reinfused into the child intravenously.

Because the child's own stem cells are used with this method, the child does not develop GVHD. Because GVHD suppresses the immune system and decreases resistance to infection, severe or fatal infections are less common after autologous transplants than allogeneic transplants. However, children who undergo autologous transplants have higher relapse rates because of residual leukemic cells in the marrow or, perhaps, because there is no GVL effect from GVHD. Patients who develop GVHD after an allogeneic transplant and survive have lower relapse rates than children who have an autologous or syngeneic transplant.

Syngeneic transplants

Syngeneic transplants are those in which the donor is the patient's identical twin. Because the marrow exactly matches the patient's, GVHD is prevented. However, as with autologous transplants, any possible GVL benefit is absent in syngeneic transplants.

> Jeremy had a syngeneic transplant from his identical twin brother as his donor to treat his secondary AML after treatment for Ewing's sarcoma. He received Cytoxan® and radiation in his conditioning regimen. One of the worst side effects he experienced was the nausea and vomiting. He was released from the hospital on Day 9, readmitted on Day 11 because of an infection, and discharged again on Day 12. We stayed near the hospital, and then we were allowed to go home on Day 30. He has done very well.

Placental blood/umbilical cord blood SCT

Placental blood/umbilical cord blood is a rich source of stem cells. Some institutions perform transplants using the umbilical cord blood obtained during the birth of a sibling (and frozen for future use) or from preserved unrelated donor cord blood. The number of stem cells in cord blood is usually sufficient for most children, but it may not be adequate for heavier children or adults. Engraftment may take longer with this type of transplant than with SCTs from other sources, but these transplants also tend to cause less GVHD.

> Our 15-month-old son, Garrett, was diagnosed with AML M4 and had CNS (central nervous system) involvement. He relapsed on treatment, and the doctors recommended a cord blood transplant. There was one perfect match in Barcelona, Spain. It matched six out of six and was also a molecular match. I wanted to fly to Barcelona and hug everyone I could see.

He was so sick during treatment, which included a trip to the ICU (intensive care unit) and several periods of extended hospitalization for complications, that the transplant was almost anticlimactic. He had cranial radiation, TBI (total body irradiation), then chemotherapy. He engrafted on Day 12 and was out on Day 21. He did wonderfully—he only got one fever, no GVHD, no other problems. He has not been inpatient since, and it's been 4 years.

GVHD occurs less frequently and may be more delayed in cord blood transplants than in peripheral blood or marrow transplants from similarly matched related or unrelated donors. In addition, cord blood is rarely contaminated by viruses such as cytomegalovirus (CMV) or Epstein Barr virus (EBV) that can cause life-threatening complications after a BMT. Cord blood SCT is one of many promising new directions in the research efforts to improve SCT. For information about public, private, and family cord blood banks, visit the Parent's Guide to Cord Blood Foundation at *www.parentsguidecordblood. org*. For information about the availability and effectiveness of cord blood transplants visit the Cord Blood Forum at *www.cordbloodforum.org/index.html.*

Christopher received his cord blood unit after 3 days of total body irradiation, testicular radiation, and other conditioning with ATG (antithymocyte globulin), cyclophosphamide, and thiotepa. He had a feeding tube inserted during his final TBI, so we didn't have to worry about eating. However, he did have a few problems keeping fluids up on the cyclosporin, so we kept the feeds running overnight for a couple of months to keep the fluids boosted. He engrafted on day +10 with a little GVHD, which was treated with prednisone. After he was discharged from the hospital, he was readmitted a few times for fevers. Overall it went very well. Our biggest problems now are fixing his cataracts, waiting for results of his endocrine tests and bone tests, and getting educational support.

Summary

SCT protocols vary among institutions and are continually evolving. Many aspects of SCT—for example, the GVL effect—are not well understood, but they are under intense scientific scrutiny. Research is also underway to identify those children most likely to benefit from a transplant, the best time to transplant, which new drugs best reduce the likelihood of infection, and the best methods to reduce post-transplant relapse.

For more information about types of transplants, write or phone BMT InfoNet, 2310 Skokie Valley Road, Suite 104, Highland Park, IL 60035, (888) 597-7674. The Blood and Marrow Transplant Newsletter is also published electronically on the Internet at *www.bmtinfonet.org.*

Collecting stem cells

Stem cells can be obtained from an umbilical cord (described in the previous section), bone marrow, or the blood.

Bone marrow

While the donor or patient (for autologous transplant) is under general anesthesia, the doctor inserts a large needle into the bones of the hips and withdraws bone marrow. This procedure is repeated enough times (usually 50 to 150) to remove 10 to 15 cc of marrow per kilogram of patient weight. The entire process usually takes less than 1 hour. After marrow donation, some hospitals keep the donor overnight, while others discharge the same day if the donor is not in pain.

Because the amount of marrow that is removed contains less than 5 percent of the donor's developing blood cells, it only takes a few days for the body to replace the marrow. The donor is usually sore for a day or two and may feel a bit tired for several days. The recovery time varies from donor to donor. The main risk of donating marrow is from the use of anesthesia. However, in an otherwise healthy donor the risk of a severe complication is less than 1 in 1,000.

> After no match was found for Christie in the 4,000 donors that we signed up and typed, I became her donor. We were just a partial match. Being her donor was just wonderful. It was Mother's Day weekend, and I was just full of faith and love. I thought this is it; God has given me a second chance to give life to this child. I had a very powerful feeling that it was so special that I could do this for my daughter. I really felt that this was it, it was going to work.

> It was uncomfortable for a couple of days, and I was a little bruised. But the people there were wonderful, and they really followed me closely. I'm still on the registry; if someone called me tomorrow, I'd be on a plane. It's a very rewarding feeling, a gift from God.

· · · · ·

> Jody's 2-year-old brother, Christoph, was a perfect match. I stayed with him when he donated marrow, and my husband stayed with Jody. Christoph seemed to handle the marrow donation easily. Although he had some nausea in the recovery room, he was up and running around late that afternoon saying, "I the donor." He felt very proud. I knew he was somewhat sore because he said, "My diaper hurts."

Blood

When doctors aspirate bone marrow from the cavities in bones, it is full of stem cells—cells from which all types of blood cells evolve. Stem cells can also be found in the circulating (also called peripheral) blood, although in much lower numbers.

In a peripheral blood SCT (PBSCT), the child's own blood stem cells are harvested in a procedure called apheresis or leukapheresis. The apheresis is performed as the child is recovering from an intensive course of chemotherapy. As blood counts begin to improve, the number of stem cells in the blood increases. Most centers also treat the child with GCSF (granulocyte colony stimulating factor) and/or GMCSF (granulocyte–macrophage colony stimulating factor) after the chemotherapy to further increase the number of stem cells in the blood.

> Six-year-old Ethan sailed through the stem cell harvest. He was on Neupogen®
> (GCSF), which is an injectable med that stimulates white cell release from the mar-
> row. Neupogen® has been a piece of cake for Ethan. Once he had enough of the stem
> cells in his bloodstream, he had a femoral PICC (peripherally inserted central cath-
> eter) line placed because they needed a larger catheter to do the harvest. The only
> downside was that he had to lie completely flat for about 6 hours, and collection took
> 2 days. Plan a lot of quiet activities! Videos, books on tape, handheld games, cards.

When the child's peripheral blood counts rise, blood is removed through a central venous catheter or a special temporary pheresis catheter and circulated through a machine that extracts the stem cells. The blood is then returned to the child. Each pheresis session lasts 2 to 8 hours. The number of sessions required varies. Infants may need only one session, but children who have received extensive prior irradiation or chemotherapy may need six or eight sessions.

In rare cases, it is impossible to get enough stem cells from children who have recently undergone extensive chemotherapy and/or irradiation. In these children, a bone marrow harvest may be able to collect an adequate number of stem cells.

Potential complications of peripheral blood stem cell apheresis include:

- **Hypocalcemia (low calcium in the blood).** Your child may experience muscle cramps, chills, tremors, tingling of the fingers and toes, dizziness, or occasional chest pain.

- **Thrombocytopenia (low platelets).** A reduction in the number of platelets can occur if platelets stick to the tubes of the apheresis machine. Your child's platelet count will be checked before and after the apheresis, and a platelet transfusion will be given if needed.

- **Hypovolemia (low blood volume).** A reduction in blood volume can occur at any time during the procedure and is more common in small children. Symptoms can include low blood pressure, rapid heart rate, lightheadedness, and sweating.

- **Infection.** In many cases, a new and larger central venous catheter is placed prior to the apheresis procedure to reduce the likelihood of infection. If your child develops fever, chills, or low blood pressure (symptoms of infection), blood cultures will be obtained and IV antibiotics will be given.

Most apheresis procedures are performed safely on an outpatient basis or in a short-stay clinic or hospital unit. Some institutions, however, do require hospitalization for the procedure.

Finding a donor

Finding a marrow donor can be a stressful and time-consuming task. The search may begin after relapse for children with ALL, in first remission for children with AML or some types of high-risk ALL, during the chronic phase for children with CML, and soon after diagnosis for children with JMML. In some families, tests show that a sibling or parent is a partial or identical match. Other children, especially those from minority groups not well represented in the donor files, can wait months or years for a match, or a match may not be found.

> My advice to parents just beginning the process is do not rely on anyone else to make all the arrangements for a donor search and financial arrangements with the transplant center. We were focused on my son's relapse treatment and thought a donor search was ongoing. We then found out that over 2 precious months had been lost in a delay for financial approval. I foolishly relied on my doctor and his staff to make arrangements and follow through, and it just slipped through the cracks. I should have been on the phone several times a week making sure the search had begun and that the transplant center was happy with the financial arrangements. I have a lot of guilt over whether those months made a difference in my son's outcome. I'll never know.

The first step in determining if a person is an HLA match is to obtain a sample of blood and send it to a laboratory for analysis. Each full sibling and biological parent is also HLA-typed. If a match is not found, the search widens to the unrelated donor registries or placental blood banks. Appendix B, "Resource Organizations," lists registries, foundations, and programs that can help you find a donor.

> Christie had a rare HLA type, and we could not find a match in all the registries worldwide. We decided that we had to do it on our own and began a donor drive in our town, which is predominantly Italian. The Red Cross discouraged us, saying

that we probably wouldn't get a good response, that they could not process the blood without the money ($45 per person) in hand, and that it would be better to spend quality time with Christie. But when the community of Rochester found out, it just snowballed. Dave and I went on TV and advocated for Christie, stressing the importance of Christie's bone marrow drive, and told people that this might help their own child one day. The first day of the drive, people lined up outside and stood for hours in the freezing rain and cold. The response was so overwhelming that late in the day they ran out of supplies. Large corporations became involved; one did a telethon that raised over $50,000. We typed over 4,000 people from Rochester and received letters from all over the country. It was just a beautiful thing. Christie was such a powerful little person, and she came to represent so much to our community.

• • • • •

We felt it was an omen that Jody's older sister and younger brother were perfect matches. They chose Marieke because she was older; but after all of the workup and tests, they discovered that she was CMV positive, so they used 2-year-old Christoph's marrow. Marieke was very disappointed.

If a sibling or other relative is identified as the best donor, that person needs to have the risks of donation fully explained. This discussion should take place in a non-threatening setting without pressure from the child's parents. The transplant team should explain that although the transplant is the best treatment for the patient, results of the transplant cannot be predicted. The success or failure of the transplant is not the donor's fault. Some centers will have a psychologist verify that a minor donor truly understands what is being requested and has not been pressured by parents to agree.

If a child needs a marrow transplant from an unrelated donor, the national and international registries are asked to conduct a computerized search of their databases. This search will identify any donors with the same HLA type as the child. The registry then contacts the potential donor to ask if he will donate more blood samples for additional tests.

While they were trying to find a match for JaNette, the church started a fundraiser and donor sign-up drive. They signed up over 600 people in 2 days, and United Blood Service had matching funds available to offset some of the costs. Meanwhile, we found an unrelated donor who lived in Milwaukee. She donated the marrow there, and a nurse from UCLA flew out to pick it up.

If the testing shows compatibility, the donor is given an extensive explanation of the entire donation procedure and a complete medical exam. The donor must then make a final commitment to provide marrow for the child in need.

Choosing a transplant center

Choosing a transplant center is an extremely important decision. Institutions may just be starting a bone marrow or blood stem cell program, or they may have vast experience. Some may be excellent for adults, but have limited pediatric experience. Some may allow you to room in with your child; others may isolate the child for weeks. Protocols also vary among institutions. The center closest to your home may not provide the best medical care available for your child or allow the necessary quality of life options (rooming in, social workers, etc.) that you need. Additionally, your insurance plan may require you and your child to go to a transplant center with which it has an existing contract.

To obtain a list of transplant centers, visit the National Marrow Donor Program (NMDP) site at *www.marrow.org,* click on "Patients and Families," then click on "Planning Your Transplant," and then "Choosing a Transplant Center." Or call (800) 627-7692 for general information or (888) 999-6743 for patient advocacy. Asking the following questions can help you learn about the policies of different transplant centers:

• How many pediatric transplants did the institution do last year? How many of the type recommended for my child?

• How successful is your program? What are the 1-year, 2-year, and 5-year survival rates for children with the same type and severity of disease? (Remember that some institutions accept very high-risk patients, so their statistics would not compare to those of a place that only performs less risky transplants.)

• How do cure rates with immediate transplantation compare with overall cure rates using chemotherapy first and transplantation only if the child has a relapse?

• What are the antigen match requirements? (Some institutions require a six-antigen match, others require five out of six, others permit a minor mismatch at the A or B antigen site but not at other antigen sites.)

• What is the nurse-to-patient ratio? Do all the staff members have pediatric training and experience?

• What support staff is available (e.g., educator, social worker, child life therapist, chaplain, etc.)?

• Will my child be in a pediatric or combined adult-pediatric unit?

• What are the institution's rules about parents staying in the child's hospital room?

• What on-site or nearby housing is available for families of children undergoing transplants? What are the costs for this housing?

• What are the institution's anti-infection requirements? Isolation? Gown and gloves? Masks? Washing hands?

- Describe the transplant procedure in detail. Is radiation part of the pretransplant treatment?

- Explain the risks and benefits of the transplant.

- What is the average length of time before a child leaves the hospital? For a child who has been discharged from the hospital but whose home is far away, how long before he can leave the area to go home?

- What will my child's life be like, assuming all goes perfectly? What will it be like if there are problems?

- What are the long-term side effects of this type of transplant? What long-term follow-up is available?

- Explain the waiting list requirements.

- How much will this procedure cost? How much will my insurance cover?

Many transplant centers have videos and booklets for patients and their families to explain services and describe what to expect before, during, and after the transplant. Call any transplant center that you are considering and ask them to send you all available materials.

> The head of oncology at UCLA comes to our city every 2 months to follow up on the kids who have been treated there. It was a big draw to us to have post-transplant follow-up at home, rather than having to travel a great distance to get back to the center. The other thing was that children are not put in laminar air flow, and families weren't required to cap and gown, only scrub their hands. Since I'm allergic to those hospital gloves, this allowed me to stay with my daughter throughout. We did, however, call around to several centers to compare facilities, costs, and insurance coverage.

Making an informed consent is a serious decision when considering a life-threatening procedure such as a bone marrow or other type of stem cell transplant. It is very important to work closely with your oncologist and treatment team when making this decision. Do not hesitate to keep asking questions until you fully understand what is being proposed. Ask the doctors to use plain English if they are using complicated medical terms. Bring a tape recorder or friend to help you remember the information. Many centers require the assent of children 7 to 18 years old in addition to parental consent. You do not have to sign the consent form until you feel comfortable that you understand the procedure and have had every question answered.

Paying for the transplant

SCTs are expensive. Some transplants are considered standard of care, so insurers cover the procedure without problems. However, you will need to research carefully whether your insurance company considers the type of transplant proposed for your child to be experimental and therefore not covered. Most insurance plans have a lifetime cap, and many only pay 80 percent of the costs of the transplant up to the cap. Often, transplant centers will not perform the procedure without all of the money guaranteed. With time being of the essence, this can cause great anguish for families who struggle to raise funds or need to take out a second mortgage to pay the costs of SCT.

Most insurance companies will assign your child's care to a transplant coordinator or case manager whose responsibility it is to make arrangements with the transplant center and handle financial issues. Getting to know your coordinator and letting that person know your needs and concerns may provide an additional valuable resource for you during this stressful time.

> Our first quote from the transplant center was $350,000, but we were able to negotiate a lower price.

· · · · ·

> My son died soon after the transplant. I hate to talk about the money, because I don't want people to think I begrudge spending it. I know that I would feel differently if the transplant had been successful, but I honestly think that we were misled about the real chance of success for his type of disease. We spent the equity on our house, plus took out a second mortgage. We will be paying it off for the rest of our lives.

If you are having difficulty getting your insurance company to pay for the transplant, the *Blood and Marrow Newsletter* provides a free referral service to attorneys and not-for-profit organizations who may be able to help you. Fill in the form at *www.bmtinfonet. org/attorney.html* or phone (888) 597-7674.

> When our son needed a transplant for AML, the insurance company kept refusing to pay because they said it was "experimental." So my wife became good friends with the catastrophic caseworker. The caseworker was extremely helpful. When it was disallowed again, she was upset and called my wife and said, "I'm going to tell you how to get this thing approved." She dictated two letters to my wife: one for unrelated transplant and one for cord blood. The doctor sent them in, and they quickly approved the unrelated transplant but denied the cord blood again as experimental, although our doctor thought cord blood was his best hope. With some more coaching from the caseworker, a third attempt at a cord blood approval was successful. The caseworker even called my wife with the good news before she alerted the hospital. Her help most likely saved my son's life.

If you are not insured (or are underinsured) and must raise all or part of the necessary funds, you can contact the organizations listed in Appendix C, "Books, Websites, and Videotapes," that provide financial assistance. They may be able to offer financial help and provide advice about how to raise funds quickly and effectively. Before working with any of these organizations, ask for all printed information available about them and ask questions about any fees or costs associated with their services. Make sure that when the treatment is completed, or if the child dies, any remaining funds will be applied to outstanding medical debts.

In Canada, each province and territory has a provincial health plan that covers the medical costs of transplantation. However, there are still expenses that will need to be covered by the family. Children will often have to travel long distances to facilities that are capable of performing a transplant. Travel, accommodations, and related costs have to be paid for by the parents. SCTs place financial burdens on all families, even if their country has a standardized healthcare system.

> Our HMO (health maintenance organization) refused to pay for our daughter's bone marrow transplant because it required an unrelated donor, which they considered to be "experimental." Her oncologist and several doctors from the transplant center gathered data and presented it to the insurance board. The HMO reversed its position and paid for the transplant, but not for the donor search, donor fees, donor harvest, or having the marrow transported from London. It cost us approximately $25,000.

The transplant

Prior to the actual transplant, the patient's bone marrow is destroyed or suppressed using high-dose chemotherapy with or without radiation. This portion of treatment is called conditioning. The purpose of the high doses of chemotherapy and radiation is to kill most or all of the remaining cancer cells in the body and to make room in the bones for the new bone marrow or stem cells. For allogeneic transplants, the conditioning also suppresses the patient's immunity in order to give the donor marrow a better chance to grow.

Conditioning regimens vary according to institution and protocol; they also depend on the medical condition and history of the child. Typically, the chemotherapy is given for 2 to 6 days, and radiation (if part of conditioning) is given in multiple small doses over several days.

> They got JaNette into her second remission in December, then gave her maintenance drugs to keep her there until they were ready to start transplant conditioning in April. So, unlike some of the other kids, she went to transplant healthy and strong. JaNette had 1,200 cGy of total body radiation in five increments—two the first day,

two the second day, and one the third day. Then she had 2 days of incredibly strong chemotherapy, 1 day of rest, then the transplant.

The transplant itself consists of simply infusing the stem cells through a central venous catheter, just like a blood transfusion. The marrow or stem cells travel through the blood vessels, eventually filling the empty marrow spaces in the bones. When the new marrow begins to produce healthy white cells, red cells, and platelets, it is called engraftment. This typically occurs from 2 to 6 weeks after transplantation but may vary according to the source and number of stem cells given. Complete recovery of all components of immune function can take from 1 to 2 years.

I couldn't believe how beautiful the bone marrow was—a bag of shimmering red liquid. It just glistened. It meant life.

• • • • •

My dad donated marrow for my transplant. He said he was sore and doing the "bone marrow hop," but he made it to my room that day to see his marrow transfused into me. I really felt different as I was getting the bone marrow, like I was getting so much more energy.

• • • • •

I cannot say enough good things about the transplant center. They were very family-oriented, allowed us in the room 24 hours a day. I was allowed to sleep in bed with her (I just told the nurses to make sure to poke her and not me). The nurses were wonderful, and I still think of them as family. We didn't get very close to the other families; we tended to stay in our own child's room. One day a family would be there, then the next day they would be gone. I got to the point where I just didn't want to know.

• • • • •

We were prepared to stay 5 months in or near the transplant center, but we went home after only 2 ½. She had the normal nausea, so she was on TPN (total parenteral nutrition) from her transplant on May 5 until the end of June. Until she could take her medications by mouth, I did some IVs at home. She had her last platelet transfusion in July. It took until the following June for her counts to normalize and for her to start producing T cells. We feel lucky that things went so well.

Donor and patient confidentiality are closely guarded. The NMDP allows letter exchanges or meetings if both donor and recipient express a strong desire to do so, but only after a year has passed since the transplant.

Emotional responses

SCT can take a heavy emotional toll on the child, parents, and siblings. It can be a physically and mentally grueling procedure, with the possibility of months or years of after effects. Most transplant team members are extensively trained to meet the needs of the patient and family during the transplant and long convalescence. The team includes physicians and nurses, psychiatrists, social workers, chaplains, educators, nutritionists, and child life therapists.

> Christie had many painful complications after the unmatched allogeneic transplant. I remember lying next to her and saying, "Christie, if Mommy could take this away from you I would." She looked at me and said, "Mommy, I love you so much, I would never want you to go through this." But then she went on to say, "It's not so bad. I met a lot of people; we got to travel; Daddy didn't have to work; Danielle and Nicole got to spend time with Daddy." She just saw something positive in everything, even this terrible disease.

> Christie was also very, very funny. She loved having me be the donor, and she started calling me her "blood sister." She kept saying, "Ma, when am I going to start being funny like you?" And I'd tell her that she was way beyond me. Her humor was contagious.

· · · · ·

> Leah was feeling good and was very healthy when she went into the laminar air flow room. We lived near the transplant center, and she had many visitors. I think the visits and the nonstop telephone conversations really kept her spirits up.

· · · · ·

> What helped me the most were the decorations and having a positive attitude. My mom decorated the area outside the LAF (laminar air flow) room with balloons, cards, and posters. It was hard to take the medicine, so my mom made a huge poster to mark off how well I did. Every time I took my medicine, I got a sticker. When I got 100 stickers, I got some roller blades.

· · · · ·

> I felt great during the transplant and at the center, but when we came home it was very, very difficult. We had just moved before my daughter was transplanted, so we didn't have a good support system in place. She had been in the hospital and the transplant center for almost a year, and then we had to stay at home for another year. For a few months she would spike a fever every time someone who was not in the family came in the house. So my young son could never have friends over. We just stayed home. It was very hard, and we all felt very isolated.

Often so much time and energy is focused on the child who needs the transplant that the needs of the siblings are overlooked. Siblings need careful preparation for what is about to occur, and all their questions need to be answered and concerns addressed. If a sibling is the stem cell donor, parents need to assure him or her that the results of the transplant are out of everyone's control. That is, the sibling is not responsible for the brother or sister's life or death. Studies have shown that regardless of transplant outcome, the vast majority of donors feel that their donation was one of the best things they have ever done.

Organizations that can offer emotional support to families during the transplant are listed in Appendix B, "Resource Organizations."

Complications

Some children have a smooth journey through the transplant process, while others bounce from one life-threatening complication to another. Some children live, and some children die. There is no way to predict which children or teens will develop problems, nor is there any way to anticipate whether the new development will be merely an inconvenience or a catastrophe. This section will present some of the major complications that can develop after a transplant, along with the experiences of several families who faced these problems.

Failure to engraft

Engraftment means that the donated stem cells take up residence in the child's bones and begin to produce healthy blood cells. When a child has received HLA-matched marrow from a sibling, engraftment failure (graft rejection) occurs in less than 5 percent of these children. In contrast, when children have received marrow from partially HLA-matched family members or unrelated donors, engraftment failure is more frequent, unless more intensive conditioning regimens are used. The pace of engraftment depends upon the stem cell source, stem cell dose, and medical complications that may be present.

Infections

Most infections following transplant come from organisms within the body (e.g., cytomegalovirus (CMV), mouth and gut bacteria). Good hand washing by parents, visitors, and healthcare workers can help decrease infection risks from bacteria and fungi.

The immune systems of healthy children quickly destroy any foreign invaders; this is not so with children who have undergone a transplant. The immune systems of these children have been destroyed by chemotherapy and radiation to allow the healthy stem cells to grow. Until the new stem cells engraft and begin to produce large numbers of functioning white cells, children post-transplant are in danger of developing serious infections.

During conditioning and until recovery of neutrophil counts, children are at high risk for developing bacterial infections. Fungal infections can also occur. The use of growth factors (such as GCSF) that stimulate and accelerate white blood cell recovery has decreased the time it takes for neutrophil engraftment, thus decreasing the incidence of serious infections. Your child may receive this medication 1 to 2 days following the transplant procedure. Additionally, your child will be evaluated carefully each day for signs and symptoms of infection. Potential sites for problems include the skin, mouth, perirectal area, and central venous catheter exit site. Immediately report to the nurses any new symptoms such as cough, shortness of breath, abdominal pain, diarrhea, pain with urination, vaginal discharge, or mental confusion. Antibiotics will be started promptly for any signs of infection. Some centers will use prophylactic (preventive) antibiotics even without signs of infection.

> Leah had so many problems with infections and getting her counts back up that she spent 2 years on steroids, cyclosporin, and monthly gammaglobulin.

· · · · ·

> During the related mismatched allogeneic transplant, I developed no mouth sores, no infections, no GVHD. Just a headache the whole time. I do miss being an athlete, I do miss the friends that I lost, and I do miss my blond hair. (It came back in brown, so I tried to dye it blond, and it turned bright, fluorescent red.) But I can deal with those things. To survive I think you need luck, a positive attitude, and a decorated room to help you stay cheery.

After the first month post-transplant, children are also susceptible to serious viral infections, most commonly herpes simplex virus, CMV, and varicella zoster virus, particularly if they have GVHD. These infections can occur up to 2 years after the transplant. Viral infections are notoriously hard to treat, so many centers use prophylactic acyclovir, granciclovir, or immunoglobulin to prevent them. The most common organisms that cause infections are CMV and pneumocystis carinii. CMV is usually preventable if the patient and donor are both CMV-negative and all transfused blood products are CMV-negative or filtered to remove white blood cells. The risk of pneumocystis carinii infection can be decreased by using prophylactic trimethoprim/sulfamethoxazole once engraftment has occurred.

Interstitial pneumonitis, a sometimes fatal form of pneumonia, is most common the second or third month post-transplant. It is uncommon after autologous transplants and is most often associated with GVHD after allogeneic transplants.

Immunity is not carried over from the donor to the patient. Therefore, the patient has to redevelop her immune system. If there is no GVHD, the immune recovery process will require at least 6 to 12 months. If GVHD is present, the recovery period may take years. During immune recovery, a patient must redevelop immunity to the common organisms that infect all children, which will require redoing the usual childhood immunizations. Live virus vaccines should be avoided, however, because the immune system after transplantation is very fragile and may not be able to handle a large viral load.

Preventing infections is the best policy for children who have had a bone marrow or stem cell transplant. The following are suggestions to minimize exposure to bacteria, viruses, and fungi:

- Medical staff and all family members must wash their hands before touching the child.

- Keep your child away from crowds and people with infections.

- Do not let your child receive live virus inoculations until the immune system has fully recovered. Your child's oncologist will determine the appropriate date for reinitiating immunizations.

- Keep your child away from anyone who recently has been inoculated with a live virus (e.g., chicken pox, polio).

- Keep your child away from barnyard animals and all types of animal feces.

- Have all carpets shampooed before the child returns home from the transplant.

- Avoid home remodeling while your child is recovering.

- Call the doctor at the first sign of a fever or infection.

For more information about infections, read Chapter 10 of *Bone Marrow Transplants: A Book of Basics for Patients*, by Susan Stewart. (These and other useful resources are listed in Appendix C.)

Graft-versus-host disease

Graft-versus-host disease (GVHD) is a frequent complication of allogeneic BMTs. It rarely occurs with autologous or syngeneic transplants. In GVHD, the bone marrow or stem cells provided by the donor (graft) attack the tissues and organs of the child receiving the transplant (host). This attack may occur because of HLA (or other) antigen differences between the donor and the patient. Toxicities from conditioning and infections may also contribute to the development of GVHD. Approximately 30 to 50 percent of children who have a related HLA-matched transplant develop some degree of GVHD. The incidence and severity of GVHD are increased for children who receive unrelated or mismatched marrow, but are decreased if cells that cause GVHD are reduced prior to infusion. The majority of GVHD cases are mild, although some can be life-threatening or fatal.

There are two types of GVHD: acute and chronic. Children can develop one type, both types, or neither. Acute GVHD usually occurs at the time of engraftment or shortly thereafter. Donor cells identify the patient's cells as foreign, and may attack the patient's skin, liver, or intestines. This immune reaction may result in fevers, skin rash, diarrhea, and liver problems. Allogeneic SCT patients are given immunosupressive drugs (such as methotrexate, cyclosporine, steroids, and others) before and after transplant in an attempt to prevent GVHD. Acute GVHD is treated with cyclosporin and steroids (prednisone, dexamethasone).

> JaNette's transplant was on May 5 and her ANC was up to 1,000 on May 30. That's when her graft-versus-host started. It doesn't look like a regular rash, more like pinpoint red dots under the skin. It's very itchy, and then it starts to peel. She looked like she had leprosy! She had very little internal graft-versus-host disease. She's a year and a half post-transplant, and she still broke out in a rash the last time they tried to taper her off the cyclosporin.

• • • • •

> Ryan died from acute graft-versus-host disease. It destroyed his liver. It was a hard death, and we felt that it robbed us of whatever time he would have had left if he hadn't had the BMT.

Chronic GVHD usually develops after the third month post-transplant. It primarily affects the skin (itchy rash, discoloration of the skin, tightening of the skin, hair loss), eyes (dry, light-sensitive), mouth and esophagus (dry, tooth decay, difficulty swallowing), intestines (diarrhea, cramping, poor absorption of foods, weight loss), liver (jaundice), lungs (shortness of breath, wheezing, coughing), and joints (decreased mobility). This list may seem overwhelming, but remember that only some patients develop chronic GVHD, and those who do may experience all, a few, or only one of these symptoms.

> A year and a half after the transplant, they tried to taper my daughter off the cyclosporin. Her liver function counts went way up, and she broke out in a rash all over her body. The bottoms of her feet were so blistered that she couldn't walk. She has permanent dark splotches all over her torso, but the ones on her face and neck gradually faded away.

• • • • •

> I wasn't supposed to go out in the sun after my transplant, but I did anyway. The sun aggravated the mild GVHD that I had, and I turned blotchy. I had itchy light and dark patches on my stomach and face. I had to go back on steroids.

Bleeding

Bleeding may occur throughout your child's post-transplant recovery phase until adequate engraftment occurs. Nosebleeds, bruising, and bleeding from the gums, urinary tract, or gastrointestinal tract are all common problems. Generally, these problems are handled with platelet transfusions. Most transplant centers strive to keep children's platelet counts at a safe level until bone marrow recovery occurs. Generally speaking, platelets are the last type of blood cell to fully recover following a stem cell transplant.

Hemorrhagic cystitis

Hemorrhagic cystitis (bleeding from the bladder) may result from the use of certain chemotherapy drugs in your child's conditioning regimen. Occasionally, the bleeding is caused by a bacterial or viral bladder infection. Symptoms of hemorrhagic cystitis include blood in the urine (which may be obvious to the eye or microscopic), blood clots in the urine, pain with urination, and bladder discomfort. If your child receives a chemotherapy drug that has the potential to cause this problem, the drug mesna may be used to decrease the risk of bladder damage due to cyclophosphamide and related drugs. If your child develops hemorrhagic cystitis or a urinary tract infection, she will receive antibiotics, IV fluids, and pain medication as needed.

Mucositis

Mucositis (inflammation of the mucous membranes lining the mouth and gastrointestinal tract) and stomatitis (mouth sores) are common complications following SCTs. Symptoms include reddened, discolored, or ulcerated membranes of the mouth, pain, difficulty swallowing, taste alterations, and difficulty speaking. The majority of children undergoing transplants experience this problem.

If mucositis occurs, your child will require frequent mouth care, modifications in diet, and pain medications. It is important to coordinate your child's required mouth care with the administration of appropriate pain medications. Likewise, make sure your child receives pain medication before eating, drinking, or taking oral medication. When white blood cells return, your child's mouth will heal.

> High-dose chemo kills your taste buds, and I wanted to only eat sweet or spicy food. Anything else tasted like cardboard. I'd eat ribs with BBQ sauce. KFC® mashed potatoes and gravy was great. Drinking was hard. I used to suck on ice cubes. It's gross when the lining of your mouth comes out. It just pulls out; it's white, and it doesn't hurt. It comes out during bowel movements, too, but you don't realize it. But, you can't swallow because of the sores, so you have to spit a lot.

Eating difficulties

The vast majority of children undergoing SCTs require IV nutrition during their convalescence. Some centers feed children using tubes inserted through the nose into the stomach or small intestine. Various factors can contribute to feeding problems, including pre-existing nutritional problems, side effects of conditioning chemotherapy, nausea and vomiting, mouth sores, and infections of the gastrointestinal tract. Your child may experience a few, some, or all of these problems before engraftment occurs. Most transplant centers initiate IV nutrition promptly after transplant and continue until your child's appetite and ability to take in adequate calories by mouth have returned.

Your child may require prophylactic ulcer medications to coat the lining of the stomach or to decrease the amount of stomach acid produced. Nausea may persist for a long time after completion of the conditioning chemotherapy. Ask to speak to the transplant unit dietitian and keep accurate records of your child's eating. As with mucositis, your child's ability to eat and drink more normally is closely correlated with the recovery of blood counts.

Veno-occlusive disease

Veno-occlusive disease (VOD) is a complication in which the flow of blood through the liver becomes obstructed. Children who have had more than one transplant, previous liver problems, or past exposure to intensive chemotherapy are more at risk of developing VOD. It can occur gradually or very quickly. Symptoms of VOD include jaundice (yellowing of the skin), enlarged liver, pain in the upper right abdomen, fluid in the abdomen, unexplained weight gain, and poor response to platelet transfusions. Treatment includes fluid restriction, diuretics (such as Lasix®), anti-clotting medications, and removal of all but the most essential amino acids from IV nutrition (hyperalimentation).

> *Every day I wake up, I am lucky. I kiss my kids good morning, yell at them to get dressed, make breakfast, pack lunches, and drive them to school. I get home and smile and say I am SO lucky. You see, leukemia has taught me to appreciate each and every day. I have learned so much about myself, and I am a much better person for it. Little things that might bug others just flow in one ear and out the other. My kids get so many hugs and kisses every day that they whine about it—OH MOM, not another one.*

> *Leukemia and cancer are part of our lives, but they are not our whole life. I remember so many bits and pieces of treatment, but our positive attitude is the thing I remember the most, and what others always commented on. During transplant, when things were really tough, I would turn on the music loud and all of us, including Robby hooked up to 10 different med lines, would get up and dance and sing.*

The nurses would come in and start dancing, and people would watch through the windows, wondering why they didn't get invited to our party.

What else did I get? I have a teenaged son who is the most gentle soul. Despite missing 60 percent of third grade for BMT, as well as many other missed days, he is in a school that is for the academically advanced and is in the top third of his class. He has three game balls from this baseball season, which are given to the player of the game. During basketball, his coach was amazed at his gift of never giving up, despite having virtually no talent for it. I have a child who helps the third graders carry their backpacks because they are too heavy. I have a child who opens doors for women and who gives up his seat to grown-ups. I have a child who loves playing with babies and making them laugh. I have a child who has his college picked out. I have a child who, when told he had relapsed, was concerned I would have to miss work so much.

I can remember, after the shock of hearing about our second relapse was gone, Robby made the comment, "I know I'm not going to die; look at all of the chemo that would have been wasted." Am I lucky—YOU BET.

Long-term side effects

Increasing numbers of children are being cured of their disease and surviving years after SCT. The intensity of the treatment before, during, and after transplant can have major effects that do not become apparent for months, or even years. This section will describe a few of the major long-term side effects that sometimes develop after SCT.

The transplant center was very clear about all of the potential problems. That was good, for it prepared me. My attitude is watch for them, hope they don't happen, but if they do, then live with them. JaNette has lost about 50 percent of her lung capacity, probably from the radiation. She has to do daily treatments to keep her lungs from tightening up. She still is on cyclosporin 1 ½ years later and flares up with the GVHD rash periodically. She can no longer tolerate gamma globulin, so her counts go down sometimes and she gets pneumonia. I know that she may get cataracts, develop heart problems, and many other things. But she had an easy time with the transplant, she's a happy third-grader, she's alive, and we feel so, so very lucky.

Relapse

Despite the intensive chemotherapy and/or radiation given prior to SCT, some children suffer a recurrence of the original disease. Relapse is most likely to occur in the first 2 years post-transplant.

Jody had his transplant in October, and we thought he was doing wonderfully. In June he just started getting tired and slowing down. We brought him in and found out that he had relapsed. They said there was no hope for a cure, but they thought that they could get him into remission again. He lived for another 15 months.

Eye problems

Some children treated with TBI develop cataracts. How the radiation is administered affects the child's chance of developing this complication. If the TBI is given in one dose, approximately 80 percent of children develop cataracts. If the TBI is given in smaller doses over several days (fractionated), the chance of developing cataracts is much lower (20 percent). Almost all protocols now use fractionated TBI.

> *My 8-year-old daughter is 6 years out from the full body radiation used to prepare her for bone marrow transplant. She had the first of two cataract surgeries Tuesday. It was an outpatient procedure, and she was a real trooper. The doctor was able to insert a permanent replacement lens, which is a good thing since it means we don't have to do the contact lens thing. I can't wait for the day when radiation is no longer a treatment for cancer. Until then I have to acknowledge begrudging thanks, because it saved my baby's life.*

Decreased tear production is common in children with chronic GVHD, but it is also sometimes seen in patients with no GVHD.

Dental development

Chemotherapy drugs, administered in high doses prior to SCT, may result in improper tooth development and blunted or absent tooth roots in children less than 5 years of age. Your child will likely have a comprehensive dental examination before the transplant and should have regular dental follow-up after recovery.

Growth and development

Children who receive TBI or radiation to the brain may have altered growth and development. All children who have had an SCT should get periodic evaluations from a pediatric endocrinologist to monitor growth and development. Growth hormone is sometimes necessary, especially for children who received radiation therapy.

Puberty and sterility

Children who had only chemotherapy during the conditioning regimen usually have normal sexual development, though not always. Those who had TBI, however, are particularly at risk for delayed puberty. (The incidence is lower if the radiation is fractionated.) All children receiving an SCT should be followed closely by a pediatric endocrinologist, who can prescribe hormones (testosterone for boys, estrogen and progesterone for girls) to assist in normal pubertal development. Girls are more likely to need hormonal replacement; boys usually produce testosterone but not sperm.

Children who receive TBI usually (but not always) become sterile; that is, after growing up, girls will not be able to become pregnant, nor will boys be able to father children. The ability to have a normal sex life is not affected. Some children treated only with chemotherapy have remained fertile, and their offspring are almost always healthy. Teenaged boys should bank sperm prior to beginning their conditioning regimen. The banking of eggs is more experimental and takes a much longer time to accomplish, so it is done infrequently.

Thyroid function

Children who receive only chemotherapy do not develop thyroid deficiency as a result of treatment. Children who receive TBI have a 25 to 50 percent chance of having low thyroid function due to a decreased production of thyroid hormone. Tablets containing thyroid hormone usually are effective in treating the problem.

Avascular necrosis

Long-term use of high-dose steroids can cause a problem called avascular necrosis. This condition is caused by the death of the small blood vessels that nourish the bones, resulting in pain and loss of mobility.

> Leslee was an athlete who played three sports prior to her AML diagnosis and bone marrow transplant. The steroids saved her life but destroyed her bones. She has had surgery on her shoulders, hips, and knee joints. Her shoulders and hips are much better, but her knees are still painful, and she has trouble getting around. The surgeon is hoping that soon he will be able to use live bone in experimental surgery to help her.

Second cancers

Children who receive SCT have a small risk of developing a second malignancy (cancer), particularly if TBI was used during conditioning. Because transplants are relatively new treatments for children and teens with cancer, the overall impact and long-term effects are not yet clear. Your doctor can explain known risks given your child's disease and treatment.

> At the age of 7, I was diagnosed with AML. After countless rounds of chemotherapy followed by total body radiation, I received a life-saving bone marrow transplant

from my older brother, Nathan. I consider myself to be incredibly lucky to be alive today. Yet, despite this medical miracle, my battle is not over.

As a result of the intensive cancer treatment, I experience chronic health issues such as a cardiomyopathy, endocrine dysfunction, and cataracts in both eyes. When I was 24, I was diagnosed with a secondary cancer—papillary thyroid cancer—a result of the total body radiation I received.

Due to the total body radiation and the cyclophosphamide that I received as a child, I was told that I would be sterile. Coming from a large family, I had always dreamed of having a child of my own. On April Fool's Day, when I was 28 years old, I was taking a routine pregnancy test prior to a medical procedure to scan for thyroid cancer and discovered I was pregnant! Twelve weeks pregnant!

I was fortunate to have both a fabulous oncologist and OB/GYN who managed my high-risk pregnancy. My cardiomyopathy was exacerbated by the pregnancy, leading to increased hypertension which was controlled by beta blockers. The total body radiation I received led to impaired uterine growth and a shortened cervix. Despite a cervical cerclage being placed in addition to being on bed rest, at 25 weeks gestation my daughter—Hope Isabella—arrived weighing 1 pound 7 ounces.

After 111 days in the NICU (neonatal intensive care unit) fighting for her life, she came home and continues to grow strong. To me, Hope is the epitome of a medical miracle. She is a wonderful example of how far we have come scientifically. She was born from an early BMT survivor who wasn't supposed to live to see her 8th birthday, and who was certainly not expected to be able to bear children. But, she also represents how far we have left to go to maintain cure rates while reducing late effects of treatments.

Chapter 22

Death and Bereavement

The loss of my son has illuminated for me the true definition of love: the giving of oneself, body and spirit, to another. His death, like that of any child, is a story of withered hopes and unfulfilled dreams. In this book I have tried to capture a few remembered strains of the brief, glad music of his life. These are all I have of him now, and they comfort me even as they break my heart.

— Gordon Livingstone, MD
Only Spring

THE DEATH OF A CHILD CAUSES almost unendurable pain and anguish for loved ones left behind. Death from cancer comes after months or years of debilitating treatments, emotional swings, and financial stress. The family begins the years of grief already exhausted from the years of fighting cancer. It is truly every parent's worst nightmare.

In this chapter, parents share their innermost thoughts and feelings about deciding to end treatment, dying at home or in the hospital, and grief. It didn't matter whether these parents had recently lost their child, or whether it had happened decades ago—tears flowed when they talked about their child's death. Family members and friends can be strong sources of support, but they can also become casualties of the grieving process. Here parents describe what really helped them, and they make suggestions about what to avoid. Grief has as many facets as there are grieving parents; what follows are the experiences of a few.

Transitioning from active treatment

For children who have had a series of relapses, medical caregivers and parents need to decide when to end active treatment and begin working toward making the child comfortable during his remaining days. This is an intensely personal decision. Some families want to try every available treatment and exhaust all possible remedies. Others reach a point where they feel they have done all they can, and they simply do not want their child to suffer any more. They hope for time to share memories, express love, and prepare for death.

After Christie came home from the transplant center, she started to perk up and feel a bit better. But she had pretty massive problems with graft-versus-host disease, infections, fragile bones, and a very weak heart. She had a stomach abscess that they thought was causing her vomiting and eating problems, so they decided to biopsy it. They came out and said they found a cluster of tumors on her ovary, which turned out to be malignant leukemic cells. In my rational mind, I knew it was time to stop. I could imagine stopping the treatment, but I just couldn't picture life without her.

Dr. Arthur Ablin, Director Emeritus of Pediatric Clinical Oncology at the University of California, San Francisco, wrote in the Spring 1995 Candlelighters newsletter about the difficulties of deciding to end active treatment:

All too often, the decision to abandon the goal for cure and, reluctantly, accept the reality of the inevitable death of a child is too painful and, therefore, never made. This paralyzing pain occurs with equal frequency, perhaps, for the family and the doctor. We of the medical profession have no equal in our ability to prolong dying. We have a powerful array of mechanical, electronic, pharmaceutical, and biotechnical interventions at our command. We can keep people from dying for months and even years. Applying or withholding this armamentarium is an awesome responsibility and it requires infinite wisdom to know how to manage wisely and correctly. We can do great good by applying these tools correctly but can also do incalculable harm through over-utilization. Physicians and families alike must work together to avoid the possible pitfalls…When cure is beyond all of us, then the challenge is to make the rest of life as worthwhile and rich as possible. There is much to do for the terminally and critically ill child and his or her family. They have that right, and we have the privilege to be of service.

One of the most difficult tasks parents will face is sharing the news with their child that treatments have stopped working. Older children and teenagers need to be an integral part of these discussions with the healthcare team. Their thoughts and feelings are crucial during the decision-making process. Honest, thorough communication between the ill child or teen, family members, and involved professionals helps everyone work together.

The history of Jody's battle with leukemia is long, and to me, marked with his resilience, strength, and incredibly strong spirit. He was diagnosed with ALL shortly after his second birthday. He relapsed just before he turned 3, then not again until he was 5 ½, 7 months after he went off chemotherapy treatment. He underwent a bone marrow transplant approached with the good omen of having a perfect match with both his older sister and younger brother, and thrived until another relapse at age 6 ½. Realistic hope for Jody's long-term survival was dashed at that time. Jody achieved another remission, which lasted for several months, then experienced a bone marrow relapse. We realized that the disease was systemic, and all conventional means of treating the leukemia were, finally, hopeless.

While the doctor was ready to present us with medical options that Thursday after-noon, we already knew our decision. It was rational: Jody should go off all chemo-therapy treatment. Jody's leukemia was clearly very resistant to chemotherapy drugs. It was ethical: With no chance of further good health and high-quality living, allow-ing death to come naturally was surely the best choice. It was humane: Jody would be treated for pain, and we would bring him home to die in familiar surroundings with his family. And it was sad: Jody's laughter wasn't to be heard again, he wasn't to feel good again, he was to become sicker and sicker and die. The unfathomable real-ity of life without Jody's presence was marching to meet us without reprieve.

Often, children take the lead in making the decision to stop treatment. In the Spring 1995 issue of the Candlelighters newsletter, Grace Monaco describes how her 4-year-old daughter told her, "I don't think I can come home, Mommy! All my machinery is worn out, and I don't think they have any more parts."

A 6-year-old shared how he felt with his parents:

When my 6-year-old son, Greg, was in the hospital in intensive relapse treatment, he would repeat over and over again, "I want to go home." When he was finally well enough to come home for awhile, he kept saying, "I want to go home." In frus-tration, I said, "Greg, you are home; why do you keep saying that?" He looked up and quietly said, "I want to go to my heavenly home. I want to go to God." I said, "Honey, please don't say that," and, knowing how much we loved him, he replied, "Okay, Mom, I'll fight, I won't go." And he did fight hard for several more months. But he was way ahead of us in acceptance, he was at peace, and he knew it was time to let go.

When it is clear that death is inevitable, parents struggle with the thought of how to discuss it with the ill child and siblings. All too often in our culture, children are per-ceived as having to be protected from death, as if this somehow makes their last days better. On the contrary, any pediatric nurse practitioner or social worker can tell you that children, often as young as 4, know they are dying. If the parents are trying to spare the child, an unhealthy situation develops. The child pretends everything is okay to please the parents, and the parents try to mask their deep grief with false smiles. Everyone loses.

Denial may keep children and parents alike from finishing up business—distributing belongings, telling each other how much they love one another, saying goodbye. It also strips parents of their ability to prepare their child for the journey from life to death. Children need to know what to expect. They need to know they will be surrounded by those they love and that their parents will be holding them. They also need to know what the family's beliefs are about what happens after death.

Jennifer contracted a respiratory fungal infection that resulted in her being hospital-ized on a ventilator. She was given lots of morphine so she wouldn't feel air hungry. She was alert off and on for a few days. We read to her and played tapes. After 1 week on the respirator she took a turn for the worse. She didn't respond to me after that. Her kidneys were ceasing to function, and she started to get puffy. Her liver was deteriorating, and her painful pancreatitis had come back. After 10 days on the respirator, I couldn't bear it any longer. I lay down in her bed, took her in my arms, and kissed her at least 200 times. I talked to her for a long time and told her that we would take care of her cats, and that I was sorry that she had to suffer so much, and how beautiful Heaven is. I told her to go be with Jesus, her Grandpa, and her dog. I also told her how much we all loved her and how proud we were of her. I got off the bed to change positions, and the nurse rushed in. Her heart had suddenly stopped the second I got up. I believe she heard me and just needed to know it was okay to go. She didn't want to leave until she knew her Mommy was ready.

She had told me that she wasn't afraid to die, and this has been a great source of comfort to us. I believe she was preparing for her death, even as we hoped for her remission. Before she went to the hospital, she spent all her money, gave away some of her possessions to her sisters, and said a final goodbye to her home, cats, teachers, and friends.

· · · · ·

After Caitlin decided she wanted no more treatments, we brought her home. She asked me to give her clothes to the poor, and her special things to her brothers. She gave them the last of her money, saying she no longer had any use for it. She had already bought them Christmas presents for the coming Christmas and had given them ahead of time. Her affairs were oh so in order. She asked my friend to make me laugh after she died. She told me that it wasn't dying she minded, because her friend who had already died had come in a dream and told her that heaven was a good place, but she did not want to leave her father and me. They were agonizing conversations, yet I am so glad that we were able to have them.

Supportive care

In the United States and Canada, there is a very active and effective hospice system. Hospices ease the transition from hospital to home and provide support for the entire family. Hospice personnel ensure adequate pain control, allow the patient to control the last days or weeks of his life, and provide active bereavement support after death.

Usually, if the family prefers that the child die at home, a smooth transition occurs from the oncology ward to hospice care. Unfortunately, pediatric patients are not always referred to hospice, and the parents are left to deal with their child's last days at home with no experienced help and no clear idea of what is to come. Your nurse practitio-ner, case manager, or hospital social worker can refer you to or help you find pediatric hospice care in your area. Before you leave the hospital, it is wise to find out the name of a contact person at the agency who will be supporting the home care of your child.

> *When Jody came home, he was assigned both a pediatric visiting nurse and a hospice nurse. On their first visits, I was handed a great deal of literature to read, including a whole notebook from hospice. I lacked both the desire and energy to read the literature and learn a whole new medical system—let alone two. I just wanted one phone number to call for help, with two or three consistent people to answer.*

> *In actuality, the care we received was wonderful. The primary nurse would call, offer to visit if we wanted it, assess Jody's condition over the phone, handle any questions we had, and would ask if we wanted a call the next day. She would tell us who would be calling if she was not working at the appointed time. Interestingly, the service that I found most beneficial at that time was the nurse running interference for us with the doctor. The pain medications needed to be adjusted and changed at times; advice was needed about his intake, his mouth sores, and his hand and foot inflammation. As I, along with Jody, became quieter and more removed from outside activities, even the thought of calling the clinic and being made directly aware of the bustle and demands of that world was very unappealing.*

Hospice not only provides home-based assistance in physically caring for your child, it can also provide emotional support for your child, you and your spouse, and any other children or family members in your home. If you have questions about hospice or what support is available, you can contact Children's Hospice International online at *www. chionline.org* or by phone at (800) 242-4453 (800-24-CHILD).

Dying in the hospital

Some children die in the hospital suddenly, while others slowly decline for weeks or months. If your child is dying slowly, you may have choices about where your child will spend her last days. There are no right or wrong choices. Much depends on the number of people available to provide care at home, and how comfortable they are doing so. Many parents ask their child where he or she would prefer to be. Some children and teens like to be with the nurses in a hospital environment, while others want to stay at home with brothers, sisters, friends, and pets.

Parents, children, and staff need to talk honestly to decide on the appropriate place for the child, and then obtain the support (e.g., hospice, private nurses in the hospital, family members) needed to make the choice a comfortable reality. Remain flexible so that as the situation changes, options remain open.

> *Although we had been advised that it didn't look good for Greg, we were trying one last time to get him to transplant. He was sleeping quietly in his hospital bed. He*

had been complaining of severe head pain, and was on a low morphine drip. The afternoon nurse woke him to take vitals, and he chatted with her. He told me, "Mom, I'm going to go back to sleep, I love you." Two hours later the night nurse tried to wake him up to give him some medicine, and she couldn't wake him. They called the doctor in from his home, and he ordered a CAT scan. When the film came up to the floor, the doctor took me out in the hall and said, "He's not going to live through the night." He held up the film showing a massive cerebral infarction; Greg was bleeding into the brain. He quietly died less than an hour later. Family and staff were in total shock. Nobody expected it. But, looking back, Greg had decided he had had enough; he was ready to go. I am grateful that he didn't die on a transplant floor in a strange city. We were able to call in friends and family, and we were surrounded and supported by the wonderful nurses whom we knew so intimately. I couldn't leave him until three nurses promised to stay with him and escort him to the morgue. They are still dear friends.

· · · · ·

I felt bad for my daughter, because like any good child, she wanted permission, even to die. My husband had promised her that he would never give up. He kept on saying, "Fight. Fight. Don't give up; don't leave me. We'll do another transplant; we'll try different medicine. It's too early to give up." I looked at him and said, "She's not going anywhere until you tell her that it's okay." Then he told her, and she took her last breath. He still feels guilty to this day because of his promises. He just doesn't understand that it was time; that she needed to know that it was okay with us.

Parents of children who died in the hospital stressed the importance of clear communication. Parents need to be strong advocates for adequate pain control, and they need to clearly describe their wishes to the staff .

In most hospitals, if a patient's heart stops or if he stops breathing, the staff immediately begins cardiopulmonary resuscitation (CPR) and electric shocks to the heart—this is called a "code." If the parents have decided they are ready to let their child die naturally, they need to discuss their wishes with the oncologist and ensure an order of "NO CODE" is put in the chart and on the child's door. A No Code order is also called a DNR, or "Do Not Resuscitate" order. Family members should understand that a DNR does not mean "Do not care for my child." On the contrary, it allows the medical team to provide comfort measures, such as:

- Allowing the child to sleep during the night without interruptions for checks of temperature and blood pressure

- Providing adequate pain medications

- Allowing family and friends open visitation without restrictions as to length and time of stay and number of people in the room

- A private room.

Dying at home

A child's death at home can be a peaceful or a frightening experience, depending on the preparation and support provided to the family.

It was scary to be taking Caitlin home to die, but she was so happy to be there. Her brother was 14 years old, six-foot-three, and he carried her everywhere she wanted to go. We let her be in charge; whoever she wanted to see would be allowed in. My parents bought her a television and a VCR, each with remotes. She'd sit in bed with a remote in each hand, glad not to have to compete with her brothers, and say, "I got the power."

The night of her death her vomiting was too bad for us to stay at home. We brought her to the hospital in our car; we fixed a bed for her in the back with me and her aunt on the floor and her dad driving. She was taken directly to the pediatric floor, where they started an IV and gave her something to stop the vomiting. My husband and I were in such denial that we had packed enough for at least a 2-week stay. No one on the staff had told us that her death was very near.

Ten days after her death we had to return to the pediatric floor with our son, and one of the doctors asked me if I had known Caitlin was dying when we came in with her. I said, "No, did you?" He replied, "Yes, because her breathing had changed." This new information hurt me deeply. It would have been good to have been told that her death was near and been given some choices about how we would like to handle it. I truly believe this could have been done quickly and as gently as all of her care had been given. I would like to have had the chance to hold Caitlin in my arms as she left our world, cradling her as closely as possible for the last time. Instead, I was hanging over the railing, holding her hand.

• • • • •

We decided to bring Jody home to die for several reasons. First of all, the medical profession was offering no more realistic hope. Secondly, Jody was young enough and small enough to be easily held, carried, and cared for by us. Thirdly, nothing violent or terrifying happened at home, which made us seriously debate whether to go back in the hospital with him.

I saw many life values in a new way from the experience of Jody dying at home. What comes to my mind is a sunny, breezy afternoon, September 13. Only Jody and I were home. I held him outside under the plum tree for perhaps an hour and a half or longer. I couldn't support him well and read to him at the same time, so we didn't do anything. I spoke to him some, but mostly just held him quietly. I was aware as I looked up into the sky that my normal reaction on such a day would be to want to be hiking, biking, "doing" something. A surprise recognition burst and spread gently through my consciousness: I was exactly where I wanted to be and no doing of anything could mean as much as being there with Jody.

Jody's last day, September 16, was peaceful. A spiritual healer, whom Jody had known for 2 years, came and spent time with him. A massage therapist/healer/ friend, who had visited him several times during the 5 weeks he was home, gave him a long, gentle massage. My husband, Tom, stayed home from teaching that day (by chance?). Jody lay in his arms or on my lap most of the day. The visiting home nurse came by briefly and offered to stay, but we preferred to be alone. I was holding Jody; Tom was next to me holding his feet. Jody's breathing became labored and irregular. His eyes were unblinking long before he took his last breath, then a heartbeat, then another, then silence.

Involving siblings

Whether your child is dying at home or in the hospital, if there are siblings, they should be included in the family response and preparations. Being part of things and having jobs to do helps brothers and sisters provide valuable contributions to the family. Young children can answer the doorbell, go on errands, or make tapes to play for the sibling. Older children can help with meals, stay with the ill child to give parents a break, answer the phone, or help make funeral arrangements. These jobs should not be "make-work"—children should truly be helping. This allows them to clarify their role in the family, prepare for the death, and say goodbye.

> *We had given our children free rein to pick out the clothes Jesse would be buried in. They made very thoughtful choices: her favorite, very comfortable pajamas with little tea cups on them, and her teddy bear. The service was very special: a celebration, a testament to her faith and ours.*

The Compassionate Friends (see Appendix B, "Resource Organizations") has dozens of resources to help all members of the family.

The funeral

Funerals and related rituals (e.g., memorial services, wakes, burial, shiva) are important not only as a time to say goodbye and begin to accept the reality of death, but also to provide an opportunity to recognize the child or teen's relationships with, and impact on, others. Funerals allow a gathering together to share memories and show support for the remaining family members. A funeral is a tangible demonstration of love.

> *We had Greg's minister, godparents, and kindergarten teacher come to our house to help plan the service. We did not want it to be scary, because we wanted all of his young friends to come. They needed to say goodbye, too, and above all, we wanted them to be comfortable. During the service, several songs were sung, and the minister didn't stand up at a pulpit. He stood on our level with his hand on Greg's casket*

and talked about Greg's life. It was simple and good. On the way to the cemetery it rained lightly, and the sky was filled with three rainbows. Sadness and hope.

Children of all ages should be allowed to attend the ceremony if they wish, but only after they have been prepared for what to expect. They need an explanation of what the event is for, where they will be going, and what will happen. They need to know what death is, what type of room they are going to, if the casket will be there, if it will be open, if there will be flowers, who will be there, how the mourners will behave, who will stay with them, what they will be expected to say or do, how long they will be there, and what will happen after the service (e.g., burial, reception). All questions should be answered honestly and children's feelings respected.

Many siblings also benefit from giving one last gift to the departed, such as a private note they have written to drop into the casket, or some of their sister's favorite flowers to put in her hands.

> *As the car drove us to Guildford Cathedral, the rain started to come down in torrents; even the angels were crying. It got darker and darker, and I felt lower and lower.*
>
> *As we walked around the corner into the Nave, we were absolutely amazed. There were 700 people in the Cathedral. 700. I could not believe my eyes. Michael obviously touched a lot of hearts.*
>
> *When the service started, the singing was just out of this world. And right next to me our son Christopher shut his eyes and sang along with his friends from St. George's who had come along to bolster the Guildford Choir. And that was quite something, to see the boys from the two choirs sitting side by side in the choir stalls, together with the men of two choirs. Michael had always wanted to sing with his brother when he was still a chorister. He finally got the two Choral Foundations together.*
>
> *The tribute from his godfather was perfect: funny, witty, poignant, and included a wonderful tribute to Christopher as well. The sermon from Canon Maureen told everyone what a strong faith Michael had and how he was so sanguine in living and in dying. "Here was someone who was alive from top to toe!" she said. And he WAS.*
>
> *The anthem was moving, the prayers touching, and then the undertakers moved in to pick up the coffin, and Graham, Christopher, and I moved behind it to take that long, long walk down the Nave. By now I was in tears—and walking past 700 people, most of whom were also in tears, was not easy. As we got to the Great West Door, the pallbearers turned round so that Michael was facing the altar, and everything was so quiet you could hear a pin drop. Suddenly, over the speakers, came the sound of Michael singing, "In the morning when I rise ..."*
>
> *Christopher and I stood with our arms around each other and tears pouring down our cheeks. As it finished, the organ swung into action and Michael's body was*

turned around and carried out for the last time of his beloved Cathedral, just as the sun came out.

For families that are involved in a spiritual community, their clergy have a unique opportunity to provide support, love, and comfort to the grieving family and friends. They usually know the family well and can evoke poignant memories of the deceased child or teen during the service. Members of the clergy often have excellent counseling skills and can visit the family after the funeral to provide ongoing help during mourning.

The role of family and friends

Family members and friends can be a wellspring of deep comfort and solace during grieving. Some people seem to know just when a hug is necessary or when silence is most welcome. Unfortunately, in our society there are few guidelines for handling the social aspects of grief. Many well-meaning people voice opinions concerning the time it is taking to "get over it" or question the parents' decision to not give away their child's clothing. Others do not know what to say, so they are silent, pretending that one of life's greatest catastrophes has not occurred. Many friends never again mention the deceased child's name, not knowing that this silence, as if the cherished child never existed, only adds to parents' pain. Holidays can become uncomfortable, as they bring sadness as well as joy.

In an attempt to alleviate these difficulties, bereaved parents helped compile the following lists of what helps, and what does not, in the hope that their suggestions may guide those family members and friends who deeply care, but just don't know how to help. These suggestions are offered with the understanding that what works for one person may not work for another. Try to use your knowledge of the bereaved family to choose options you think will make them comfortable. If in doubt, ask them.

What not to say

Please do not say to the parents:

- I know exactly how you feel.
- It's a blessing her suffering has ended.
- Thank goodness you are young enough to have another child.
- At least you have your other children.
- Be brave.
- Time will heal.

- God doesn't give anyone more than they can bear.

- It was God's will.

- He's in a better place now.

- God must have needed another angel.

- It's lucky this happened to someone as strong as you.

- Don't worry, in time you'll get over it.

- Why did you decide to cremate him?

- How is your marriage holding up?

- You need to be strong for your other children.

Please do not say to the siblings:

- You need to be strong for your mom and dad.

- Don't cry; it upsets your parents.

- You're the man of the house now.

- How does it feel to be the big sister?

Even if a bereaved parent has deep religious faith, it is often tested by the child's death. Parents are not comforted by well-meaning friends who assume faith is making the grief bearable; indeed, many parents find it to be infuriating. It's better to just say "I'm sorry."

In the months and years following the child's death, any of the following comments are unlikely to be appreciated and may, in fact, be hurtful:

- Don't you think it's time to get over it?

- It's been 6 months; it's time to put the past behind you.

- You need to get on with your life.

- You shouldn't be feeling that way.

- Don't you think you should give away all his clothes?

- Don't cry.

- Don't be sad.

- Doesn't it bother you to have her pictures around?

- Please don't talk about Johnnie, it just stirs up all those memories.

- It's not good to just sit around; you need to get out and have some fun.

Don't let your own sense of helplessness keep you from reaching out, even if you are unsure about what to say or do. It hurts the grieving family members when others pretend nothing is wrong or avoid (or refuse) talking about the child who has died.

What not to do

The following are suggestions from parents about what not to do:

- Don't remove anything that belonged to the child who died, unless specifically asked to by the parents.

    One family member took my son's toothbrush out of the bathroom and threw it away. I missed it immediately. She probably felt she was doing me a favor, but it made me so angry. I needed to keep things. I have his hair from the second time it fell out, because he wanted to save it, and I've kept his teeth that had to be pulled during treatment. I just need to have those things, and I resent people who insist you must clear out a child's things. Parents should be able to keep things or get rid of them—whichever is comfortable—regardless of others' opinions.

- Don't offer advice.

    Christie's room is still her room. We still refer to it as Christie's room. People just don't have the right to say you shouldn't leave that room empty: it's not empty, it's full of her life. I know that they are not trying to hurt us. It just bothers them to see that room. Sometimes it is just a reminder of death; yet, there are times when being in there and surrounded by all her things brings us closer to her and her time with us.

- Don't say anything that in any way suggests the child's medical care was inadequate.

    I can't tell you how many people said things like "If only you had gone to a different treatment facility," or "If only you had used this or that treatment." What people need most is support for what they are doing or did do.

- Don't look on the bright side or find silver linings.

    I became unexpectedly pregnant the month after my daughter died. I can't tell you how many people said things like "The circle of life is complete," or "God is taking one and giving you another," or "God is replacing her." She can never be replaced. It was horrible to hear those things, and I felt it was unfair to both the unborn baby and to my daughter who died.

- Don't drop bereaved parents from the support group. Talk about your options; grief-stricken parents have enough silence in their lives.

Our support group was run by two social workers from the two local hospitals. The rule was that bereaved parents could come for one visit after the funeral to say goodbye, and that was it. They were out. Two parents in our group lost their children, and we had a struggle with the social workers about changing the rules. They were adamant that the two groups of parents should not mingle, that it would be too upsetting for the parents of kids on treatment. My son was on treatment, and I felt strongly that we shouldn't abandon our friends in their time of greatest need and that we would all benefit from sharing their experiences and grief. In the end, we compromised by having the bereaved parent/s stay in the group for a year, then they would become a member of the new bereaved group. Both groups meet at the same time and place, so we socialize together after the meetings.

· · · · ·

We don't have a support group or a bereaved group per se, we just have frequent gatherings. So we all see each other almost monthly, and there is no issue of losing your friends if your child dies.

· · · · ·

When my daughter was terminal, in really bad shape, I went to the support group. We had all bonded and were very close. I felt guilty because I really wanted to cry and was trying to hold it back because I didn't want to upset everybody else. All of a sudden, I felt like I was the alien, like you feel when your child is diagnosed. Here I was in a room full of people I loved, where I had felt safe. Now I was alone again, this time with no hopes of Christie's recovery. It was truly the end. I never felt more scared or alone.

- Don't make comments about the parents' strength.

  People would say things to me like "You're so strong," or "I just couldn't live through what you have." It makes me want to scream. Do they mean I loved my child less than they love theirs because I have physically survived?

Things that help

Chapter 12, "Family and Friends," includes long lists of practical ways to help, such as helping to run the household, pay the bills, and feed the family. The following lists are specific suggestions to help people deal with grief.

Helpful things to say:

- I am so sorry.

- I cannot even imagine the pain you are feeling, but I am thinking about you.

- I really care about you.

- You and your family are in my thoughts and prayers.
- We would like to hold a memorial service at the school for your son if you think it would be appropriate.
- I will never forget John's sunny smile.
- I will never forget Jane's gentle way with children and animals.

Parents also offer a list of helpful things to do:

- Go to the funeral or memorial service.

  We were overwhelmed and touched by all of the people who came to the funeral. Even people that I had not seen in years—like some of my college professors—attended. Her oncologist and nurse drove 100 miles to be there.

- Show genuine concern and caring by listening.

  What has helped me the most is for people to just listen. Finding time to remember and reminisce is sometimes very difficult and painful, yet other times I feel much pride and happiness. Friends whose children also have cancer have been the greatest help to me during my daughter's illness and after her death.

- Help the siblings.

  When Jody was dying, his two well siblings, ages 9 and 4, presented concerns. I witnessed extremely tender moments, also flares of anger and hurt feelings. I assumed they felt neglected as I spent more and more time with Jody, just being his companion and caretaker. Christoph, 4, wanted to be near, to talk, to play. His energetic pace and my feelings of guilt became nearly intolerable to me the last 10 days or so. I decided to get the help of close friends and relatives to play with and lovingly attend to Christoph as many hours as possible when Tom was not home. Often they were in the same room with Jody and me.

  · · · · ·

  We had friends just call and say, "We will pick up Nick on Saturday and take him to Water World, then to our house for dinner. We were hoping he could spend the night. Will that be all right?" They did this many times, and it not only was fun for him, but it gave us a chance to be alone with each other and our grief.

  · · · · ·

  The day my daughter died, a close friend—herself a bereaved parent—did something wonderful. She took over my three kids, and prepared them for the funeral. She sat down with them and they read a book entitled, Today My Sister Died, and talked about it. She described in great detail what would happen at the funeral, and more importantly, she prepared them for some of the not-so-helpful comments that they would hear. So, when the first person said, "You're the big sister now," they had a response. She listened to them and prepared them and it truly helped them cope.

- Write the parents a note instead of just sending a preprinted sympathy card with your signature. Include special things you remember about their child or your feelings about their child. Letters, poems, or drawings from classmates and friends allow children to share their feelings with the family of the deceased, as well as provide poignant testimonials that the family will cherish.

- Talk about the child who has died. Parents forever carry in their heart cherished memories of their child and enjoy hearing others' favorite recollections.

    Months after the funeral, we gathered family members and some close friends to share memories on tape. We did a lot of laughing, as well as shed a few tears. But I will always cherish those tapes.

    · · · · ·

    I think, most of all, parents want their child to be remembered. It really comforts me to go to Greg's grave and find flowers, notes, or toys left by others.

- When parents express guilt over what they did or did not do, reassure them that they did everything they could. Remind them that they provided their child with the best that medicine had to offer.

- Remember anniversaries and birthdays. Call or send a card or flowers on the anniversary of the child's death.

- Respect the family's method of grieving.

- Give donations in the child's name to a favorite charity of the child or parents, for instance, the child's school library, Candlelighters, the local children's camp, the Leukemia and Lymphoma Society, or U.S. Children's Hospice International.

    Every year we still get a card saying that Caitlin's occupational therapist donated money to Camp Goodtimes. It makes me feel good that she is remembered so fondly and that the money will help other kids with cancer and their brothers and sisters.

- Commemorate the child's life in some tangible way. Examples are planting trees, shrubs, or flowers; erecting a memorial or plaque; or displaying a picture of the child.

    One of our Candlelighters fathers was on the city council. He encouraged the city to dedicate a new park to the children who had never grown up. They agreed, and named it "Children's Memorial Park." A local nursery offered to sell trees at a special discount for families or groups to buy and dedicate to a deceased child. A kiosk was built at the front of the park with the location of each tree and the name of the child to whom it is dedicated. Our Candlelighters board bought a grove of trees and a plaque with the names of the more than 70 children from our organization who have died since 1978 when we were founded. Last summer, we reserved the park for a "memorial picnic" and remembered and celebrated our departed children.

- Be patient. Acute grief from the loss of a child lasts a long, long time. Expectations of a rapid recovery are unrealistic and hurtful to parents.

- Encourage follow-up from medical personnel.

Caitlin had a very kind, very gentle radiation oncologist. I went back to see her after Caitlin died; she said, "We were so happy when we saw the progress that Caitlin made, from a stretcher to sitting to talking and walking again; and then our hearts broke when she relapsed. I wept." It was so human and so wonderful for her to let me know that she cared.

· · · · ·

We have had several phone calls from Jesse's oncologist, surgeon, and primary nurse. They were so wonderful to our entire family for years, and we miss them. We also had one call from the grief counselor at Children's, but we never heard from her again. We named our cat after one of the doctors, and it had been a running joke at the hospital. He wrote my children a funny letter about that. But, after the death of my child, I realized that they were busy and we really didn't have a relationship left. It is hard, after such intimacy. But my job now is grieving, and their job is trying to save other kids.

Sibling grief

Siblings are sometimes called the "forgotten grievers" because attention is typically focused on the parents. Children and teens may hesitate to express their own strong feelings in an attempt to prevent causing their parents additional distress. Indeed, adult family members and friends may advise the brothers and sisters to "be strong" for their parents or to "help your parents by being good." These requests place a terribly unfair burden on children who have already endured months or years of stress and family disruption. Siblings need continual assurance that each of them is an irreplaceable member of the family and that the entire family has suffered a loss. They have the right, and need, to mourn openly and in their own way.

The family requires such reorganization after a child's death, and there is nowhere to look for an example. Each person in the family constellation has different feelings and different ways of grieving; there is just no way to reconcile all of this when the supposed leaders of the group are totally out of it. Not to mention the fact that both my husband and I wanted more understanding and compassion from each other than we were possibly able to give.

Children express grief in many ways. Some children develop physical manifestations, such as stomach aches, a loss of appetite or voracious eating, or changes in sleeping or toileting habits. Many younger children regress; they may revert to diapers or baby talk, stop walking, or stop talking. Fears and phobias, such as a fear of the dark or of being alone, are common responses to loss. Children may develop unpredictable or disruptive behaviors, such as tantrums, crying, sadness, anxiety, withdrawal, or depression. Older children and teens may appear nonchalant, angry, withdrawn, or engage in risky behaviors, such as sexual promiscuousness, alcohol abuse, and drug use.

Parents need to engage siblings of different ages at their appropriate developmental levels. Private time together, or individual outings with the parents, can be very helpful for siblings.

Families can pull apart when individuals within the family have incompatible ways of expressing grief. Men and women tend to express grief in profoundly different ways that may seem intolerable or inexplicable to one another. In these situations, family therapy or some other form of counseling may be advisable.

Some parents worry that if they start talking about their feelings, they will "break down" in front of the children. But the children know their parents are grieving and it hurts them to feel excluded. They are grieving, too, and if they see their parents pulling away from them, they are likely to feel that their parents do not love them as much as they loved the child they lost. Here are suggestions from families about ways to pull together while mourning:

- Let the siblings go to the funeral. They have suffered a loss; they need to say good-bye and they need support for their grief just as much as adults do.

  I grew up going to my relatives' funerals. Having those positive experiences really helped me deal with the loss of my son. There is nothing more natural than to take a child to the funeral, where they are part of families loving each other, crying together, and laughing at some of the memories. Too many people try to protect kids from death, and it does them a great disservice.

- Children and teens experience the same feelings as adults. Sharing your feelings can encourage them to identify and share their own emotions. (For example, "I'm really feeling sad today. How do you feel?")

- Some families establish a regular meeting time to talk about their feelings and/or memories. Both tears and laughter erupt when family members talk about funny or touching memories of the departed child.

- Jointly discuss how holidays and anniversaries should be observed. For example, some families hang a Christmas stocking every year for the departed child, while others simply mention her name during a blessing. Each family devises different ways to handle holidays, the child's birthday, and the anniversary of her death.

Parental grief

Losing a child is one of life's most horrific and painful events. There is no "right way" to grieve. There is no timetable, no appropriate progression from one stage to the next, and no time when parents should "be over it." The death of a child shatters the very order of the universe—children are not supposed to die before their parents. It seems unnatural, incomprehensible. Losing a child, especially after such a long and grueling battle to save her, seems cruel and unjust. When a child dies, parents mourn not only the child herself, but all of the hopes, dreams, wishes, and needs relating to her. When you lose a child, you lose part of yourself and an important part of your future.

This book will not go through the numerous psychological descriptions of the grieving process. Many excellent reference books are available, several of which are listed in Appendix C, "Books, Websites and Videotapes." Below, the parents themselves tell you about grief.

> I truly think that it is the worst thing in the entire world. Nothing worse can happen than losing your child. There is no reprieve. None.

· · · · ·

> My life is void of the very essential magic of Elena, the stories, the brightness of her being. Her giggles, her sweet kisses, her calling me cupcake and giving me the nosie "uggamuggums." She would be in fourth grade Tuesday, and instead she is dead! The school planted flowers by the memorial that they gave last year on her birthday. Yes, it was hard to shop for two instead of three of my kids. I miss the games and the playing school and the calls between her friends. I miss sitting with her on my lap; I miss touching her smooth skin, touching her curly hair, and smelling her scent. I miss looking at her long fingers. But I feel that I was blessed with her life, her love of life, her friends and passions, her angels, and her beauty. I will carry her life with honor in my heart for my lifetime.

· · · · ·

> I was having a very hard time grieving when a wonderful therapist that I was seeing said to me, "You are beating yourself up about grieving. Think about it: When you enter marriage, what are you called? A wife. When your spouse dies, what are you called? A widow. When you don't have a home and you are living on the street, what is the name for that? A homeless person. When you lose a child, what's it called, what's the name?" I said, "I don't know." She said, "Exactly. There is not even a word in our vocabulary. That's how terrible it is. It doesn't even have a name."

The biggest thing I had to learn was just to cope with whatever I was feeling on that particular day. When I feel angry, I just need to let myself be angry. If I need to cry all day, I do. I still have plenty of those days. If someone calls me and wants to take me out to lunch to cheer me up, I have learned to say no when I'm not feeling like going out. I know that it hurts other people to see me cry, but I need to do that sometimes. I just miss her so much.

. . . . .

Every day when I walk out of my house I tell myself to grab the mask. I feel like I walk different than everybody and talk different than everybody and look different than everybody. It's the worst part of bereavement, the isolation caused by people who just don't know how to talk to you, when really all they need to do is listen and remember with you.

. . . . .

I found myself getting busier and busier, thinking that I could outrun the pain. I realized that I couldn't avoid the hurt; I just had to grit my teeth, cry, and live through it.

. . . . .

My daughter was our firefly; she lit the whole scene up. When she died, that spirit was gone, and there was just a hole left. We just didn't feel like a family anymore.

. . . . .

I feel jealous when I hear about people who lose their fear when their child dies. I became more fearful, of everything. I am a very strong person, but I really picked up a lot of fear, and, 4 years later, I still have it.

. . . . .

I felt like our sick daughter was the center of our universe for so long, that now I need to start feeling some responsibility for my other kids whom I've been away from for so long, both physically and emotionally. I told my husband the other night that I didn't even know if I loved the three kids anymore. I cannot feel a thing. Pinch me, I don't feel it. Hug me, I don't feel it. I'm numb.

. . . . .

It's hard to admit, but there was an element of relief when my daughter died. Not relief for myself, but for her. I was almost glad that she wouldn't face a life full of disabilities. That she wouldn't face the numerous orthopedic surgeries that would have been required to repair the damage from treatment. That she wouldn't face the pain of not having children of her own. I just felt relief that she would no longer feel any pain.

• • • • •

At first we didn't feel like a family anymore. Now it's better, but it's still not the family that I was used to, that I want. I still feel like the mother of four children, not three. I find it very hard to answer when someone asks me how many children I have. I also can't sign cards like I used to, with all of our names, so now I just write "from the gang." I guess that's not fair to the boys, but I just can't bear to leave her name off.

• • • • •

I had a visual image of our family of five. When Jody died, it became this physical square thing with only mom, dad, boy, girl, and it bothered me so much.

• • • • •

I thought this morning of how I used to listen to Jesse breathe. Now I can't hear her breathe or laugh. I can't feel her arms around me. I remember missed kisses and late-night times. I ache. Heaven seems so far away.

• • • • •

It seems that sometimes she is still so near that during conversations I can hear her comments or answers, and yet I fear the memories might fade and I so cherish the nearness. We each wear articles of her clothes or jewelry every day. One daughter is sleeping on the floor in our room, and the other two are sleeping in her bed.

• • • • •

The worst times were the first two Christmases. We had to grit our teeth, put our heads down, and just get through it. We had to keep moving, never stop moving. I would have ignored it altogether if I didn't have another child.

• • • • •

Birthdays are hard for us. Greg's birthday was June 10, and his brother's is June 9. So it's pretty hard to ignore. On Greg's birthday and the anniversary of his death, we blow up balloons, one for every year he would have been alive, write messages on them with markers, and release them at his grave.

• • • • •

It seems like just about every holiday has some difficult memory attached to it now. He was diagnosed on Easter, and then relapsed the next year on Valentine's Day. I hate them both now. Christmas is always hard. And Halloween is tough because he so loved to dress up. I see all those little ones in their costumes and I'm just flooded with pain.

• • • • •

I keep wondering if I should have put a stop to the bone marrow transplant, because I had no peace about it. I felt such fear and dread about her platelets and liver. And what I feared happened. I still pray to have peace over making that choice. To have peace over giving a teenager the weight of deciding all that herself. I still feel so guilty and know I'd still be kissing her goodnight if we hadn't gone forward—and how I miss those kisses.

· · · · ·

I feel like Job 3:25-26: What I feared has come upon me; What I dreaded has happened to me; I have no peace, no quietness; I have no rest but only turmoil.

· · · · ·

This evening my heart was so saddened. I paced up and down in front of the mantel, pausing to look at each picture of my daughter. Something that I cannot describe catches in my chest, and I can't breathe right. I look at her face and try to will it to life for a kiss and a touch, for softly spoken endearments at night. How we love all of our children, yet one missing leaves such a stabbing pain.

· · · · ·

I worry that missing one child so desperately pervades my very ability to be a good mom to my other three. I so wish to find joy again, to find things in life to smile about. I so wish my children could see me smile again. I pray that God will give me this thing, because it is beyond my finding in this world.

· · · · ·

I had always heard that time heals all things. I was afraid of healing, because I didn't want to feel any farther away than I felt when he died. It's been 7 years, and he still feels really close—a presence. But I still ache to touch his body so, that little back and fat tummy.

· · · · ·

It's been 2 years, and I still feel a lot of rage. I walk down the street and see kids hanging out, smoking, doing drugs, being rude, wasting themselves, and I am filled with rage that my son—such a straight arrow, so decent, so strong—is gone.

· · · · ·

I feel strongly that parents should seek out other parents who have lost children. Nobody else understands as well. Nobody else is as comfortable with it. We have our own sense of humor, and we often laugh hard about things that make other people uncomfortable.

· · · · ·

It's hard when people I have just met ask, "How many children do you have?" In the beginning, I always felt I had to explain that I had two but one died. Now I just say one. I don't want their sympathy, I don't want their pity, but most of all I just don't want to have to explain. After 2 years or so, I started to feel uncomfortable giving out my life history and then having to deal with other people's discomfort. So now I just say one, and yet it still feels like I'm betraying him every time I do it.

· · · · ·

That 1-year rule, when you are supposed to start feeling better, I've found to be true. Not that any of the pain is lessened, but I realized I had managed to live through a year of holidays and anniversaries. I knew it was possible to do it a second, then a third time. One year isn't magic, but it does prove to you that you can survive.

· · · · ·

On the anniversary of Ryan's death we all went to the cemetery, and his girlfriend's parents planted a cherry tree at the foot of his grave. That was on a Sunday. I woke up on Monday feeling just as bad as I did the day before. All I could think was, "Oh hell, I have to go through that whole cycle again." The first year did not bring me any peace.

· · · · ·

This morning was the 4-year anniversary of my daughter's death. While I was at church I wanted to write in the intentions book, "I want my daughter back," but then I didn't because nobody would understand. I guess I'm pretty unreal in my thoughts a lot of the time.

· · · · ·

From the minute I turn the calendar over to August, I'm on a knife edge. The twentieth of August just pulses on the calendar. I become depressed, spacey; I'm just in a very bad mood. I get sick a lot those first 3 weeks of August. But when it's over, I begin to relax and look forward to fall.

· · · · ·

At church, we always sit with the same group of close friends who helped us through Jesse's illness and are helping us grieve her death. If they begin to sing a hymn that reminds one of us of Jesse, we all start to cry, and someone produces a box of tissues, which gets passed down the aisles. People must wonder at the group that sobs through services. But it has helped me so much to have a community of grievers, it's been a very cleansing thing. It has spread out the tears.

· · · · ·

I think parents need to know that it hurts like hell and they will feel crazy. But it is a normal craziness. If they talk to other bereaved parents, they will know that pain, guilt, rage, and craziness are how normal human beings feel when their child dies.

Bereaved parents are frequently reassured that "time will ease the pain." Most find this is not the case. Time helps them understand the pain; the passage of time reassures them that they can adjust and they will survive. The acute pain becomes more quiescent, but it still erupts when parents go to what would have been their child's graduation, hear their child's favorite song, or just go to the grocery store. Grief is a long, difficult journey, with many ups and downs. But, with time, parents report that laughter and joy do return. They acknowledge that life will never be the same, but it can be good again.

Looking back after many years

Four parents whose children died many years ago share their thoughts about grief and how they changed:

My 15-year-old son was diagnosed with leukemia in 1962, and he lived until February 1963. He was tall, sturdy, wonderful. He inspired us all. Although it was very painful when he died, I truly felt that I had done all that I possibly could. I had four younger children, and I'd parceled myself out as best I could. Jennifer was born in October 1965, and my mother always said David had asked Our Lord to send her "to help me mend my heart."

I felt I had done my best for David, he was at peace, and I also needed peace. Our deep faith greatly helped. David was strong enough to tell me, "I don't want you to worry, Mom, God knows what he is doing." I also had a flock of kids who were hurting and needed me. So I threw myself back into life and carried on.

There are many imponderables that I think of. What would David be like if he had survived? Would the lives of his brothers and sisters have been different if they had not lived through his illness and death? How would my marriage have been different? What would I be like if he was still alive? These thoughts serve no purpose; you just have to give yourself credit for doing your best and leave it at that. But at times when I feel desperate, I simply look up at the night sky, and I know that one of those stars is mine.

• • • • •

My daughter died in March 1971. That feeling that I had a hole in my solar plexus and was walking around with a heart literally broken in two lasted for over a year. I didn't go to a movie for 4 years, and it was very difficult for me to find pleasure in anything. But I have healed and am again a fully functional person. I have fun, tell jokes, play guitar, make speeches, and love my children.

There are many things I did to heal. I linked up with another bereaved parent. Our relationship worked wonderfully; we clung to each other and we helped each other survive the holidays. During my daughter's illness and a catastrophic diagnosis of mental illness in my other daughter, I began to take too many tranquilizers. So I entered a 12-step program, and think that it literally saved my life. I gave up pills, quit smoking, rediscovered faith, and learned a new way to live.

At that time I also became very involved in a church, which was perhaps the most comforting, healing thing of all. I decided never to visit my daughter's grave. I know it comforts some people, but not me. I never thought for a second that she was there, just her bones. She and I will meet again. And finally, I had more children. I caution newly bereaved parents to think long and hard about the timing of the next child. But I look at my children, and I thank God for them.

Grieving was such hard work. For years her birthday was a black time for me, but that has faded away with the years. For a long time I felt like I was only going through the motions of life. But I just decided to act cheerful, force myself to go out, count my blessings, and reach out to people who were less fortunate than me. It worked.

· · · · ·

Life does go on after the death of someone you love…even if it's your child. It isn't always easy or fun or purposeful, but it's like anything else…life is what you make of it.

My son Cory died on Mother's Day 1985 after 5½ years of battling leukemia. When he left this existence a big part of my heart died with him. At first, the sky wasn't as blue as it once was…the mountains weren't as majestic…the ocean wasn't as magnificent, and yeah, it was hard to get out of bed and put one foot in front of the other. But I had to do it. I had to go on, not only for my daughter, but for myself, too.

One day the fog lifted, and I knew in what remained of my heart that my little boy wanted me to continue on loving life and all it has to offer. Before he died, Cory told me, "Don't weep for me, Mama. Just remember me and all the love I brought with me. I chose this life to be with you, but I was never meant to grow up."

I will never stop missing him. Thankfully he gave me the strength to move forward. Cory loved life so much and fought so courageously during the short time he was here, it would be an insult to his memory if I didn't cling to and enjoy life as tenaciously as he taught me to. The memories of the fun we had, the love we shared, and the vision of him dancing on the stars sustain me.

· · · · ·

The old adage that "time heals" is a myth. You need to choose to heal and then find out how to help yourself. As I look back on our journey, our first instinct was to huddle as a family; to bask in what was left. We were hurting together; we loved him; we missed him; we needed to celebrate who he was. We intuitively knew that we were going to make it, we just didn't know how.

When Donny died 13 years ago, we didn't know much about grief. There wasn't as much written about it then as there is now. But we were committed to healing individually and as a family. One of the important things we did for one another was to give each other lots of space. My husband and I knew the distancing was necessary but temporary. We were on a teeter-totter. We each had a different schedule, a different way of handling pain. He allowed me my "craziness," and I respected his silence. I found that it helped me to wallow in it, to feel it all, to cry. I've grieved clean.

If you have children, learn about how kids grieve. They revisit their grief at each developmental stage. Keep the door open so they can talk about it. After Donny's death, I found that I just had to be with kids. I volunteered at the school, and followed all of his friends until they graduated from high school. A friend carried his cap and gown, and they made a speech about how a very important person was missing from the ceremony. I cried, but it was good.

I think it is very important for people to choose to feel. If you attend a grief support group or Compassionate Friends, or read about the grief process, you will quickly realize that your feelings are normal and that each person goes through grief differently. Another good reason to go to a group is that other people can give voice to your feelings when you just don't have any words. In the beginning you are just a ball of pain. You learn that every person feels that way; that it is normal, human. Many people come to group and never speak, but they are comforted. I found it was far better for me to be in the same room with real people who had walked down the same road, rather than just to read about it in books. Feel the pain and you will heal.

I just wish that I had armfuls of time.

— Four year old with cancer
Armfuls of Time

Blood Counts and What They Mean

KEEPING TRACK OF THEIR CHILD'S BLOOD counts becomes a way of life for parents of children with leukemia. Unfortunately, misunderstandings about the implications of certain changes in blood values can cause unnecessary worry and fear. To help prevent these concerns, and to better enable parents to help spot trends in the blood values of their child, this appendix explains the blood counts of healthy children, the blood counts of children being treated for leukemia, and what each blood count value means.

Values for healthy children

Each laboratory and lab handbook has slightly different reference values for each type of blood cell, so your lab sheets may differ slightly from those that appear later in this appendix. (See figure A-1.) There is also variation in values for children of different ages. For instance, in children from newborn to 4 years old, granulocytes are lower and lymphocytes are higher than the numbers listed below. The following table lists blood count values for healthy children.

Blood Count Type	Values for Healthy Children
Hemoglobin (Hgb)	11.5 to 13.5 g/100 mL
Hematocrit (HCT)	34 to 40%
Red blood cell count (RBC)	3.9 to 5.3 million/cm^3 or 3.9 to 5.3 x 10^{12}/L
Platelets	160,000 to 380,000/mm^3
White blood cell count (WBC)	5,000 to 10,000/mm^3 or 5 to 10 K/uL
WBC differential:	
Segmented neutrophils	50 to 70%
Band neutrophils	1 to 3%
Basophils	0.5 to 1%
Eosinophils	1 to 4%
Lymphocytes	12 to 46%

Blood Count Type	Values for Healthy Children
Monocytes	2 to 10%
Bilirubin (total)	0.3 to 1.3 mg/dL
Direct (conjugated)	0.1 to 0.4 mg/dL
Indirect (unconjugated)	0.2 to 1.88 mg/dL
AST (SGOT)	0 to 36 IU/L
ALT (SGPT)	0 to 48 IU/L

Values for children on chemotherapy

Blood counts of children being treated for leukemia fluctuate wildly. WBCs can go down to zero or be above normal. RBCs go down periodically during treatment, necessitating transfusions of packed red cells. Platelet levels also decrease, sometimes requiring platelet transfusions. Absolute neutrophil counts (ANC) are closely watched, as they give the physician an idea of the child's ability to fight infections; ANCs vary from zero to in the thousands. Doctors try to keep the ANC around 1,000 for children being treated for leukemia.

Oncologists consider all of the blood values to get the total picture of a child's reaction to illness, chemotherapy, radiation, or infection. Trends are more important than any single value. For instance, if the values were 5.0, 4.7, and 4.9, then the second result (4.7) was insignificant. If, on the other hand, the values were 5.0, 4.7, and 4.3, then the trend would indicate a decrease in the cell line.

The explanations below describe each blood cell type and value. If you have any questions about your child's blood counts, ask your child's doctor for a clear explanation. Especially in the beginning, many parents agonize over whether the rapid changes in blood counts (often requiring transfusions, changes in chemotherapy dosages, or restrictions to the child having visitors) are normal and expected. The only way to address your worries and prevent them from escalating is to ask what the changes mean.

What do these blood values mean?

The following sections explain each line of the previously listed blood values. See Figure A-1 to get an idea of the different ways these values might be displayed on actual lab reports prepared for your child.

TEST	RESULTS	UNITS	REFERENCE RANGE	
Collection Cmt. -				
*CBC**				
White Blood Count	1.7	L x10-3	3.8 - 12.5	JK
Red Blood Cnt	3.02	L x10-6	3.90 - 5.30	JK
Hemoglobin	8.9	L g/d1	11.5 - 13.5	JK
Hematocrit	26.1	L %	34.0 - 40.0	JK
MCV	86.0	um3	75.0 - 87.0	JK
MCH	29.4	uug	24.0 - 30.0	JK
MCHC	34.1	%	32.0 - 36.0	JK
Segs	33	%	30 - 70	JK
Bands	1	%	0 - 5	JK
Lymphocytes	19	L %	20 - 70	JK
Monocytes	42	H %	0 - 6	JK
Eosinophiles	5	H %	0 - 3	JK
Morphology Cmt 1 Anisocytosis		2+		
Platelets	34	L x10-3	250 - 550	JK

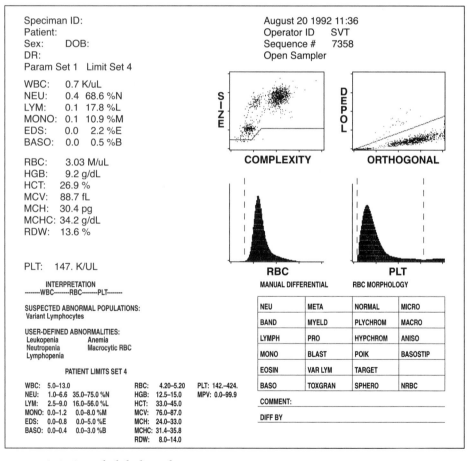

Specimen ID:
Patient:
Sex: DOB:
DR:
Param Set 1   Limit Set 4

August 20 1992 11:36
Operator ID   SVT
Sequence #   7358
Open Sampler

WBC: 0.7 K/uL
NEU: 0.4 68.6 %N
LYM: 0.1 17.8 %L
MONO: 0.1 10.9 %M
EDS: 0.0   2.2 %E
BASO: 0.0   0.5 %B

RBC: 3.03 M/uL
HGB: 9.2 g/dL
HCT: 26.9 %
MCV: 88.7 fL
MCH: 30.4 pg
MCHC: 34.2 g/dL
RDW: 13.6 %

PLT: 147. K/UL

INTERPRETATION
------WBC-------RBC-------PLT------

SUSPECTED ABNORMAL POPULATIONS:
Variant Lymphocytes

USER-DEFINED ABNORMALITIES:
Leukopenia   Anemia
Neutropenia   Macrocytic RBC
Lymphopenia

PATIENT LIMITS SET 4

WBC: 5.0–13.0
NEU: 1.0–6.6 35.0–75.0 %N
LYM: 2.5–9.0 16.0–56.0 %L
MONO: 0.0–1.2 0.0–8.0 %M
EDS: 0.0–0.8 0.0–5.0 %E
BASO: 0.0–0.4 0.0–3.0 %B

RBC: 4.20–5.20   PLT: 142.–424.
HGB: 12.5–15.0   MPV: 0.0–99.9
HCT: 33.0–45.0
MCV: 76.0–87.0
MCH: 24.0–33.0
MCHC: 31.4–35.8
RDW: 8.0–14.0

COMPLEXITY   ORTHOGONAL

RBC   PLT
MANUAL DIFFERENTIAL   RBC MORPHOLOGY

NEU	META	NORMAL	MICRO
BAND	MYELD	PLYCHROM	MACRO
LYMPH	PRO	HYPCHROM	ANISO
MONO	BLAST	POIK	BASOSTIP
EOSIN	VAR LYM	TARGET	
BASO	TOXGRAN	SPHERO	NRBC

COMMENT:

DIFF BY

Figure A-1: Sample lab data sheets

Hemoglobin (Hgb)

Red cells contain Hgb, the molecules that carry oxygen and carbon dioxide in the blood. Measuring Hgb gives doctors an exact picture of the ability of the child's blood to carry oxygen. Children may have low Hgb levels at diagnosis and during the intensive parts of treatment; this is because both cancer and chemotherapy decrease the bone marrow's ability to produce new red cells. During maintenance, your child's Hgb level will be higher than during induction and consolidation, but may still be lower than that of a healthy child. Signs and symptoms of anemia—pallor, shortness of breath, fatigue—may occur if the Hgb gets very low.

Hematocrit (HCT)

The hematocrit is sometimes called the packed cell volume (PCV). The purpose of the HCT test is to determine the ratio of plasma (the clear liquid part of blood) to red cells in the blood. For this test, blood is drawn from a vein, a finger prick, or from a central catheter and is spun in a centrifuge to separate the red cells from the plasma. The HCT is the percentage of cells in the blood; for instance, if the child has a HCT of 30 percent, it means that 30 percent of the amount of blood drawn was cells and the rest was plasma. When the child is on chemotherapy, the bone marrow does not make many red cells, and the HCT will go down. Your child may be given a transfusion of packed red cells when the HCT goes below 18 to 19 percent. (Packed red cells are obtained by spinning whole blood until the plasma separates from the blood cells. Only the blood cells are transfused.) Even during maintenance the bone marrow is partially suppressed, so the HCT is often in the low to mid-30s. This suppression results in less oxygen being carried in the blood, and may cause your child to have less energy.

Red blood cell count (RBC)

Red blood cells are produced by the bone marrow continuously in healthy children and adults. These cells contain hemoglobin, which carries oxygen and carbon dioxide throughout the body. To determine the RBC, an automated electronic device is used to count the number of red cells in a specified amount of blood.

Red cell indices (MCV, MCH, MCHC) are mathematical relationships of hematocrit to red cell count, hemoglobin to red cell count, and hemoglobin to hematocrit. The indices give a mathematical expression of the degree of change in shape found in red cells. The higher the number (low teens are fine), the more distorted the red cell population is.

White blood cell count (WBC)

The total WBC determines the body's ability to fight infection. Treatment for cancer kills healthy white cells as well as diseased ones. Parents need to expect prolonged periods of low WBCs during treatment. To determine the WBC, an automated electronic device counts the number of white cells in a specified amount of blood. If your lab sheet uses K/uL instead of mm³, multiply by 1,000 to get the value in mm³. For example, on the lab sheet in Figure A-1, the total WBC is 0.7 K/uL, therefore, 0.7 x 1,000 = 700 mm³.

White blood cell differential

When a child has blood drawn for a complete blood count (CBC), one section of the lab report will state the total WBC and a "differential," meaning that each type of white blood cell will be listed as a percentage of the total. For example, if the total WBC count is 1,500 mm³, the differential might appear as in the following table:

White Blood Cell Type	Percentage of Total WBC
Segmented neutrophils (also called polys or segs)	49%
Band neutrophils (also called bands)	1%
Basophils (also called basos)	1%
Eosinophils (also called eos)	1%
Lymphocytes (also called lymphs)	38%
Monocytes (also called monos)	10%

You might also see cells called metamyelocytes, myelocytes, promyelocytes, and myeloblasts listed. These are immature white cells usually only found in the bone marrow. They may be seen in the blood during recovery from low counts.

The differential is obtained by microscopic analysis of a blood sample on a slide.

Absolute neutrophil count (ANC)

The ANC (also called the absolute granulocyte count or AGC) is a measure of the body's ability to withstand infection. Generally, an ANC above 1,000 means the child's infection-fighting ability is near normal.

To calculate the ANC, add the percentages of neutrophils (both segmented and band) and multiply by the total WBC. Using the example above, the ANC is 49 percent + 1 percent = 50 percent, and 50 percent of 1,500 (.50 x 1,500) = 750, so the ANC is 750.

Platelet count

Platelets are needed to repair the body and stop bleeding through the formation of clots. Because platelets are produced by the bone marrow, platelet counts decrease when a child is on chemotherapy. Signs of lowering platelet counts are bruises, gum bleeding, or nosebleeding. Platelet transfusions may be given when the count is very low (between 10,000 and 20,000 mm³) or when there is bleeding. Platelets are counted by passing a blood sample through an electronic device.

Approximately one-third of all platelets spend a great deal of time in the spleen. Any splenic dysfunction, such as enlargement, may cause the counts to drop sharply. If the spleen is removed, platelet counts may skyrocket. This transient thrombocytosis (elevated platelet count) usually declines within a month.

Alanine aminotransferase (ALT)

ALT is also called serum glutamic pyruvic transaminase (SGPT). When doctors talk about "liver functions," they are usually referring to blood sample tests that measure liver damage. If the chemotherapy is proving to be toxic to your child's liver, the damaged liver cells release an enzyme called ALT into the blood serum. ALT levels can go up into the hundreds, or even thousands, in some children on chemotherapy. Each institution and protocol has different points at which they decrease dosages or stop chemotherapy to allow the child's liver to recover. If you notice a change in your child's ALT, ask for an explanation and plan of action. (For example: "John's ALT is now 450. What is your plan to reduce or stop the chemotherapy to allow his liver to recover?")

> *I was very interested in my daughter's blood counts throughout her treatment. I also tried to get information without making people mad. If I asked a question and received an unsatisfactory answer, I would reply in a nice way: "I am worrying about this and would really appreciate a few minutes of your time to explain it to me." I found the attendings and clinic director to be the most willing to provide explanations. If you get a ridiculous reply (once a fellow patted me on the head and said, "It's our job to think about these things, not yours."), go find someone else to ask.*

Aspartate aminotransferase (AST)

AST is also called serum glutamic oxaloacetic transaminase (SGOT). AST is an enzyme present in high concentrations in tissues with high metabolic activity, such as the liver. Severely damaged or killed cells release AST into the blood. The amount of AST in the blood is directly related to the amount of tissue damage. Therefore, if your child's liver is being damaged by chemotherapy, the AST count can rise into the thousands. There are many other causes for an elevated AST, such as viral infections or reactions to an anesthetic. If your child's level jumps unexpectedly, ask the physician for an explanation and a plan of action.

Bilirubin

The liver converts hemoglobin released from damaged red cells into bilirubin. The liver then removes bilirubin from the blood and excretes it into the bile, which is a fluid released into the small intestine to aid digestion.

Normally, there is only a small amount of bilirubin in the bloodstream. Bilirubin rises if there is excessive red blood cell destruction, or if the liver is unable to excrete the normal amount of bilirubin produced.

The two types of bilirubin are indirect (also called unconjugated) and direct (also called conjugated). An increase in indirect is seen when destruction of red cells has occurred, while an increase of direct is seen when there is a dysfunction or blockage of the liver.

If excessive amounts of bilirubin are present in the body, the bilirubin seeps into the tissues, producing a yellow color in the skin and whites of the eyes that is called jaundice.

Your child's pattern

Each child develops a unique pattern of blood counts during treatment, and observant parents can help track these changes. If there is a change in the pattern, show it to your child's doctor and ask for an explanation. Doctors consider all of the laboratory results before deciding how to proceed. They should be willing to explain their plan of action so you can better understand what is happening and worry less.

If your child is participating in a clinical trial and you have obtained the entire clinical trial protocol (discussed in Chapter 4, "Choosing a Treatment"), it will contain a section that clearly outlines the actions that should be taken by the oncologist if certain changes in blood counts occur. For example, my daughter's protocol had an extensive section that listed each drug and stated when the dosage should be modified. For vincristine the protocol stated:

Vincristine
   1.5 mg/m^2 (2 mg maximum) IV push weekly x 4 doses days 0, 7, 14, 21.

Seizures
   Hold one dose, then reinstitute.

Severe foot drop, paresis, or ilius
   Hold dose(s): when symptoms abate, resume at 1.0 mg/m^2; escalate to full dose as tolerated.

Jaw pain
   Treat with analgesics; do not modify vincristine dose.

Withhold if total bilirubin >1.9 mg/dL. Administer 1/2 dose if total bilirubin 1.5–1.9 mg/dL.

Resource Organizations

Service organizations

Candlelighters Childhood Cancer Foundation (CCCF)

P.O. Box 498
Kensington, MD 20895-0498
(800) 366-CCCF / (800) 366-2223
www.candlelighters.org (will soon be *www.americanchildhoodcancer.org*)

Founded in 1970, CCCF (new name will be American Childhood Cancer Organization) has more than 40,000 members worldwide. Some of the free services provided are a toll-free information hotline, a biannual newsletter, various handbooks to help families of children with cancer, local support group chapters, and national advocacy.

American Cancer Society (ACS)

1599 Clifton Road NE
Atlanta, GA 30329
(800) ACS-2345 / (800) 227-2345
www.cancer.org

The ACS has a national network of employees and volunteers who implement research, education, and patient service programs. Although programs differ according to state, some widely available programs are patient-to-patient visitation, transportation to appointments, housing near treatment centers, equipment and supplies, support groups, literature about a variety of topics, summer camps for children with cancer, and research and educational programs.

Leukemia & Lymphoma Society (LLS)

1311 Mamaroneck Avenue, Suite 310
White Plains, NY 10605
(800) 955-4LSA / (800) 955-4572
www.leukemia.org

The LLS is an organization that provides financial assistance to families, funds research, sponsors a national education program for the public and the medical community, and publishes a large number of booklets about cancer-related topics.

Ronald McDonald House Charities (RMHC)
One Kroc Drive
Oakbrook, IL 60523
(630) 623-7048
http://rmhc.org

The RMHC is committed to creating, finding, and supporting programs that directly improve the health and well being of children. They help families of seriously ill children by providing Ronald McDonald Houses, the Ronald McDonald Learning Program, and Ronald McDonald Family Rooms within hospitals.

Canada

Candlelighters Childhood Cancer Foundation Canada
1300 Yonge St., Suite 405
Toronto, Ontario M4T 1X3
(800) 363-1062 or (416) 489-6440
www.candlelighters.ca

Provides information and monetary support for families, and advocates for healthcare policies in support of childhood cancer.

Canadian Cancer Society
National Office
Suite 200, 10 Alcorn Avenue
Toronto, Ontario M4V 3B1
(888) 939-3333 or (416) 961-7223
www.cancer.ca

The Canadian Cancer Society is a national community-based organization of volunteers whose mission is the eradication of cancer and the enhancement of the quality of life for people living with cancer.

Australia

Childhood Cancer Association
P.O. Box 1094
North Adelaide SA 5006
Australia
www.childhoodcancer.asn.au/services

This South Australia organization is dedicated to providing emotional, practical, and financial support to families in need, including peer, family, and sibling support; free accommodations for families from rural areas; respite accommodations; financial and educational assistance; and bereavement services. The Association also provides funds for pediatric oncology research and clinical trials.

Leukaemia Foundation
1 Walton Street
Isaacs ACT 2607
Australia
www.leukaemia.org.au

This organization is dedicated to the care and cure of patients and families living with leukemia, lymphomas, myeloma, and related blood disorders. The Foundation provides emotional support, education programs, information, accommodation, transport, and financial support.

Ronald McDonald Children's Charities (RMCC)
P.O. Box 392
Pennant Hills NSW 1715
Australia
www.rmhc.org.au

The RMCC is committed to helping the families of seriously ill children by providing Ronald McDonald Houses, the Ronald McDonald Learning Program, Ronald McDonald Family Rooms within hospitals, and the Ronald McDonald Family Retreat (free holiday accommodations).

Country Care Link
Sisters of Charity Outreach
438 Victoria Street
Darlinghurst NSW 2010
Australia
www.sistersofcharityoutreach.com.au

Country Care Link has been assisting rural families since 1992. It provides support and hospitality to country people visiting Sydney for medical purposes.

Organizations that provide information

The Academy for Guided Imagery
10780 Santa Monica Blvd., Suite 290
Los Angeles, CA 90025
(800) 726-2070
www.academyforguidedimagery.com

This organization trains health professionals to use interactive guided imagery with their patients and clients. Self-care books and tapes about guided imagery are available for sale. The Academy can help families locate a professional in their area to teach children visualization.

The American Society of Clinical Hypnosis
140 N. Bloomingdale Rd.
Bloomingdale, IL 60108
(630) 980-4740
www.asch.net

A membership organization for doctors, psychologists, and dentists who use hypnosis in their practices. Parents can use the member referral service to find a specialist in their area.

The Disability Rights Education and Defense Fund
2212 Sixth Street
Berkeley, CA 94710
(800) 348-4232
www.dredf.org

Answers questions about the Americans with Disabilities Act, explains how to file a complaint, and provides dispute resolution.

Job Accommodation Network (JAN)
P.O. Box 6080
Morgantown, WV 26506-6080
(800) 526-7234 or (800) ADA-WORK / (800) 232-9675
www.jan.wvu.edu

JAN's mission is to facilitate the employment and retention of workers with disabilities by providing employers, employment providers, people with disabilities, their family members, and other interested parties with information about job accommodations, entrepreneurship, and related subjects. JAN's efforts are in support of the employment, including self-employment and small business ownership, of people with disabilities.

Learning Disabilities Association of America

4156 Library Rd.
Pittsburgh PA 15234-1349
(412) 341-1515
www.ldanatl.org

Organization of parents, professionals, and individuals with learning disabilities. It has local chapters and provides educational materials.

National Cancer Institute (NCI)

NCI Public Inquiries Office
6116 Executive Blvd, Room 3036A
Bethesda, MD 20892-8322
(800) 4-CANCER / (800) 422-6237
www.cancer.gov

Physicians Data Query (PDQ)

(800) 4-CANCER / (800) 422-6237
www.cancer.gov/cancertopics/pdq

Provides a comprehensive website and a nationwide telephone service for people with cancer, their families and friends, and the professionals who treat them. The NCI answers questions and provides informational documents about a variety of cancer-related topics, including fact sheets on cancers, treatment options, and clinical trials.

PDQ is the NCI's computerized listing of accurate and up-to-date information for patients and health professionals about cancer treatments, research studies, and clinical trials.

CureSearch, National Childhood Cancer Foundation

4600 East West Highway, Suite 600
Bethesda, MD 20814-3457
(800) 458-6223
www.curesearch.org

Children's Oncology Group

Research Operations Center
440 E. Huntington Dr., Suite 400
Arcadia, CA 91006
www.childrensoncologygroup.org

Supports pediatric cancer treatment and research at approximately 235 hospitals in North America. Provides information about childhood cancers, clinical trials, and psychosocial support.

National Coalition for Cancer Survivorship
1010 Wayne Avenue, Suite 770
Silver Spring, MD 20910
(301) 650-9127 or (888) 650-9127
www.canceradvocacy.org

An organization that addresses the needs of long-term cancer survivors and advocates for change in healthcare to maximize survivor's access to optimal treatment and support. Extensive resource guide and publications list.

National Dissemination Center for Children and Youth with Disabilities (NICHCY)
1825 Connecticut Ave. NW, Suite 700
Washington, DC 20009
(800) 695-0285 or (202) 884-8441
www.nichcy.org

A clearinghouse that provides pamphlets and information about disabilities and the rights of disabled children and their parents.

Organizations that provide emotional support

Cancer Care, Inc.
275 Seventh Avenue
New York, NY 10001
(800) 813-HOPE / (800) 813-4673 or (212) 712-8400
www.cancercare.org

A national, nonprofit organization that provides referrals, one-on-one counseling, specialized support groups, and educational programs.

Center for Attitudinal Healing
33 Buchanan Drive
Sausalito, CA 94965
(415) 331-6161
www.corstone.org

A nonprofit, nonsectarian group that sponsors local and national workshops for children with catastrophic or life-threatening diseases and their siblings. The Center uses music and art in a supportive program to help children ages 6 to 16 share their feelings about their situation.

Chai Lifeline/Camp Simcha
National Office
151 West 30th Street, Third Floor
New York, NY 10001
(877) CHAI-LIFE / (877) 242-4543 or (212) 465-1300
www.chailifeline.org

A national, nonprofit Jewish organization that provides support service programs to children and their families in crisis, including medical referrals, support groups, visits to hospitalized and housebound children, financial aid, transportation, a kosher camp for kids with cancer, and more.

Child Life Council
11821 Parklawn Drive, Suite 310
Rockville, MD 20852
(301) 881-7090
www.childlife.org

Promotes the well-being of children and families in healthcare settings by supporting the development and practice of the child life profession with training conferences, publications, and information.

Coping Magazine
P.O. Box 682268
Franklin, TN 37068
(615) 790-2400
www.copingmag.com

A bimonthly publication for people whose lives have been touched by cancer.

National Children's Cancer Society
One South Memorial Drive, Suite 800
St. Louis, MO 63101
(800) 5–FAMILY / (800) 532-6459 or (314) 241-1600
www.children-cancer.com
www.beyondthecure.org

Helps children affected by childhood cancer and their families by providing financial assistance, advocacy, education, and emotional support. Beyond the Cure offers free telephone workshops about various childhood cancer issues.

Songs of Love Foundation
P.O. Box 750809
Forest Hills, NY 11375
(800) 960-SONG / (800) 960-7664
www.songsoflove.org

A nonprofit organization with a volunteer group of more than 200 artists who produce personalized musical portraits for children with chronic or life-threatening diseases.

Starlight Foundation
5757 Wilshire Boulevard, Suite M100
Los Angeles, CA 90036
(310) 479-1212
www.starlight.org

Starlight brings together experts from pediatric healthcare, technology, and entertainment to create programs that educate, entertain, and inspire seriously ill children. Whether it's finding friends online, learning more about a disease, or just spending time together as a family, Starlight's programs help children and families cope with the challenges they face daily.

Australia

CanTeen, The Australian Organization for Young People Living with Cancer
National Office
GPO Box 3821
Sydney NSW 2001
Australia
www.canteen.org.au

CanTeen provides support services to its members, who are young people aged 12 to 24 and living with cancer.

Challenge Foundation
529-535, King Street
West Melbourne VIC 3003
Australia
www.challenge.org.au

Challenge is a nonprofit organization that was established in 1983 to provide children living with cancer with the opportunity to interact with other children in similar circumstances. Challenge offers services for families 365 days a year, including camps, hospital support, respite and holiday accommodations, parent support, family activity days, and extensive ticketing programs.

Childhood Cancer Support (CCS)
P.O. Box 295
Red Hill Qld 4059
Australia
www.ccs.org.au

CCS is a charity with a big heart, which has, for more than 30 years, kept its focus where it's needed—on sick children and their families. CCS provides counseling, financial assistance, recreational therapy activities, and most importantly, love and support.

Humour Foundation
Unit 6, 17-19 Mooramba Road
Dee Why NSW 2099
Australia
www.humourfoundation.com.au

The Humour Foundation's core project is Clown Doctors, which touches the lives of more than 100,000 people every year. The focus is children's hospitals, and Clown Doctors are now part of hospital life in all major children's hospitals around Australia.

Bone marrow and stem cell transplantation

BMT InfoNet
2310 Skokie Valley Road, Suite 104
Highland Park, IL 60035
(888) 597-7674
www.bmtinfonet.org

The BMT InfoNet (Blood & Marrow Transplant Information Network) is a not-for-profit organization dedicated to serving the needs of people facing a bone marrow, blood stem cell, or umbilical cord blood transplant. BMT InfoNet provides high-quality medical information in easy-to-understand language so patients can be active, knowledgeable participants in their healthcare planning and treatment.

Children's Organ Transplant Association (COTA)
2501 West COTA Drive
Bloomington, IN 47403
(800) 366-2682
www.cota.org

Provides fundraising help.

National Bone Marrow Transplant Link
20411 W. 12 Mile Road, Suite 108
Southfield, MI 48076
(800) LINK-BMT / (800) 546-5268 or (248) 358-1886
www.nbmtlink.org

Provides educational booklets, peer support, a library, clearinghouse, and suggestions for financial assistance.

National Marrow Donor Program (NMDP)
3001 Broadway Street, NE, Suite 100
Minneapolis, MN 55413
Patient Advocacy: (888) 999-6743
Business Line: (800) MARROW-2 / (800) 627-7692
www.marrow.org

The NMDP has the world's largest computerized listing of potential bone marrow donors. The NMDP, which in 2009 renamed the registry "Be The Match," has cooperative search arrangements with many other registries worldwide, providing access to more than 12 million donors and 300,000 umbilical cord units. It also provides information about transplant centers in the United States.

The National Transplant Assistance Fund
150 N. Radnor Chester Road, Suite F-120
Radnor, PA 19087
(800) 642-8399 or (610) 353-9684
www.transplantfund.org

Provides fundraising assistance and donor awareness material to transplant and catastrophic injury patients nationwide.

Camps

For a comprehensive list, visit *www.acor.org/ped-onc/cfissues/camps.html*.

Camp Simcha
151 West 30th Street, Third Floor
New York, NY 10001
(877) CHAI-LIFE / (877) 242-4543 or (212) 465-1300
www.chailifeline.org

A kosher camp from the national, nonprofit Jewish organization Chai Lifeline.

Children's Oncology Camping Association International
P.O. Box 41433
Des Moines, IA 50311
(515) 669-4580
www.coca-intl.org

Umbrella organization of groups that provide camps for children with cancer.

Australia

Camp Quality
P.O. Box 400
Epping, NSW 1710
Australia
www.campquality.org.au

Organization that provides fun therapy for children and families of children with cancer, including camps for ill children and their siblings, family camps, fun days, pamper days for moms and daughters, and fishing weekends for fathers and sons. It also has interactive puppets that visit the children at clinic, and puppets that go into schools to educate children about living with cancer and acceptance of those who are different.

Drug reimbursement

Partnership for Prescription Assistance
950 F Street NW
Washington, DC 20004
(888) 477-2669
www.phrma.org/searchcures/dpdpap

The Partnership is sponsored by America's pharmaceutical research companies. It helps find companies and agencies that provide prescription medicines free of charge to physicians whose patients might not otherwise have access to necessary medicines.

RxHope
P.O. Box 42886
Cincinnati, OH 45242
(877) 267-0517
www.rxhope.com

A resource for patient-assistance programs that are offered by federal, state, and charitable organizations.

PatientAssistance.com, Inc.
11608 Darryl Drive
Baton Rouge, LA 70815
www.patientassistance.com

Helps uninsured patients get free medication.

NeedyMeds, Inc.
P.O. Box 219
Gloucester, MA 01931
www.needymeds.org

NeedyMeds is a nonprofit with the mission of helping people who cannot afford medicine or healthcare costs. The information at NeedyMeds is available anonymously and free of charge.

Financial help

Cancer Fund of America
2901 Breezewood Lane
Knoxville, TN 37921
(800) 578-5284
www.cfoa.org

Helps with cancer-related expenses not covered by insurance.

Sparrow Clubs USA
906 NE Greenwood Ave., Suite 2
Bend, OR 97701
(541) 312-8630
www.sparrowclubs.org

Promotes youth compassion by establishing and supporting Sparrow Clubs to help local children in medical crises. Provides a grant for the ill child that local children/schoolmates/friends earn by doing community service or fundraising.

Australia

Kids with Cancer Foundation
P.O. Box 135
Westmead NSW 2145
Australia
www.kidswithcancer.org.au

Provides funds to assist doctors, nurses, families, and support groups involved in caring for children suffering with childhood cancer.

Insurance help

Patient Advocate Foundation
700 Thimble Shoals Boulevard, Suite 200
Newport News, VA 23606
(800) 532-5274
www.patientadvocate.org

Provides publications, help with insurance problems, and referrals to attorneys.

The National Association of Insurance Commissioners (NAIC)
2301 McGee Street, Suite 800
Kansas City, MO 64108-2662
(816) 842-3600
www.naic.org

The NAIC is an organization of insurance regulators from the 50 states, the District of Columbia, and the four U.S. territories. The NAIC website links to each state's insurance regulator.

Insure Kids Now!
(877) KIDS NOW / (877) 543-7669
www.insurekidsnow.gov

The U.S. Department of Health and Human Services began the Insure Kids Now! Program to link the nation's uninsured children with free or low-cost health insurance.

Free air services

Air Charity Network
4620 Haygood Road, Suite 1
Virginia Beach, VA 23455
(877) 621-7177
http://aircharitynetwork.org

Air Charity Network is made up of independent member organizations identified by specific geographical service areas. These organizations are groups of volunteer pilots, or groups that coordinate free airline tickets or reduced-price ambulatory services.

Air Care Alliance
2060 State Hwy 595
Lindrith, New Mexico 87029
(888) 260-9707
www.aircareall.org

A nationwide association of humanitarian flying organizations that provide flights for healthcare, compassion, and community service.

Angel Flight America
Administrative Office
4620 Haygood Road, Suite 1
Virginia Beach, VA 23455
(800) 296-3797
www.angelflightmidatlantic.org

Provides free transportation to medical treatment for people who cannot afford public transportation or who cannot tolerate it for health reasons. (A member of Air Charity Network.)

Miles For Kids In Need (American Airlines)
(817) 963-8118
www.aa.com/kids

Provides free travel for ill children and their families. A third party, such as a charitable organization, hospital, or other tax-exempt organization, must submit travel requests.

CAREFORCE (Continental Airlines)
(281) 261-6626

Provides nearly free travel for ill children and one accompanying adult to or from any destination serviced by Continental Airlines. A third party, such as a doctor, social worker, or lawyer, must submit requests.

Corporate Angel Network, Inc. (CAN)
Westchester County Airport
One Loop Road
White Plains, NY 10604
(866) 328-1313
www.corpangelnetwork.org

A nationwide, nonprofit program designed to give patients with cancer the use of available seats on corporate aircrafts to get to and from recognized cancer treatment centers. Patients must be able to walk and travel without life-support systems or medical attention. A child may be accompanied by up to two adults. This service will also fly donors. There is no cost or financial-need requirements.

Mercy Medical Airlift
4620 Haygood Road, Suite 1
Virginia Beach, VA 23455
(800) 296-1217
http://mercymedical.org

Dedicated to serving people in situations of compelling human need through the provision of charitable air transportation. (A member of Air Charity Network.)

Miracle Flights for Kids
2756 N. Green Valley Parkway, #115
Green Valley, NV 89014-2120
(800) FLY-1711 / (800) 359-1711 or (702) 261-0494
www.miracleflights.org

An organization that purchases commercial airline tickets, utilizes private aircrafts, and combines resources from individual donors to provides free transportation to medical treatment centers all across America.

PatientTravel.org
24-hour hot line: (800) 296-1217
www.patienttravel.org

Specialists refer callers to the most appropriate, cost-effective charitable or commercial services, including volunteer pilot organizations and special airline transport programs. (A member of Air Charity Network.)

Canada

Hope Air
4711 Yonge Street, Suite 703
Toronto, ON Canada M2N 6K8
(877) 346-HOPE / (877) 346-4673
www.hopeair.org

An organization that provides free air transport to Canadians in financial need who must travel from their communities to recognized facilities for medical care.

Australia

Angel Flight Australia
P.O. Box 1201
Fortitude Valley, QLD 4006
Australia
www.angelflight.org.au

Angel Flight is a charity that coordinates non-emergency flights to help people trying to deal with bad health, poor finances, and daunting distance. All flights are free and may involve patients traveling to medical facilities anywhere in Australia.

Wish-fulfillment organizations

In addition to the large organizations listed below, there are many smaller and local organizations that grant wishes to seriously ill children. A more comprehensive list of wish fulfillment organizations can be found online at *www.acor.org/ped-onc/cfissues/maw.html.*

Children's Wish Foundation International
8615 Roswell Road
Atlanta, GA 30350
(800) 323-WISH / (800) 323-9474
www.childrenswish.org

Organization in the United States and Europe that fulfills the wishes of terminally ill children.

The Dream Factory, Inc.
200 W. Broadway, Suite 504
Louisville, KY 40202
(800) 456-7556
www.dreamfactoryinc.com

This organization has chapters in 30 states and grants the wishes of children ages 3 to 18 who are critically or chronically ill.

Make-a-Wish Foundation of America
4742 N. 24th St., Suite 400
Phoenix, AZ 85016
(800) 722-WISH / (800) 722-9474
www.wish.org

The Foundation has U.S. and international chapters and affiliates. It grants wishes to children under the age of 18 with life-threatening illnesses.

Sunshine Foundation
1041 Mill Creek Drive
Feasterville, PA 19053
(215) 396-4770
www.sunshinefoundation.org

This Foundation has no geographic boundaries and grants wishes to chronically or terminally ill children ages 3 to 18.

Canada

The Children's Wish Foundation of Canada
350-1101 Kingston Road
Pickering, ON L1V 1B5
(905) 839-8882 or (800) 700-4437
www.childrenswish.ca

This group's goal is to provide a once-in-a-lifetime experience for children ages 3 to 18 with high-risk, life-threatening diseases. There are chapters throughout Canada.

Australia

Make-A-Wish Foundation of Australia National Office
P.O. Box 5006
Burnley VIC 3121
Australia
www.makeawish.org.au

Grants seriously ill children in Australia their most-cherished wish.

Starlight Children's Foundation Australia
www.starlight.org.au

Brightens the lives of seriously ill and hospitalized children and their families throughout Australia by granting wishes, providing vans that travel to remote hospitals to cheer children's lives, and offering activities, entertainment, and engagement in hospital Starlight Rooms. In 2009, Starlight launched Livewire (*www.livewire.org.au*), an online community connecting children and young people aged over 10 and under 21 who are living with a serious illness, chronic health condition, or disability. The community helps reduce the isolation and loneliness these young people often experience.

Hospice and bereavement

The Centering Corporation
7230 Maple Street
Omaha, NE 68134
(402) 553-1200 or (866) 218-0101
www.centering.org

Publishes a free catalog that contains an extensive listing of books, cards, audiotapes, and videotapes about death and grieving.

Children's Hospice International
1101 King Street, Suite 360
Alexandria, VA 22314
(800) 24-CHILD / (800) 242-4453 or (703) 684-0330
www.chionline.org

Provides resources and referrals for families of children with life-threatening conditions.

The Compassionate Friends National Office
900 Jorie Blvd., Suite 78
Oak Brook, IL 60523
(877) 969-0010 or (630) 990-0010
www.compassionatefriends.org

A self-help organization that offers understanding and friendship to bereaved families through support meetings at local chapters and telephone support (they match people with similar losses). Publishes a newsletter for parents and one for siblings.

Australia

Bear Cottage
P.O. Box 2500
Manly NSW 1655
Australia
www.bearcottage.chw.edu.au

NSW's only children's hospice, located on the grounds of St Patrick's Estate, Manly, in Sydney. It offers both respite and palliative care to children and young people with life-limiting illnesses and their families.

The Compassionate Friends New South Wales
4th Floor, Room 404
32 York Street
Sydney NSW 2000
Australia
www.thecompassionatefriends.org.au

Assists families in the positive resolution of grief following the death of a child and provides information to help others be supportive.

Palliative Care Australia
P.O. Box 24
Deakin West ACT 2600
Australia
www.palliativecare.org.au

National organization representing the interests and aspirations of all who share the ideal of quality care at the end of life for all.

Books, Websites, and Videotapes

A WEALTH OF INFORMATION about childhood leukemia is available through libraries and computers. This appendix briefly describes how to get the most from these resources and lists specific books, videotapes/DVDs, and websites that you might find helpful when researching your child's medical condition or treatment.

You might find there are some books you wish to own. If they are not in stock at your local or online bookstore, ask if they can be special-ordered for you—most bookstores are happy to do this. Copies of out-of-print books can often be located on the Internet through used bookstores or private sellers on sites such as Amazon.com.

How to get information from your library or computer

Most libraries have a computerized database of all materials available in their various branches, although some libraries may still use a manual card catalog system. If you need help learning how to use these book-locating systems, ask a librarian. You can also learn how to request a book from another branch and how to put a book on hold if it is currently checked out.

If a book is not in your library's collection, ask the librarian if she can obtain it from another library via an inter-library loan. This is a common practice, and you might be able to get medical texts from university or medical school libraries. Some areas/counties also have online databases that list all publications available at regional libraries; this way, you can look up a book on the Internet, find out which library has it, and request that it be sent to your local library for pick up.

In addition to books, you can find relevant magazine and medical journal articles at the library. The librarian can show you how to use the database to search for articles and where to find the periodicals. Public libraries usually subscribe to only the most popular medical journals, such as the *New England Journal of Medicine* and *Journal of the American Medical Association.* If you are able to visit a university or medical school library, you will find many more medical journals available. To find the nearest medical library open to the public, call the National Network of Libraries of Medicine at (800) 338-7657. If you do not live close to one of these libraries, ask your local librarian to help you obtain copies of the articles you want.

An astonishing amount of information is available through the Internet. Libraries from all over the world can be accessed, and you can download information in minutes from huge databases such as MedLine or Cancerlit. Obtaining information from large medical databases, established journals, or large libraries is exceedingly helpful for parents at home with sick children. However, the huge numbers of people using the Internet has spawned chat rooms, bulletin boards, and thousands of lists of FAQs (frequently asked questions) that may or may not contain accurate information. You may want to adopt the motto: "Let the buyer beware."

If you do not have a home computer, many libraries provide Internet access. Ask the librarian to help you connect to MedLine, Physician's Data Query (PDQ), or other databases you wish to search.

Information provided in this appendix has been organized by topic. If you cannot find a book in your bookstore, library, or online bookseller, the following organizations may have copies available, as well as additional resources for all age groups:

- **Candlelighters Childhood Cancer Foundation.** Books and articles about childhood cancer, coping skills, death and bereavement, effects on family, and long-term side effects. Excellent resource. Available by calling (800) 366-2223 (CCCF) or visiting *www.candlelighters.org.*

- **Centering Corporation's Creative Care Package.** Lists more than 350 books and videos about coping with serious illness, loss, and grief. Available at (402) 553-1200 or by visiting *www.centering.org.*

General

Reading for adults

Bearison, David J. *"They Never Want to Tell You": Children Talk About Cancer.* Cambridge, Massachusetts: Harvard University Press, 1991. Several children and teenagers living with cancer candidly discuss their feelings. Written by a developmental psychologist.

Bombeck, Erma. *I Want to Grow Hair, I Want to Grow Up, I Want to Go to Boise.* New York: Harper & Row Publishers, 1989. Funny, touching book about children surviving cancer. This book is out of print, but it may be in your local library or a used bookstore.

Connolly, Harry. *Fighting Chance: Journeys Through Childhood Cancer.* Baltimore: Woodholm House, 1998. Contains more than 200 pictures of patients, families, and caregivers battling childhood cancer.

Cousins, Norman. *Head First: The Biology of Hope and the Healing Power of the Human Spirit.* New York: E.P. Dutton, 1990. After 25 years as editor of Saturday Review, Cousins spent a decade on the medical staff of University of California Los Angeles (UCLA) researching the biological basis for hope. He presents the mounting volume of evidence that positive attitudes help combat disease. Also contains excellent information about enhancing the doctor/patient relationship.

Johnson, Joy, and S. M. Johnson. *Why Mine? A Book for Parents Whose Child Is Seriously Ill.* Omaha, Nebraska: Centering Corporation, 1981. To order, call (402) 553-1200. Quotes from parents across the country make this a valuable book for families of seriously ill children. Addresses fears, feelings, marriages, siblings, and the ill child.

Krueger, Gretchen. *Hope and Suffering: Children, Cancer, and the Paradox of Experimental Medicine.* Baltimore: John Hopkins University Press, 2008. This narrative explores how doctors, families, and the public viewed the experience of childhood cancer from the 1930s through the 1970s, a period in which cancer was transformed from a killer to a curable disease.

Krumme, Cynthia. *Having Leukemia Isn't So Bad. Of Course It Wouldn't Be My First Choice.* Winchester, Massachusetts: Sargasso Enterprises, 1993. Personal story of Catherine Krumme, who was diagnosed with leukemia at age 4, relapsed at age 7, and finished treatment at age 10.

Kushner, Harold. *When Bad Things Happen to Good People,* revised ed. Boston: G.K. Hall, 1997. Rabbi Kushner wrote this comforting book about how people of faith deal with catastrophic events.

Laszlo, John. *The Cure of Childhood Leukemia: Into the Age of Miracles.* Piscataway, NJ: Rutgers University Press, 1996. Fascinating book that describes researchers and scientific developments that contributed to the high rate of cures for childhood leukemia.

Lerner, Michael. *Choices in Healing: Integrating the Best of Conventional and Complementary Approaches to Medicine.* Cambridge, Massachusetts: The MIT Press, 1996. A comprehensive overview of both conventional and complementary approaches to cancer treatment, including nutritional therapies, physical therapies, psychological and spiritual approaches, traditional medicines from around the world, and methods for living with cancer. Compassionate and objective. Available online at *www. commonweal.org/pubs/choices-healing.html.*

National Cancer Institute. *Young People with Cancer: A Handbook for Parents.* A 67-page booklet. To obtain a free copy, call (800) 422-6237 / (800-4-CANCER), or go to *www.cancer.gov/cancertopics/youngpeople.* This booklet describes the different types of childhood cancer, medical procedures, dealing with the diagnosis, family issues, and sources of information.

Woznick, Leigh, and Carol D. Goodheart. *Living With Childhood Cancer: A Practical Guide to Help Families Cope.* Washington, DC: American Psychological Association, 2001. Written by a mother–daughter team, this guidebook draws on the authors' experiences with cancer, as well as their professional expertise and stories from others to help families address the psychological impact of childhood cancer.

General online resources

National Cancer Institute
www.cancer.gov

Detailed descriptions of types of cancers, treatment, and clinical trials.

CANSearch
www.canceradvocacy.org

A guide to cancer resources on the Internet, produced by the National Coalition for Cancer Survivorship (NCCS).

Granny Barb and Art's Leukemia Links
www.acor.org/leukemia

Includes leukemia-specific information, leukemia organizations, and links to useful resources such as CancerNet, abstracts, cancer literature, Internet support groups, bone marrow transplant sites, and cord blood transplant sites.

Pediatric Oncology Resource Center
www.acor.org/ped-onc

Edited by Patty Feist-Mack, this site is the best single source of information about pediatric cancers on the Internet. Contains detailed and accurate material about diseases, treatment, family issues, activism, and bereavement. Also provides links to other helpful cancer sites.

Squirreltales
www.squirreltales.com

An uplifting and practical website that encourages and empowers parents of children with cancer when they are feeling discouraged and powerless.

Reading for children

Crary, Elizabeth. *Dealing with Feelings. I'm Frustrated; I'm Mad; I'm Sad Series.* Seattle: Parenting Press, 1992. Fun, game-like books to teach preschool and early elementary children how to handle feelings and solve problems.

Hautzig, Deborah. *A Visit to the Sesame Street Hospital.* New York: Random House, 1985. Grover, his mother, Ernie, and Bert visit the Sesame Street Hospital in preparation for Grover's upcoming operation.

Keene, Nancy, and Trevor Romain. *Chemo, Craziness & Comfort: My Book About Childhood Cancer,* 2002. A 200-page resource that provides practical information for children diagnosed with cancer between 6 and 12 years of age. Warm and funny illustrations and easy-to-read text help the child (and parents) make sense of cancer and its treatment. Available from the Candlelighters website at *www.candlelighters.org.*

Klett, Amy, and Dave Klett. *The Amazing Hannah.* This 28-page picture book is written for the preschool (1 to 5 years) child who has been diagnosed with cancer. Through real-life photos, children will be able to identify with Hannah's hospital stay, special friends, tests, treatment, and germ care. Also available in Spanish. Order from Candlelighters website at *www.candlelighters.org.*

Krisher, Trudy. *Kathy's Hats: A Story of Hope.* Concept Books, 1992. (800) 255-7675. A charming book for ages 5 to 10 about a girl whose love of hats comes in handy when chemotherapy makes her hair fall out.

Nessim, Susan, and Barbara Wyman. *Draw Me a Picture.* Los Angeles, 1993. A coloring book for children ages 3 to 6 who have cancer. Marty Bunny talks about how it was when he was in the hospital for cancer and invites readers to draw pictures about their experiences. Available for $15 on the Internet at *www.cancervive.org.*

Richmond, Christina. *Chemo Girl: Saving the World One Treatment at a Time.* Sudbury, MA: Jones and Bartlett Publishers, 1996. Written by a 12-year-old girl with rhabdomyosarcoma, this book describes a superhero who shares hope and encouragement.

Rogers, Fred. *Going to the Hospital.* New York: G.P. Putnam's Sons, 1997. With pictures and words, TV's beloved Mr. Rogers helps children ages 3 to 8 learn about hospitals.

Romain, Trevor. *Bullies are a Pain in the Brain.* Minneapolis: Free Spirit Publishing, 1997. Full of warmth and whimsy, this book teaches children skills to cope with teasing and bullying.

Schultz, Charles. *Why, Charlie Brown, Why?* New York: Topper Books, 1990. Tender story of a classmate who develops leukemia. Available as a book or video. For video availability, call the Leukemia and Lymphoma Society, (800) 955-4572 / (800) 955-4LSA.

Reading for teens

Dorfman, Elena. *The C-Word: Teenagers and Their Families Living with Cancer.* Newbury Park, CA: New Sage Press, 1998. Contains photos and the stories of five teenagers with cancer.

Gravelle, Karen, and John A. Bertram. *Teenagers Face to Face with Cancer.* New York: Julian Messner, 1986. Seventeen teenagers talk openly about their experiences with cancer, including diagnosis, dealing with doctors, chemotherapy, relationships with others, planning for the future, and relapse. A heartfelt, honest, yet comforting book. Out of print, but may be available from a library or used bookstore.

Lazar, Linda, and Bonnie Crawford. *In My World.* Omaha, NE: Centering Corporation, 1999. Available by calling (866) 218-0101 or visiting *www.centering.org.* Journal for teens coping with life-threatening or terminal illness. Includes chapters called "Things Accomplished in My Life," "I've Been Thinking," and "Questions I'd Like Answered."

Reading for siblings

American Cancer Society. *When Your Brother or Sister Has Cancer.* To obtain a free copy, call (800) 227-2345. This 16-page booklet describes the emotions felt by siblings of a child with cancer.

O'Toole, Donna. *Aarvy Aardvark Finds Hope: A Read Aloud Story for People of All Ages About Loving and Losing, Friendship and Hope.* Burnsville, NC: Compassion Books, 1988. Aarvy Aardvark and his friend Ralphie Rabbit show how a family member or friend can help another in distress.

Dodd, Mike. 2004. *Oliver's Story* is a 40-page illustrated book targeted for the 3- to 8-year old siblings of children diagnosed with cancer. Illustrated by Mike Dodd and written through the eyes of his 6-year-old son, Oliver. Available through Candlelighters by calling (800) 366-2223 or visiting *www.candlelighters.org.*

Peterkin, Allan. *What About Me? When Brothers and Sisters Get Sick.* Washington, DC: Magination Press, 1992. Describes the feelings of siblings whose brother or sister is hospitalized.

Medical treatment

Leukemia

Baker, Lynn. *You and Leukemia: A Day at a Time,* 2nd ed. Philadelphia: W.B. Saunders Company, 2002. Warm book about many aspects of childhood leukemia. Chapter 4 contains clear descriptions of procedures and treatments for both children and adults.

Leukemia and Lymphoma Society. *Acute Lymphocytic Leukemia, Acute Myelogenous Leukemia, and Chronic Mylogenous Leukemia.* Booklets that explain the three diseases, symptoms, diagnosis, prognosis, and treatments. Available at (800) 955-4572 / (800) 955- 4LSA.

Pizzo, Philip A. and David G. Poplack, eds. *Principles and Practice of Pediatric Oncology,* 5th ed. Philadelphia: Lippencott-Raven, 2005. Extremely technical medical textbook.

Pui, Ching-Hon, ed. *Childhood Leukemias,* 2nd ed. New York: Cambridge University Press, 2006. Medical textbook, extremely technical.

Coping with procedures

Benson, Herbert. *The Relaxation Response.* New York: Harper Paperbacks, 2000. This is an excellent resource for the relaxation method of pain relief.

Lewis, Sheldon, and Sheila Lewis. *Stress-Proofing Your Child: Mind-Body Exercises to Enhance Your Child's Health.* New York: Bantam Books, 1996. This book is highly recommended for all parents. It clearly explains easy ways to teach children techniques such as guided imagery, deep breathing, and meditation to decrease stress, increase a child's sense of control, and boost children's confidence. A wonderful, practical book.

Partnership with medical team

Center for Attitudinal Healing. *Advice to Doctors and Other Big People from Kids.* Berkeley, California: Celestial Arts, 1995. Book written by children with catastrophic illnesses that offers suggestions and expresses their feelings about healthcare workers. Wise and poignant, it reminds us how perceptive and aware children of all ages are, and how absolutely necessary it is to involve them in medical decisions.

Komp, Diane M. *Children Are Images of Grace: A Pediatrician's Trilogy of Faith, Hope, and Love.* Grand Rapids, Michigan: Zondervan Publishing House, 1996. Written by a Christian pediatric oncologist, this book combines three previous books that describe her feelings for her patients and her warm and loving approach to caring for children with cancer.

Hospitalization

Keene, Nancy. *Your Child in the Hospital: A Practical Guide for Parents,* 2nd ed. Sebastopol, California: O'Reilly & Associates, 2002. A pocket guide full of parent stories to help parents prepare their child physically and emotionally for hospitalizations. Also available in Spanish.

Kellerman, Johnathan. *Helping the Fearful Child.* New York: Warner Books, 1986. Although this book was written as a guide for everyday and problem anxieties, it is full of excellent advice for parents of children undergoing traumatic procedures. Chapters 7, "Going to the Doctor," and 8, "Coping with Hospitalization," are full of real-life examples and effective methods to help children. This book is out of print, but it may be available in your local library or a used bookstore.

Clinical trials

Finn, Robert. *Cancer Clinical Trials: Experimental Treatments and How They Can Help You.* Sebastopol, California: O'Reilly & Associates, 1999. Excellent guide that explains the structure, ethics, and types of clinical trials. Also covers how to evaluate a clinical trial and deal with financial issues.

The Centerwatch Clinical Trials Listing Service. This service contains a searchable database of 7,500 current clinical trials in all areas of medicine, including cancer. Available at *www.centerwatch.com.*

Chemotherapy

Dodd, Marylin J. *Managing the Side Effects of Chemotherapy & Radiation Therapy: A Guide for Patients and Their Families,* 2nd ed. University of California San Francisco Nursing, 2001. This book contains thorough explanations of possible side effects of chemotherapy and radiation and suggestions for managing them.

Leukemia and Lymphoma Society. *Understanding Drug Therapy and Managing Side Effects.* Updated 2009. To obtain a free copy, call (800) 955-4572 / (800) 955-4LSA or view it online at *www.leukemia-lymphoma.org.* The 76-page guide includes general information about side effects of chemotherapy and detailed information about drugs used to treat leukemia, lymphoma, and multiple myeloma.

National Institutes of Health. *Chemotherapy & You: Support for People With Cancer.* 2007. Booklet includes answers to commonly asked questions about chemotherapy, its side effects, emotions while on chemotherapy, and nutrition. Available online at *www.cancer.gov.*

Physicians' Desk Reference. Oradell, New Jersey: Medical Economics Data, 2009. Reference, issued yearly, which lists authoritative information about all Food and Drug Administration (FDA)-approved drugs. Technical language. Available at the reference desk in most libraries.

Pizzo, Philip A. and David G. Poplack, eds. *Principles and Practice of Pediatric Oncology,* 5th ed. Philadelphia: Lippencott-Raven, 2005. See chapters titled "General Principles of Chemotherapy" and "Symptom Management in Supportive Care." Extremely technical.

USP DI, Volume II, *Advice for the Patient: Drug Information in Lay Language.* United States Pharmacopeial Convention, Inc., 2005. Contains detailed drug information in non-medical language. Available in most libraries.

Radiation

McKay, Judith and Nancee Hirano. *The Chemotherapy and Radiation Survival Guide.* Oakland, California: New Harbinger, 1998. Basic, understandable guide to chemotherapy and radiation and their side effects.

National Cancer Institute. *Radiation Therapy and You: Support for People With Cancer.* 2007. To order a free copy, call (800) 422-6237 / (800) 4-CANCER; also available online at *www.cancer.gov.* A 52-page booklet that clearly defines radiation, explains what to expect, describes possible side effects, and discusses follow-up care.

O'Connell, Avice, and Norma Leone. *Your Child and X-Rays: A Parents' Guide to Radiation, X-Rays, and Other Imaging Procedures.* Rochester, New York: Lion Press, 1988. An 88-page book that explains x-ray treatments in easy-to-understand language.

Pizzo, Philip A., and David G. Poplack, eds. *Principles and Practice of Pediatric Oncology,* 5th ed. Philadelphia: Lippencott-Raven, 2005. See chapter titled "General Principles of Radiation Oncology." Extremely technical.

Relapse

Adams, David, and Eleanor Deveau. *Coping with Childhood Cancer: Where Do We Go From Here?* revised ed. Toronto: Kinbridge Publications, 1993. Contains an excellent chapter about relapse, which covers such topics as the impact of relapse, how relapse strikes, feelings, pain, siblings, adjustment to living, the adolescent patient, and some thoughts for single parents.

National Cancer Institute. *Advanced Cancer: Living Each Day.* To obtain a free copy, call (800) 422-6237 / (800) 4-CANCER or go to *www.cancer.gov.* This 32-page booklet provides practical information about living with advanced cancer easier.

Stem cell transplantation

Blood and Marrow Transplant Newsletter. This extremely informative and up-to-date newsletter is written and published by a former bone marrow transplant (BMT) patient. To subscribe, call (888) 597-7674. Also electronically published on the Internet at *www.bmtinfonet.org.* Free, but donations are accepted (and appreciated). Includes articles about medical aspects of BMTs, personal stories, and reviews of books and videos about the topic.

Pizzo, Philip A., and David G. Poplack, eds. *Principles and Practice of Pediatric Oncology,* 5th ed. Philadelphia: Lippencott-Raven, 2005. See chapter titled "Stem Cell Transplantation in Pediatric Oncology." Extremely technical.

Stewart, Susan. *Bone Marrow and Blood Stem Cell Transplants: A Book of Basics for Patients.* Highland Park, IL: BMT InfoNet. Available by calling (888) 597-7674, (847) 433-3313, or visiting *www.bmtinfonet.org.* A 228-page book that clearly explains the medical aspects of bone marrow and blood stem cell transplantation, the different types of transplants, emotional and psychological considerations, pediatric transplants, complications, and insurance issues. Technically accurate, yet easy to read.

Stewart, Susan. *Autologous Stem Cell Transplants: A Handbook for Patients*. Highland Park, IL: BMT InfoNet, 2000. Order by calling (888) 597-7674, (847) 433-3313, or visiting *www.bmtinfonet.org*.

General online medical resources

American Cancer Society

www.cancer.org

Provides useful information about cancer treatments, news, and research.

Canadian Cancer Society

www.cancer.ca

Provides useful information about cancer and includes a link to the Society's research partner, the National Cancer Institute of Canada.

Cancer Glossary

www.meds.com/glossary.html

Terms and definitions of words commonly used in cancer care.

Medicine Online

www.meds.com

Provides patients and professionals with in-depth educational information about specific diseases. Also includes information about reimbursement and provides a treatment guide.

Medline Plus

www.nlm.nih.gov/medlineplus/druginformation.html

A service of the U.S. National Library of Medicine and the National Institutes of Health, this site gives information about drugs, including precautions and side effects.

National Cancer Institute

www.cancer.gov

A huge, revamped site that provides accurate information about cancer, its treatments, and clinical trials.

Oncolink

www.oncolink.com

Offers a wide variety of cancer-related information, including articles, handbooks, case studies, writings by patients and their families, and visual images, including a children's art gallery.

PubMed
www.ncbi.nlm.nih.gov/PubMed

The National Library of Medicine's free search service provides access to more than 18 million citations in MEDLINE and PREMEDLINE (with links to participating online journals) and other related databases. Also includes frequently asked questions (FAQs), news, and clinical alerts.

Quackwatch
www.quackwatch.com

Site devoted to explaining questionable practices, including cancer treatments.

Rx List—The Internet Drug Index
www.rxlist.com

Information about more than 4,500 drugs. Also contains a medical dictionary. Available in Spanish and English.

TeleSCAN-Telmatics Services in Cancer
telescan.nki.nl

The first European Internet service for cancer research, treatment, and education, providing a hypermedia interface to primarily European information resources and services related to cancer.

Stem cell transplantation online resources

The Anthony Nolen Bone Marrow Trust
www.anthonynolan.org.uk

A leading research center and the United Kingdom registry for potential donors. This site references other international bone marrow transplant sites.

Blood and Marrow Transplant Newsletter
www.bmtinfonet.org

All issues of the newsletter are online, as well as the book *Bone Marrow Transplants: A Book of Basics for Patients*.

Bone Marrow Donors Worldwide
www.bmdw.org

Maintains a database of volunteer bone marrow donors and cord blood units. Participants comprise 50 bone marrow donor registries from 37 countries, and 28 cord blood registries from 18 countries. The current number of donors and cord blood units is more than 7 million.

The National Marrow Donor Program
www.marrow.org

A nonprofit, single point of access for all sources of stem cells used in transplantation: marrow, peripheral blood, and umbilical cord blood. Currently has more than 4.5 million donors registered.

Emotional support

Babcock, Elise NeeDell. *When Life Becomes Precious: A Guide for Loved Ones and Friends of Cancer Patients.* New York: Bantam Books, 1997. Written by a counselor with more than 2 decades of experience helping cancer patients, this book is full of practical advice for caregivers of cancer patients. It explains with great warmth how to be supportive, handle special occasions, explain cancer to children, and take care of yourself.

Sourkes, Barbara M. *Armfuls of Time: The Psychological Experience of the Child with a Life-Threatening Illness.* Pittsburgh: University of Pittsburgh Press, 1995. Written by a psychologist, this eloquent book features the voices and artwork of children with cancer. It clearly describes the psychological effects of cancer on children and explains the power of the therapeutic process. Highly recommended.

Support groups

Chesler, Mark A. and Barbara Chesney. *Cancer and Self-Help: Bridging the Troubled Waters of Childhood Illness.* Madison: The University of Wisconsin Press, 1995. Written for and about the parents of children with cancer, this book provides explanations of how self-help groups are formed, how they function and recruit, and why they are effective. The authors explain how, through self-help groups, parents improve their coping abilities and become better advocates for their children in an increasingly complex healthcare system.

National Cancer Institute. *Taking Time: Support for People with Cancer and the People Who Care About Them.* 2003. To obtain a free copy, call (800) 422-6237 / (800) 4-CANCER; also available online at *www.cancer.gov.* Sixty-one-page booklet includes sections about sharing feelings, coping within the family, and what to do when you need assistance.

Pizzo, Philip A., and David G. Poplack. *Principles and Practice of Pediatric Oncology,* 5th ed. Philadelphia: Lippincott-Raven, 2005. See the chapters titled "Psychiatric and

Psychosocial Support for the Child and Family" and "The Other of Side of the Bed: What Caregivers Can Learn from Listening to Patients and Their Families."

Speigel, David. *Living Beyond Limits*. New York: Random House, 1993. Dr. Speigel devised the landmark study that showed participation in support groups by women with breast cancer not only lowered rates of depression, but significantly increased their life spans. This book is an excellent guide for coping with cancer, strengthening family relationships, controlling pain, dealing with doctors, and evaluating alternative medicine claims. This book is out of print, but it may be available from your local library or a used bookstore.

Online support groups

ACOR, The Association of Cancer Online Resources, Inc.

www.acor.org

ACOR offers access to 151 mailing lists that provide support, information, and community to everyone affected by cancer and related disorders. It hosts several pediatric cancer discussion groups, including PED-ONC (a general pediatric cancer discussion group), ALL-KIDS (childhood acute lymphoblastic leukemia), ALL-KIDS-RELAPSED (for parents of children with relapsed acute lymphoblastic leukemia), and PED-ONC-SURVIVORS (for parents of survivors).

Feelings, communication, and behavior

Faber, Adele, and Elaine Mazlish. *How to Talk So Kids Will Listen…and Listen So Kids Will Talk*, 20th ed. New York: Rawson, Wade Publishers, 1999. The classic book about developing new, more effective ways to communicate with your children, based on respect and understanding. Highly recommended.

Faber, Adele, and Elaine Mazlish. *Siblings Without Rivalry: How to Help Your Children Live Together So You Can Live Too*. New York: Harper Paperbacks, 2004. Required reading for parents with fighting siblings. Offers dozens of astonishingly simple yet effective methods to reduce conflict and foster a cooperative spirit.

Kurcinka, Mary Sheedy. *Raising Your Spirited Child: A Guide for Parents Whose Child Is More Intense, Sensitive, Perceptive, Energetic*, rev. ed. New York: Harper Paperbacks, 2006. Reassuring guide about how to effectively parent children who are more intense, sensitive, perceptive, persistent, energetic, or uncomfortable with change than average children. Many of the strategies are very effective for children stressed by cancer treatment.

Nelsen, Jane. *Positive Discipline*, rev. ed. New York: Ballantine Books, 2006. Written by a psychologist, educator, and mother of seven, this book teaches parents how to promote self-discipline and personal responsibility.

Practical support

Finances

Leeland, Jeff. *One Small Sparrow: Michael's Story of Hope and Compassion in the Classroom.* Sisters, Oregon: Multnomah Books, 2000. Written by the father of a baby with leukemia, this heartwarming true story describes how a community raised the entire cost of a successful bone marrow transplant. Contains numerous ideas for methods to raise funds. Christian perspective.

Pammenter Tolley, Diane. *Finding the Money: A Guide to Paying Your Medical Bills.* Highland Park, IL: Tyndale House Publishers, 2001. Available from BMT Infonet at (888) 597-7674. A book to help families of people who need transplants. It provides information about assessing what your transplant and aftercare will cost, how to track and pay for bills, and fundraising. Includes stories from patients who succeeded in raising funds to cover the costs of medical care.

Peterson, Sheila. *A Special Way to Care.* Croton Falls, NY: Friends of Karen, 1988. A guide for those who wish to provide financial/emotional support for families of ill children. Discusses how to differentiate between interference and advocacy. Explains how to organize, manage, and perpetuate a support fund. Excellent resource. Out of print but might be available at libraries or a used bookstore.

Pizzo, Philip A., and David G. Poplack, eds. *Principles and Practice of Pediatric Oncology,* 5th ed. Philadelphia: Lippincott-Raven, 2005. See the chapter titled "Financial Issues in Pediatric Cancer."

Nutrition

National Cancer Institute. *Eating Hints for Cancer Patients,* rev. ed. Darby, PA: Diane Pub Co, 1994. To obtain a copy, call (800) 422-6237 / (800) 4CANCER, or go online to *www.cancer.gov.* This 96-page booklet covers eating well during cancer treatment, managing eating problems, special diets, family resources, and recipes.

Pizzo, Philip A., and David G. Poplack, eds. *Principles and Practice of Pediatric Oncology,* 5th ed. Philadelphia: Lippincott-Raven, 2002. See the chapter titled "Nutritional Supportive Care."

Wilson, J. Randy. *Non-Chew Cookbook.* Wilson Publishing, Inc., 1986. Contains recipes for patients unable to chew due to the side effects of chemotherapy and/or radiation.

Overview of Nutrition in Cancer Care. National Cancer Institute, 2009. General information, along with links to cookbooks and other resources. Article online at the National Cancer Institute website at *www.cancer.gov/cancertopics/pdq/supportivecare/nutrition.*

School

Anderson, Winifred, Stephen Chitwood, and Deidre Hayden. *Negotiating the Special Education Maze: A Guide for Parents and Teachers,* 3rd ed. Bethesda, Maryland: Woodbine House, 1997. Excellent, well-organized text clearly explains the step-by-step process necessary to obtain help for your child. Has resource list and a comprehensive bibliography.

Chai Lifeline. *Back to School: A Handbook for Educators of Children with Life-threatening Diseases in the Yeshiva/Day School System.* New York: Chai Lifeline/Camp Simcha, 1995. Covers diagnosis, planning for school reentry, infection control in schools, needs of junior and senior high school students, children with special educational needs, and saying good-bye when a child dies. Includes a bibliography and resource list. Available through Chai Lifeline at *www.chailifeline.org.*

Gliko-Braden, Majel. *Grief Comes to Class: A Teacher's Guide.* Omaha, NE: Centering Corporation, 1992. Comprehensive guide to grief in the classroom. Includes chapters about grief responses, the bereaved student, teen grief, developmental changes, sample letter to parents, sample teacher-parent conference, and suggestions for dos and don'ts. Available at (402) 553-1200 or by visiting *www.centering.org.*

Keene, Nancy, ed. *Educating the Child With Cancer: A Guide for Parents and Teachers.* 2003. An essential resource for families who have faced the childhood cancer diagnosis. Written by top researchers in the field and balanced with parents' personal experiences, this 322-page resource focuses on educational issues for children treated for cancer. It is intended to promote understanding and communication between parents, educators, and medical professionals so that together they can provide an appropriate education for children who have been treated for cancer. Available through Candlelighters by calling (800) 366-2223 or visiting *www.candlelighters.org.*

Levine, Mel. *All Kinds of Minds.* Cambridge, Massachusetts: Educator's Publishing Service, Inc., 1993. Highly readable book about different learning styles. Written for grade-school-aged children, but parents will also benefit from reading it.

Leukemia and Lymphoma Society (LLS). *The Trish Greene Back-to-School Program for Children with Cancer.* Designed to increase communication among healthcare professionals, parents, patients, and school officials to assure a smooth transition from active treatment back to school and daily life. Materials, videos, and other printed inventory are available at all local LLS chapters. Available at *www.leukemia-lymphoma.org* or by calling (800) 955-4572 / (800) 955-4LSA.

Levine, Mel. *Keeping a Head in School: A Student's Book About Learning Abilities and Learning Disorders.* Cambridge, Massachusetts: Educator's Publishing Service, Inc., 1991. Book about different learning styles of junior high and high school students.

Mangrum, Charles (ed.). *Peterson's Colleges With Programs for Students With Learning Disabilities or Attention Deficit Disorders,* 6th ed. Princeton, NJ: Peterson's Guides, 2003. Excellent reference that is available at most large libraries.

Pizzo, Philip A. and David G. Poplack, eds. *Principles and Practice of Pediatric Oncology.* Philadelphia: Lippincott-Raven, 2005. See chapter 50, "Educational Issues for Children with Cancer."

Silver, Larry. *The Misunderstood Child: Understanding and Coping with Your Child's Learning Disabilities,* 4th ed. New York: Times Books, 2006. Comprehensive discussion about positive treatment strategies that can be implemented at home and in the school to help children with learning disabilities. Excellent chapters about psychological, social, and emotional development; evaluation; and treatment.

The Compassionate Friends. *Suggestions for Teachers and School Counselors.* Oak Brook, IL: The Compassionate Friends, 2008. To obtain a copy, write to: P.O. Box 3696, Oak Brook, IL 60522, call (630) 990-0010, or visit *www.compassionatefriends.org.*

Federal agencies

U.S. Food and Drug Administration
www.fda.gov

Social Security Benefits for Children with Disabilities
www.ssa.gov/pubs/10026.html

Americans with Disabilities Act Homepage
www.ada.gov

Health Insurance Portability and Accountability Act
www.hhs.gov/ocr/privacy/index.html

Practical support online

Bandaids and Blackboards—When Chronic Illness Goes to School
www.lehman.cuny.edu/faculty/jfleitas/bandaides

Scholarships for Survivors of Childhood Cancer
www.acor.org/ped-onc/scholarships/index.html

Wrightslaw
www.wrightslaw.com

Accurate, up-to-date information about special educational law for parents, advocates, and attorneys.

After treatment ends

Survivorship reading

Hoffman, Barbara, ed. *A Cancer Survivor's Almanac: Charting Your Journey,* 3rd ed. Silver Spring, MD: National Coalition for Cancer Survivorship. Comprehensive guide to the issues of cancer survivorship. Includes sections about dealing with doctors and hospitals; the mind/body relationship; support services; peer support; employment, insurance, and money matters; dealing with the family; and an appendix with survivor resources. Available for $3.50 at *www.canceradvocacy.org/resources/resources-order-form.html.*

Harpham, Wendy Schlessel. *After Cancer: A Guide to Your New Life.* New York: Harper Perrennial, 1995. Written in a question and answer format, doctor and cancer survivor Harpham addresses the medical, psychological, and practical issues of recovery.

Institute of Medicine, National Research Council. *Childhood Cancer Survivorship, Improving Care and Quality of Life.* Washington, DC: 2003. Comprehensive coverage of survivorship issues, including late effects of treatment and how to obtain survivorship care. Available as full text online or as a paperback ($29.70) through the National Academies Press website at *www.nap.edu.*

Keene, Nancy, Wendy Hobbie, and Kathy Ruccione. *Childhood Cancer Survivors: A Practical Guide to Your Future,* 2nd ed. Sebastopol, California: O'Reilly Media, 2007. A user-friendly, comprehensive guide about late effects of treatment for childhood cancer. Full of stories from survivors of all types of childhood cancer. Also covers emotional issues, insurance, jobs, relationships, and ways to stay healthy.

Leukemia and Lymphoma Society. *Coping with Survival.* To obtain a free copy, call (800) 955-4572 / (800) 955-4LSA or visit online at *www.leukemia-lymphoma.org.* This 32-page booklet includes information about diagnosis, communicating with physicians, treatment, life after treatment, and services and support.

Pizzo, Philip A. and David G. Poplack, eds. *Principles and Practice of Pediatric Oncology,* 5th ed. Philadelphia: Lippincott-Raven, 2005. See chapter 49, "Late Effects of Childhood Cancer and Its Treatment," and the chapters titled, "Pediatric Cancer: Advocacy, Legal, Insurance, and Employment Issues" and "Preventing Cancer in Adulthood: Advice for the Pediatrician."

Survivorship resources online

Childhood Cancer Guides' Survivor Resource Center

www.childhoodcancerguides.org/sresource.html

Contains portions of the book Childhood Cancer Survivors and links to important resources.

Ped-Onc Resource Center Survivor Issues

www.acor.org/ped-onc/survivors

Articles about the late effects of childhood cancer, a bibliography of journal articles of interest to survivors, links to resources and online articles, and a list of survivors' clinics.

Children's Oncology Group Long-term Follow-up Guidelines

www.childrensoncologygroup.org/disc/LE/default.htm

Downloadable document that details current knowledge about the late effects of childhood cancer. The late effects are listed by treatment (chemotherapy drug or radiation dose/site). Guidelines for diagnostic tests are detailed. Includes individual "Health Links" for more than 30 specific late effects issues.

Beyond the Cure

www.beyondthecure.org

Articles about late effects issues, teleconference series, and free publications.

LiveStrong

www.livestrong.org

A resource for cancer survivors.

Survivor Alert Website

www.survivoralert.org

A project created in association with the film "The Lion in the House." Survivor Alert offers information about survivorship issues.

Terminal illness and bereavement

Callanan, Maggie, and Patricia Kelley. *Final Gifts: Understanding the Special Awareness, Needs, and Communications of the Dying.* New York: Bantam Books, 1997. Written by two hospice nurses with decades of experience, this book helps families understand and communicate with terminally ill patients. Compassionate, comforting, and insightful, *Final Gifts* movingly teaches us how to listen to and comfort the dying. Highly recommended.

Kubler-Ross, Elisabeth. *On Children and Death.* New York: Scribner, 1997. In this comforting book, Dr. Kubler-Ross offers practical help for living through the terminal period of a child's life with love and understanding. Discusses children's knowledge about death, visualization, letting go, funerals, help from friends, and spirituality.

Morse, Melvin. *Closer to the Light: Learning from Near Death Experiences of Children.* New York: Villard Books, 1990. Dr. Morse, a pediatrician and researcher into children's near-death experiences, writes about the startlingly similar spiritual experiences of children who almost die.

Stacy Orloff and Susan M. Huff, ed. *Home Care for the Seriously Ill Child: A Manual for Parents.* Alexandria, VA: Childrens' Hospice International, 2003. Available for $18.00 from Children's Hospice International by calling (800) 2-4-CHILD / (800) 242-4453 or going online to *www.chionline.org.* Helps parents explore the possibility of home care for the dying child. Contains practical information about what to expect, methods of pain relief, and control of medical problems. Appendices on medications, bibliographies, and dos and don'ts for helping bereaved parents.

Pizzo, Philip A., and David G. Poplack, eds. *Principles and Practice of Pediatric Oncology,* 5th ed. Philadelphia: Lippincott-Raven, 2005. See chapter 51 titled "Palliative Care for the Child with Advanced Cancer."

Parental grief

Bereavement: A Magazine of Hope and Healing. For a free copy or to subscribe, call: Bereavement Publishing, Inc., (888) 604-4673 / (888) 604-HOPE; online at *www.bereavementmag.com.*

Bernstein, Judith R. *When the Bough Breaks: Forever After the Death of a Son or Daughter.* Kansas City, Missouri: Andrews & McMeel, 1998. A serious and sensitive look at how to cope with the loss of a child.

Rando, Therese, ed. *Parental Loss of a Child.* Champaign, Illinois: Research Press, 1986. Thirty-seven articles about death cover such topics as serious illness; guilt; grief of fathers, mothers, siblings, single parents; professional help; advice to physicians, clergy, funeral directors; and support organizations.

Wild, Laynee. *I Remember You: A Grief Journal,* 2nd ed. San Francisco: HarperCollins, 2000. A journal for recording written and photographic memories during the first year of mourning. Beautiful book filled with quotes and comfort.

Sibling grief (adult reading)

Doka, Kenneth, ed. *Children Mourning, Mourning Children.* New York: Hemisphere Publications, 1995. A collection of chapters (first presented at the Hospice Foundation of America conference) written by many healthcare professionals who work with grieving children. Topics include children's understanding of death, answering grieving children's questions, the role of the schools, and many others.

Grollman, Earl. *Talking About Death: A Dialogue Between Parent and Child,* 3rd ed. Boston: Beacon Press, 1991. One of the best books for helping children cope with grief. Contains a children's read-along section to explain and explore children's feelings.

In very comforting language, the book teaches parents how to explain death, understand children's emotions, understand how children react to specific types of death, and know when to seek professional help. Also contains a resource section.

Schaefer, Dan, and Christine Lyons. *How Do We Tell the Children? A Step-by-Step Guide for Helping Children Two to Teen Cope When Someone Dies,* 3rd ed. New York: Newmarket Press, 2002. If your terminally ill child has siblings, read this book. In straightforward, uncomplicated language, the authors describe how to explain the facts of death to children and teens, and show how to include the children in the family support network, laying the foundation for the healing process to begin. Also includes a crisis section for quick references about what to do in a variety of situations.

Sibling grief (young child reading)

Buscaglia, Leo. *The Fall of Freddy the Leaf: A Story of Life for All Ages.* New York: Holt, Rinehart and Winston, 1982. This wise yet simple story about a leaf named Freddy explains death as a necessary part of the cycle of life. This book is out of print, but it may be available in your local library or a used bookstore.

Hickman, Martha. *Last Week My Brother Anthony Died.* Abingdon, Tennessee: 1984. Touching story of a preschooler's feelings when her infant brother dies. The family's minister (a bereaved parent himself) comforts her by comparing feelings to clouds—always there but ever changing.

Mellonie, Bryan, and Robert Ingpen. *Lifetimes: The Beautiful Way to Explain Death to Children.* New York: Bantam Books, 1983. Beautiful paintings and simple text explain that dying is as much a part of life as being born.

Sibling grief (school-aged children)

Romain, Trevor. *What on Earth Do You Do When Someone Dies?* Minneapolis: Free Spirit Publishing, 1999. Warm, honest words and beautiful illustrations help children understand and cope with grief.

Temes, Roberta. *The Empty Place: A Child's Guide Through Grief.* Far Hills, New Jersey: New Horizon Press, 1992. To order, call (402) 553-1200. Explains and describes feelings after the death of a sibling, such as the empty place in the house, at the table, and in a sibling's heart.

White, E. B. *Charlotte's Web.* New York: Harper, 1952. Classic tale of friendship and death as a part of life. (A movie version is widely available for rent; there are animated and live action versions available.)

Sibling grief (teenagers)

Gravelle, Karen and Charles Haskins. *Teenagers Face to Face with Bereavement*. Englewood Cliffs, NJ: J. Messner, 2000. The perspectives and experiences of 17 teenagers comprise the heart of this book, which focuses on teens coping with grief.

Grollman, Earl. *Straight Talk About Death for Teenagers: How to Cope with Losing Someone You Love*. Boston: Beacon Press, 1993. Wonderful book that talks to teens, not at them. Discusses denial, pain, anger, sadness, physical symptoms, and depression. Charts methods to help teens work through their feelings at their own pace.

Videotapes/DVDs

Some of the videotapes/DVDs listed in this section are available free from national organizations. Others can be purchased for a modest fee. Some, however, are quite expensive. You might consider asking your hospital social worker or resource room librarian to purchase it for their collection.

Children/Teens

Hairballs on My Pillow. Produced by CARTI. Interviews children with cancer and their friends about friendship and returning to school. Cost is $35 for the video, along with newsletters for students, exercises and activities for students, and a teacher's notebook of information about cancer, its treatment, and dealing with returning students. Available by calling (800) 482-8561 or (501) 664-8573.

Mr. Rogers Talks About Childhood Cancer. Two videos, a guidebook, and a storybook. The videos are 45 minutes. Available free from some local American Cancer Society chapters and Children's Hospitals. Mr. Rogers talks to children and uses characters from the "Land of Make Believe" to stress the importance of talking about feelings.

Why, Charlie Brown, Why? 1990. Tender story of a classmate who develops leukemia. Available as a book or video. For video availability, call the Leukemia and Lymphoma Society at (800) 955-4572 / (800) 955-4LSA.

You Don't Have to Die: Jason's Story. A 27-minute video of Jason Gaes' book, *My Book for Kids With Cansur: A Child's Autobiography of Hope*. To order, call Ambrose Video Publishing at (800) 526-4663.

Parents

CancerEd: Necessary Pictures Film and Media. A workshop presentation kit for schools or communities designed to engage, empower, and enlighten students and teachers about the social, emotional, physical, and psychological aspects of childhood cancer. The video and workbook are designed to connect students and teachers, schools, families, and communities. Available by calling (800) 221-3170.

Cancervive Back to School. Two award-winning documentary videos: "Emily's Story: Back to School After Cancer" and "Making the Grade: Back to School After Cancer for Teens." Available at *www.cancervive.org/dvd.html*. ($40 each)

Coping with Childhood Cancer. A 28-minute video. Five family portraits covering issues such as guilt, sibling rivalry, divorce, the adopted child, and involvement of other family members in the care of the child. Introduction and closing by Bob Keeshan (Captain Kangaroo). Purchase from: Films for the Humanities and Sciences, at *http://ffh.films.com* or by calling (800) 257-5126. Item No. 2519. ($99.95)

Talking about Death with Children. A 13-minute video by Dr. Earl Grollman explains what death means, how it happens, and why there is a funeral. Includes a tour of a funeral home. Available from Batesville Management Services at (800) 446-2504, ext. 7788. ($99)

No Fears, No Tears. Fanlight Distributors, 1986. A 27-minute video by Leora Kuttner, PhD. Documentary about eight young children with cancer and their parents learning how to manage the pain of cancer treatment. Distributed by Fanlight Distributors at (800) 937-4113 or *www.fanlight.com*.

No Fears, No Tears—13 Years Later. Fanlight Distributors, 1998. A 47-minute video by Leora Kuttner, PhD. Thirteen years after learning how to manage their painful cancer treatments, seven survivors of childhood cancer make sense of their early traumatic experiences and demonstrate the power of mind-body pain relief. Distributed by Fanlight Distributors at (800) 937-4113 or *www.fanlight.com*.

When a Child Has Cancer: Helping Families Cope. Discusses marriage, siblings, finances, and other topics. Available at some chapters of the American Cancer Society. Available by calling (800) 227-2345.

Teachers

Drying Their Tears. Produced by CARTI. For information, call (800) 482-8561. Video and manual to help counselors, teachers, and other professionals help children deal with the grief, fear, confusion, and anger that occur after the death of a loved one. Has three segments: one about training facilitators, one for children ages 5 to 8, and one for children ages 9 to teens. Each section includes interviews with children and videos from children's workshops.

The Learning Disabilities Association of Massachusetts has several videos about different aspects of coping with learning disabilities including: "Einstein & Me: Talking About Learning Disabilities"; "Meeting with Success: Ten Tips for a Successful I.E.P"; "Planning for Success: The College Application Process for Students with Learning Disabilities"; "Portraits of Success: Fostering Hope and Resilience in Individuals with Learning Disabilities"; and "Stop and Go Ahead with Success: An Integrated Approach to Helping Children Develop Social Skills." For more information, visit *www.ldam.org*.

Grief

The Healing Path. The Compassionate Friends' video for siblings addresses concerns of surviving siblings, such as sadness, pain, anger, and fear. Video explores eight topics: facing the reality of death, who will listen, changed family life, special days, visiting the cemetery, parental overprotection, feelings and expectations, and looking to the future. For information, call (877) 969-0010 or (630) 990-0010.

Understanding Grief: Kids Helping Kids. A 14-minute video appropriate for children ages 9 to 14. Children who lost a parent or a loved one discuss their feelings. Offers advice about the four Ts (talk, touch, teach, time). Developed by Dr. Earl Grollman. Available from Batesville Management Services at (800) 446-2504, ext. 7788. ($99)

Several videos about grief are available from the Centering Corporation. Go to *www. centering.org* and search for "video" to get a complete list of the products available.

Index

A

Absolute neutrophil count (ANC), 186–189, 339, 438, 441

Accepting help, 232

Acupressure for pain, 70

Acupuncture for pain, 70

Acute lymphoblastic leukemia (ALL), 20–24
 cell types in, 22–23
 chromosome number in, 23
 CNS prophylaxis for, 42–43
 consolidation therapy for, 43
 follow-up care, 363
 induction phase of treatment, 41–42
 maintenance for, 43–44
 newest treatment options, 44–45
 online support groups for, 477
 prognosis for, 21–23
 relapse, treatment of, 377–381
 response to treatment, 23
 standard treatment for, 40–45
 stem cell transplantation for, 44, 386
 thymus enlargement, 16
 translocations in, 22

Acute myeloid leukemia (AML), 24–27
 chloromas, treatment for, 48
 CNS prophylaxis for, 47
 induction phase of treatment, 46
 newest treatment options, 48
 prognosis for, 25
 relapse, treatment of, 381–382
 standard treatment for, 45–48
 stem cell transplantation for, 48,
 subtypes of, 25

Acyclovir, 191
 stem cell transplantation and, 402

Adhesives, 129–130

Adjunctive treatments, 178

Adolescents
 assent to treatment, 59–60
 avascular necrosis, 203
 diagnosis, 31
 pill-taking, 85–86
 school, 37
 support groups, 308
 talking with, 243–246
 withdrawal, 248

Adriamycin (doxorubicin), 148–149
 risks of smoking after, 365

Adversarial relationships with doctors, 93

Advocating for child, 110–113

AIDS virus, 77, 366

Air services, free, 457–460

Alanine aminotransferase (ALT), 442

Alkaloids, 134

Alkylating agents, 134

Allogeneic transplants, 387–388

All-trans-retinoic acid (ATRA), 46, 50, 140

Alternative treatments, 178–180

American Childhood Cancer Organization. *See* Candlelighters Childhood Cancer Foundation

Americans with Disabilities Act (ADA), 368, 448

Anemia, 13, 77, 140

Anesthesia. *See* Sedation

Anger. *See also* Temper tantrums
 acceptable outlets for, 258
 of children, 246
 at diagnosis, 7–9
 at healthcare team, 8, 101
 relapse and, 375
 of siblings, 267

Animals, living with, 204–205

Anniversaries, observing, 425

Anthracyclines, 220, 378

Antibiotics, 134

    dental work and, 198

    lactose intolerance, 321

    prophylactic antibiotics, 166

    stem cell transplantation, 393, 402

    infections in catheters, 117

Antidepressants, 314

Antimetabolites, 134

Antinausea drugs, 146, 167–172

Apheresis, 392–393

APL differentiation syndrome, 140

Appetite

    increased appetite, 320

    loss of, 319–320

    stem cell transplant, after, 406

ARA-C. *See* Cytarabine

Art therapy, 316

Asparaginase, 139, 143–145

Aspartate aminotransferase (AST), 442

Aspirin, 180, 189

Assent, to clinical trial, 59

Atarax, 167

Ataxia telangiectasia, 15

Ativan, 168

ATRA, 46, 50, 140

Attending physicians, 90

Attorneys

    for insurance matters, 350

    National Organization for Social Security Claimant's Representatives (NOSSCR), 350

    stem cell transplantation issues, 397

Australia

    camps, 455

    emotional support organizations, 452–453

    financial help, 456

    free air service, 460

    hospice and bereavement, 462–463

    service organizations, 447–448

    wish fulfillment, 461

Autologous stem cell transplants, 388–390

Avascular necrosis (osteonecrosis), 141, 203–204, 409

B

B-cell ALL, 22–23

Bacterial infections, stem cell transplantation and, 402–403

Bactrim, 85, 166

Bag Balm, 193

Beckwith-Wiedemann syndrome, 15

Bed wetting, 195–198

Behavioral issues

    of children, 246–251

    of parents, 251–255

    stressed children, parenting, 260

Benadryl, 77, 168

Benzene exposure, 16

Bereavement. *See* Death

Bilirubin, 141, 438, 442–443

Biofeedback, 178

    for pain management, 70

Blast, defined, 14

Blended families, 240

Blood, 13–14

    transfusions, 77–78

Blood cell counts, 2, 74

    children on treatment, values for, 438

    healthy children, values for, 437

    low blood counts, 215–219

    pattern, 443

    sample lab data sheets, 439

Blood and Marrow Newsletter, 397

Blood draws, 74

Blood patch, 82

Bloom syndrome, 15

Body surface area (BSA), 135

Bone marrow aspiration, 78–80

    on last day of treatment, 355

    relapse diagnosis at, 374

    sedation for, 70–73

Bone marrow transplant (BMT). *See* Stem cell transplantation

Breads, servings of, 323

Broviac lines. *See* External catheters

Bruising, 1, 15

C

Immune system
GVHD suppresses, 389
redevelop after transplant, 402–403
stem cell transplantation and, 387–388
Immunizations,
after transplant, 403
after treatment, 365
during treatment, 188
Individual Education Program (IEP), 296–308
in Canada, 299
placement options, 296–298
related services under, 297
transition services, 299
Individualized Family Service Plan (IFSP), 290–291
Individuals with Disabilities Education Act (IDEA), 291
Induction therapy
for acute lymphoblastic leukemia (ALL), 41–42
for acute myeloid leukemia (AML), 45–46
Infections
external catheters and, 117
from peripherally inserted central catheters, 127
reducing risk of, 187–189
stem cell transplantation and, 401–403
from subcutaneous ports, 124
Informed consent
to clinical trials, 57–59
to stem cell transplantation, 396
Insurance. *See also* HMOs (health maintenance organizations)
challenging denials, 348–349
contact persons, locating, 347
coping with, 345–346
explanations of benefits (EOBs), 343
Health Insurance Portability and Accountability Act of 1996, 370
hospital billing, 342–345
insurance plans (CHIPS), 369
investigational treatments, 56
negotiating with company, 347–348
second opinions, obtaining, 59, 99
state-sponsored supplemental insurance programs, 351
stem cell transplantation, paying for, 397

survivorship issues, 369
understanding policy, 345–347
Interns, 90
Interstitial pneumonitis, 402
Intrathecal medication, 42
IRS Publication 502 (medical expenses), 342
IV infusion ball, 118
IV (intravenous) lines
feedings, 334–335
starting, 76

J

Jealously of siblings, 35, 265
Job Accommodation Network (JAN), 368–369
Job issues. *See* Employment issues
Journals, keeping, 338
Juvenile myelomonocytic leukemia (JMML), 27, 49–50
stem cell transplantation for, 386

K

Kaopectate, 192
Karyotyping, 23
Ketamine, 72
Klinefelter's syndrome, 15
Kytril (granisetron), 168–170

L

Lactose intolerance, 321
L-ASP, 139, 143–145
L-Asparaginase, 139, 143–145
Lawyers. *See* Attorneys
Learning disabilities, 234. *See also* Special education
acceptance of, 300
Canada, legal rights in, 299
identifying, 293
legal rights, 291–299
radiation therapy and, 218–219
referral for services, 291–292
Leucovorin, 157
Leukapheresis, 41, 392

N

O

P

Relief Band, 185
Religious organizations. *See also* Clergy
Remission, 3
Residents, 90
Resource organizations, 445–463
Resource rooms at hospitals, 310

S

Sadness. *See also* Grief
  at diagnosis, 9
  of siblings, 266–267
Safe sexual practices, 366
School issues, 281–312. *See also* Learning
  disabilities; Special education
    cognitive late effects, identifying, 293
    communicable diseases, 289
    communication with schools, 281
    involving school and classmates, 282–283
    keeping up with work, 284
    legal rights, 291–292
    preschoolers, 290–291
    resources for, 479–480
    returning to school, 285–289
    sibling issues, 285
    terminally ill children, 300–302
    videotape resources, 485–486
Schoolmates. *See* Classmates
Scopolamine patch, 167
Secondary cancers
  cranial radiation and, 220
  stem cell transplantation and, 409
Second opinions, 75
  obtaining, 59, 99–100
  on relapse, 382
Sedation
  drugs used for pain control, 70–73
  for radiation therapy, 211–212
Septra, 85, 166
  methotrexate and, 157
Serum glutamic oxaloacetic transaminase (SGOT),
  438, 442
Serum glutamic pyruvic transaminase (SGPT), 438,
  442

Service organizations, 351, 445–448
  for wigs, 182
Sexual practices, 366
Shingles, 191
Shwachman-Diamond syndrome, 15
Siblings, 263–280
  abandonment, feelings of, 266
  anger of, 267
  communication about diagnosis with, 34
  concerns, 264, 268
  death and, 413, 418, 424
  emotional responses of, 263
  experiences of, 268–276
  fears of, 264
  friends and, 226–227
  gifts for, 227, 256
  grief of, 426–428, 483–484, 487
  guilt of, 265
  household rules, application of, 253
  jealousy of, 265
  lack of time with, 254
  at memorial services, 418–419
  polio vaccinations for, 188
  positive outcomes for, 279
  resources for, 470, 477
  sadness of, 266
  school issues, 285
  stem cell transplantation and, 410
  suggestions for helping, 276–279
  summer camps for, 316
  support groups for, 309
  as transplant donors, 394
  worries of, 264, 267
Sick leave
  donating hours, 229
  using hours, 235
Side effects. *See also* Learning disabilities; Nutrition
  bed wetting, 196
  constipation, 193
  dental problems, 198
  diarrhea, 191
  fatigue, 194
  hair loss, 181–184
  intracranial hypertension, 202
  long-term side effects, 364–365

About the Author

Nancy Keene, a well-known advocate and writer, is the parent of an 18-year survivor of high-risk acute lymphoblastic leukemia. Nancy is one of the founders of Childhood Cancer Guides™, and she has written and co-authored many books for families of children with cancer. In addition to *Childhood Leukemia*, Nancy also wrote *Working with Your Doctor; Your Child in the Hospital* (currently available in its 2nd edition and in Spanish); and *Chemo, Craziness, and Comfort: Your Book about Childhood Cancer.* She is the co-author of *Childhood Cancer: A Parent's Guide to Solid Tumor Cancers* (currently in its 2nd edition) and *Childhood Cancer Survivors: A Practical Guide to Your Future* (currently in its 2nd edition). She has also edited many consumer health books, including two about childhood cancer—*Childhood Brain & Spinal Cord Tumors* and *Educating the Child with Cancer.*

Nancy is a tireless advocate for children's health issues, including pediatric clinical trials, late effects of childhood cancer treatments, pediatric pain relief, children's medical rights, and emotional support for families. She was the first chair of the patient advocacy committee of the Children's Oncology Group (COG), a consortium of researchers from more than 350 institutions that treat children with cancer. In addition, she served as the first public member of the U.S. Food and Drug Administration (FDA) pediatric subcommittee of the FDA Oncologic Drug Advisory Committee.

Nancy has been interviewed on National Public Radio about childhood cancer survivorship, frequently speaks to professional and parent groups, and has participated on national online pediatric cancer support groups (*www.acor.org*) since they began in 1996.

Childhood Cancer Guides™

Questions Answered
Experiences Shared

When your life is turned upside down, your need for information is great. You have to make critical medical decisions, often with what seems like little to go on. Plus, you have to break the news to family, quiet your own fears, help your ill child and your other children, figure out how you are going to pay for things, and sometimes get to work or put dinner on the table.

Childhood Cancer Guides provide authoritative information for the families and friends of children with cancer or survivors of childhood cancer. They cover all aspects of how these illnesses affect family life. In each book, there's a mix of:

- **Medical information**
  Dozens of experts on childhood cancer and survivorship contributed to these books to provide state-of-the-art information to help you weigh treatment options. Modern medicine has much to offer. When there are treatment controversies, we present differing points of view.

- **Practical information**
  After making treatment decisions, life focuses on coping with treatment and any late effects that develop. We cover day-to-day practicalities, such as those you'd hear from a helpful nurse or a knowledgeable support group.

- **Emotional support**
  It's normal to have strong reactions to a condition that threatens your child's life. It's normal that the whole family is affected. We cover issues such as the shock of diagnosis, living with uncertainty, and communicating with loved ones.

Each book contains stories from parents, children, and siblings—medical "frequent flyers" who share, in their own words, the lessons they have learned and what truly helped them cope.

We provide information online, including updated listings of some of the resources that are listed in our books. This is freely available for you to print out and share with others, as long as you retain the copyright notice on the printouts.

www.childhoodcancerguides.org

Other Books for Families

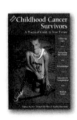

Childhood Cancer Survivors
A Practical Guide to Your Future, 2nd Edition

By Nancy Keene, Wendy Hobbie & Kathy Ruccione
ISBN 0-596-52851-5, Paperback, 6" x 9", $27.95, 436 pages

"An extraordinary resource for survivors of childhood cancer, as well as for their families, caregivers, and friends."

— Barbara Hoffman, JD
Editor, *A Cancer Survivor's Almanac:*
Charting Your Journey

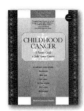

Childhood Cancer
A Parent's Guide to Solid Tumor Cancers, 2nd Edition

By Honna Janes-Hodder & Nancy Keene
ISBN 0-596-50014-9, Paperback, 7" x 9", $29.95, 537 pages

"I recommend [this book] most highly for those in need of high-level, helpful knowledge that will empower and help parents and caregivers to cope."

— Mark Greenberg, M.D.
Professor of Pediatrics, University of Toronto

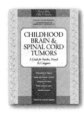

Childhood Brain & Spinal Cord Tumors
A Guide for Families, Friends, and Caregivers

By Tania Shiminski-Maher, Patsy Cullen, & Maria Sansalone
ISBN 0-596-50009-2, Paperback, 7" x 9", $29.95, 546 pages

"A must read for both parents and professionals."

— Henry Friedman, M.D.
Co-Director, The Clinical Neuro-Oncology
Center of the Brain Tumor Center at Duke

Childhood Cancer Guides™

Our helpful guides are available at
an online bookseller or a bookstore near you.

www.childhoodcancerguides.org
P.O. Box 31937 Bellingham WA 98228